Skin Lymphoma: The Illustrated Guide

Skin Lymphoma: The Illustrated Guide

Lorenzo Cerroni MD

Associate Professor of Dermatology
Medical University of Graz
Graz, Austria

Kevin Gatter BM DPhil FRCPath

Head of Department and Professor of Pathology
Nuffield Department of Clinical Laboratory Sciences
University of Oxford
Oxford, UK

Helmut Kerl MD

Professor Emeritus of Dermatology
Medical University of Graz
Graz, Austria

THIRD EDITION

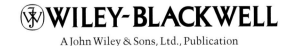

WILEY-BLACKWELL

A John Wiley & Sons, Ltd., Publication

This edition first published 2009, © 2009 by L. Cerroni, K. Gatter and H. Kerl
Previous editions: 1998, 2004

Blackwell Publishing was acquired by John Wiley & Sons in February 2007. Blackwell's publishing program has been merged with Wiley's global Scientific, Technical and Medical business to form Wiley-Blackwell.

Registered office: John Wiley & Sons Ltd, The Atrium, Southern Gate, Chichester, West Sussex, PO19 8SQ, UK

Editorial offices: 9600 Garsington Road, Oxford, OX4 2DQ, UK
        The Atrium, Southern Gate, Chichester, West Sussex, PO19 8SQ, UK
        111 River Street, Hoboken, NJ 07030-5774, USA

For details of our global editorial offices, for customer services and for information about how to apply for permission to reuse the copyright material in this book please see our website at www.wiley.com/wiley-blackwell.

Library of Congress Cataloging-in-Publication Data
Cerroni, Lorenzo.
  Skin lymphoma : the illustrated guide / Lorenzo Cerroni, Kevin Gatter, Helmut Kerl. – 3rd ed.
    p. ; cm.
  Rev. ed. of: Illustrated guide to skin lymphoma / Lorenzo Cerroni, Kevin Gatter, Helmut Kerl. 2nd ed. 2004.
  Includes bibliographical references and index.
  ISBN 978-1-4051-8554-7
  1. Skin–Cancer. 2. Lymphomas. I. Gatter, Kevin. II. Kerl, Helmut. III. Cerroni, Lorenzo. Illustrated guide to skin lymphoma. IV. Title.
  [DNLM: 1. Skin Neoplasms–diagnosis. 2. Skin Neoplasms–therapy. 3. Lymphoma–pathology. WR 500 C417s 2009]
  RC280.S5C47 2009
  616.99'477–dc22

                                           2008049864

ISBN: 978-1-4051-8554-7

A catalogue record for this title is available from the British Library

Set in 9/12pt Meridien by Graphicraft Limited, Hong Kong
Printed and bound in Singapore by Fabulous Printers Pte Ltd

1 2009

To Ninetta Ferrazzi,
whose dedication, generosity, and obstinate love permeate and enrich the lives
of her son Lorenzo and of her grandchildren Luca and Livia

CONTENTS

Contents

Preface

The field of cutaneous lymphomas is continuously evolving, mainly due to the application of new techniques and to the identification of precise diagnostic and prognostic categories. One of the consequences is that classifications are changing, too. Shortly after the publication of the second edition of this book, a classification of primary cutaneous lymphomas was proposed by the World Health Organization (WHO) and the European Organization for Research and Treatment of Cancer (EORTC). This classification is a major step forward and provides a better basis for diagnosis and management of patients with cutaneous lymphomas. In addition, in 2008 the WHO published an updated classification of tumors of hematopoietic and lymphoid tissues, including most of the entities recognized in the WHO-EORTC scheme. In short, in the last few years major changes in the nomenclature and diagnostic criteria of cutaneous lymphomas have been made. Bearing this in mind, we decided to prepare a third edition of this book that would provide readers with up-to-date information about cutaneous lymphoproliferative disorders. The positive response to the first and second editions gave us the necessary enthusiasm to plan a third one.

The outline of the book has changed, reflecting modifications in classification of some entities. In addition, diagnostic criteria have been refined, thanks to the introduction of new markers or new techniques. In addition to updating diagnostic features and management options of all disease entities, we have also added completely new chapters, including entities that were only briefly mentioned or not covered at all in the first two editions of the book. In addition, in many chapters we have added a section on "Teaching cases" where one or more clinicopathologic cases with particular teaching value are presented and briefly discussed. In short, as we stated for the second edition, this is more a new book than a third edition of the old one.

The number of references has been greatly expanded, adding mainly relevant articles published in the last 5 years. As the great strength of the first two editions of this book was the high quality and large number of illustrations, in this third edition we have greatly increased the amount of illustrations and replaced some of the old ones. This was possible due to the efforts of those working at Blackwell: we are greatly indebted to Rob Blundell and Martin Sugden for the help and support provided in the preparation of this third edition.

Whether our efforts have been worth the time and energies spent will be decided by the readers. We hope that the information contained in this book will be helpful for students of the field of cutaneous lymphomas, and will be useful for the management of these elusive disorders.

Lorenzo Cerroni
Helmut Kerl
Kevin Gatter
Graz and Oxford, June 2009

Acknowledgments

We would like to thank the many clinicians who provided the essential material and information necessary to prepare the book. A particular thank you goes to those who send us unusual, interesting and challenging cases in consultation.

We would like to express special thanks to Uli Schmidbauer, who prepared superb histopathologic and immunohistochemical sections, and to Werner Stieber, who is responsible for the excellent quality of the clinical pictures.

We would also like to thank the team of engaged and competent physicians that is helping us in taking care of patients with cutaneous lymphoma, and in particular Regina Fink-Puches and Ingrid Wolf.

Finally, we would like to express our deep gratitude to our patients. We have followed many of them for decades, learning from them as much as from scientific publications. Even from those who succumbed to their lymphoma, we are still learning by virtue of continuously studying their disease according to new information and techniques that are becoming available. We thank all of them, and hope that the information included in this book will help in improving the life of their fellow human beings affected by cutaneous lymphomas.

1   Introduction

Since completion of the last edition of this book, many advances have been made in the field of lymphomas in general and of cutaneous lymphomas in particular. Thanks to the efforts of the lymphoma groups of both the World Health Organization (WHO) and the European Organization for Research and Treatment of Cancer (EORTC), a joint WHO-EORTC classification for primary cutaneous lymphomas has been proposed [1], allowing different centers in various countries to speak one and the same language in the field of cutaneous lymphomas (Table 1.1). This may seem a trivial fact, something that should be obvious in medicine, but until a few years ago we were stuck with different terminologies, definitions, and classifications.

The WHO-EORTC classification is based for the most part on the original EORTC classification of cutaneous lymphomas published in 1997 [2]; this classification (as well as the WHO-EORTC one) was really a milestone in the history of cutaneous lymphomas, as for the first time we had precise definitions of entities that had been categorized differently in different centers. The WHO-EORTC classification has been absorbed virtually unchanged into the new WHO classification of tumors of hematopoietic and lymphoid tissues published in 2008 (Tables 1.2 and 1.3) [3], thus implying that the same language will be used by hematologists, dermatologists, and pathologists. Of course, this is not the end of the story, as a) cases are still published that are classified without the necessary ancillary studies and that are therefore questionable – and confusing; and b) continuous progress, particularly in the field of molecular pathology, is bringing an incredible number of new informations that will have to be integrated with the actual knowledge and that, indubitably, will change this field again in the near future.

It is accepted now that primary cutaneous lymphomas represent distinct clinical and histopathologic subtypes of extranodal lymphomas [2,4–9]. Although in some cases the corresponding extracutaneous entities have similar morpho-

Table 1.1 WHO-EORTC classification of primary cutaneous lymphomas [1]

Cutaneous T-cell and NK cell lymphomas
Mycosis fungoides
  MF variants and subtypes
  Folliculotropic MF
  Pagetoid reticulosis
  Granulomatous slack skin
Sézary syndrome
Adult T-cell leukemia/lymphoma
Primary cutaneous CD30[+] lymphoproliferative disorders
  Primary cutaneous anaplastic large cell lymphoma
  Lymphomatoid papulosis
Subcutaneous panniculitis-like T-cell lymphoma
Extranodal NK/T-cell lymphoma, nasal type
Primary cutaneous peripheral T-cell lymphoma, unspecified
  Primary cutaneous aggressive epidermotropic CD8[+] T-cell lymphoma (provisional)
  Cutaneous γ/δ T-cell lymphoma (provisional)
  Primary cutaneous CD4[+] small/medium-sized pleomorphic T-cell lymphoma (provisional)

Cutaneous B-cell lymphomas
Primary cutaneous marginal zone B-cell lymphoma
Primary cutaneous follicle center lymphoma
Primary cutaneous diffuse large B-cell lymphoma, leg type
Primary cutaneous diffuse large B-cell lymphoma, other
  Intravascular large B-cell lymphoma

Precursor hematologic neoplasm
CD4[+]/CD56[+] hematodermic neoplasm (blastic NK cell lymphoma)

logy, phenotype, genetic features, and prognosis, in most cases tumors that look identical under the microscope or on phenotypic grounds are profoundly different biologically, depending on the organ of origin. Primary cutaneous lymphomas can be defined as neoplasms of the immune system, characterized by a proliferation of either T or B lymphocytes which show a particular tropism for the skin. Extracutaneous spread with lymph node involvement can be observed during the course of the disease. The definition of primary cutaneous lymphomas has been changed to "no extracutaneous

Skin Lymphoma: The Illustrated Guide. By L. Cerroni, K. Gatter and H. Kerl. Published 2009 Blackwell Publishing. ISBN: 978-1-4051-8554-7.

Table 1.2 WHO classification of tumors of hematopoietic and lymphoid tissues [3]

MYELOPROLIFERATIVE NEOPLASMS
Chronic myelogenous leukemia, *BCR-ABL1* positive
Chronic neutrophilic leukemia
Polycythemia vera
Primary myelofibrosis
Essential thrombocythemia
Chronic eosinophilic leukemia, NOS
Mastocytosis
   Cutaneous mastocytosis
   Systemic mastocytosis
   Mast cell leukemia
   Mast cell sarcoma
   Extracutaneous mastocytoma
Myeloproliferative neoplasm, unclassifiable

MYELOID AND LYMPHOID NEOPLASMS WITH EOSINOPHILIA AND ABNORMALITIES OF *PDGFRA*, *PDGFRB* OR *FGFR1*
Myeloid and lymphoid neoplasms with *PDGFRA* rearrangement
Myeloid neoplasms with *PDGFRB* rearrangement
Myeloid and lymphoid neoplasms with *FGFR1* abnormalities

MYELODYSPLASTIC/MYELOPROLIFERATIVE NEOPLASMS
Chronic myelomonocytic leukemia
Atypical chronic myeloid leukemia, *BCR-ABL1* negative
Juvenile myelomonocytic leukemia
Myelodysplastic/myeloproliferative neoplasm, unclassifiable
Refractory anemia with ring sideroblasts associated with marked
   thrombocytosis (provisional)

MYELODYSPLASTIC SYNDROMES
Refractory cytopenia with unilineage dysplasia
   Refractory anemia
   Refractory neutropenia
   Refractory thrombocytopenia
Refractory anemia with ring sideroblasts
Refractory cytopenia with multilineage dysplasia
Refractory anemia with excess blasts
Myelodysplastic syndromes associated with isolated del(5q)
Myelodysplastic syndrome, unclassifiable
Childhood myelodysplastic syndrome
Refractory cytopenia of childhood (provisional)

ACUTE MYELOID LEUKEMIA (AML) AND RELATED PRECURSOR NEOPLASMS
AML with recurrent genetic abnormalities
AML with t(8;21)(q22;q22); *RUNX1-RUNX1T1*
AML with inv(16)(p13.1q22) or t(16;16)(p13.1;q22); *CBFB-MYH11*
Acute promyelocytic leukemia with t(15;17)(q22;q12); *PML-RARA*
AML with t(9;11)(p22;q23); *MLLT3-MLL*
AML with t(6;9)(p23;q34); *DEK-NUP214*
AML with inv(3)(q21q26.2) or t(3;3)(q21;q26.2); *RPN1-EVI1*
AML (megakaryoblastic) with t(1;22)(p13;q13); *RBM15-MKL1*
AML with mutated NPM1 (provisional)
AML with mutated CEBPA (provisional)

AML with myelodysplasia-related changes

Therapy-related myeloid neoplasms

Acute myeloid leukemia, not otherwise specified
AML with minimal differentiation
AML without maturation
AML with maturation
Acute myelomonocytic leukemia
Acute monoblastic and monocytic leukemia
Acute erythroid leukemia
Acute megakaryoblastic leukemia
Acute basophilic leukemia
Acute panmyelosis with myelofibrosis

Myeloid sarcoma

Myeloid proliferations related to Down syndrome
Transient abnormal myelopoiesis
Myeloid leukemia associated with Down syndrome

Blastic plasmacytoid dendritic cell neoplasm

ACUTE LEUKEMIAS OF AMBIGUOUS LINEAGE
Acute undifferentiated leukemia
Mixed phenotype acute leukemia with t(9;22)(q34;q11.2); *BCR-ABL1*
Mixed phenotype acute leukemia with t(v;11q23); *MLL* rearranged
Mixed phenotype acute leukemia, B/myeloid, not otherwise specified
Mixed phenotype acute leukemia, T/myeloid, not otherwise specified
Natural killer (NK) all lymphoblastic leukemia/lymphoma (provisional)

PRECURSOR LYMPHOID NEOPLASMS
B-lymphoblastic leukemia/lymphoma
B lymphoblastic leukemia/lymphoma, not otherwise specified
B lymphoblastic leukemia/lymphoma with recurrent genetic abnormalities
B lymphoblastic leukemia/lymphoma with t(9;22)(q34;q11.2); *BCR-ABL1*
B lymphoblastic leukemia/lymphoma with t(v;11q23); *MLL* rearranged
B lymphoblastic leukemia/lymphoma with t(12;21)(p13;q22); *TEL-AML1*
   (*ETV6-RUNX1*)
B lymphoblastic leukemia/lymphoma with hyperdiploidy
B lymphoblastic leukemia/lymphoma with hypodiploidy
   (hypodiploid ALL)
B lymphoblastic leukemia/lymphoma with t(5;14)(q31;q32); *IL3-IGH*
B lymphoblastic leukemia/lymphoma with t(1;19)(q23;p13.3);
   E2A-PBX1; (*TCF3-PBX1*)

T-lymphoblastic leukemia/lymphoma

MATURE B-CELL NEOPLASMS
Chronic lymphocytic leukemia/small lymphocytic lymphoma
B-cell prolymphocytic leukemia
Splenic B-cell marginal zone lymphoma
Hairy cell leukemia
Splenic lymphoma/leukemia, unclassifiable (provisional)
   Splenic diffuse red pulp small B-cell lymphoma (provisional)
   Hairy cell leukemia-variant (provisional)
Lymphoplasmacytic lymphoma
   Waldenström macroglobulinemia
Heavy chain diseases
   α Heavy chain disease
   γ Heavy chain disease
   μ Heavy chain disease

Table 1.2 *(cont'd)*

Plasma cell myeloma	Subcutaneous panniculitis-like T-cell lymphoma
Solitary plasmacytoma of bone	Mycosis fungoides
Extraosseous plasmacytoma	Sézary syndrome
Extranodal marginal zone lymphoma of mucosa-associated lymphoid tissue (MALT lymphoma)	Primary cutaneous CD30+ T-cell lymphoproliferative disorders

Plasma cell myeloma

Solitary plasmacytoma of bone

Extraosseous plasmacytoma

Extranodal marginal zone lymphoma of mucosa-associated lymphoid
    tissue (MALT lymphoma)

Nodal marginal zone lymphoma

    Pediatric nodal marginal zone lymphoma (provisional)

Follicular lymphoma

    Pediatric follicular lymphoma (provisional)

Primary cutaneous follicle center lymphoma

Mantle cell lymphoma

Diffuse large B-cell lymphoma (DLBCL), not otherwise specified

    T-cell/histiocyte-rich large B-cell lymphoma

    Primary DLBCL of the CNS

    Primary cutaneous DLBCL, leg type

    EBV-positive DLBCL of the elderly (provisional)

DLBCL associated with chronic inflammation

Lymphomatoid granulomatosis

Primary mediastinal (thymic) large B-cell lymphoma

Intravascular large B-cell lymphoma

ALK-positive DLBCL

Plasmablastic lymphoma

Large B-cell lymphoma arising in HHV8-associated multicentric
    Castleman disease

Primary effusion lymphoma

Burkitt lymphoma

B-cell lymphoma, unclassifiable, with features intermediate between
    diffuse large B-cell lymphoma and Burkitt lymphoma

B-cell lymphoma, unclassifiable, with features intermediate between
    diffuse large B-cell lymphoma and classic Hodgkin lymphoma

MATURE T-CELL AND NK CELL NEOPLASMS

T-cell prolymphocytic leukemia

T-cell large granular lymphocytic leukemia

Chronic lymphoproliferative disorder of NK cells (provisional)

Aggressive NK cell leukemia

Systemic EBV-positive T-cell lymphoproliferative disease of childhood

Hydroa vacciniforme-like lymphoma

Adult T-cell leukemia/lymphoma

Extranodal NK/T-cell lymphoma, nasal type

Enteropathy-associated T-cell lymphoma

Hepatosplenic T-cell lymphoma

Subcutaneous panniculitis-like T-cell lymphoma

Mycosis fungoides

Sézary syndrome

Primary cutaneous CD30+ T-cell lymphoproliferative disorders

    Lymphomatoid papulosis

    Primary cutaneous anaplastic large cell lymphoma

Primary cutaneous γ/δ T-cell lymphoma

Primary cutaneous CD8+ aggressive epidermotropic cytotoxic T-cell
    lymphoma (provisional)

Primary cutaneous CD4+ small/medium T-cell lymphoma
    (provisional)

Peripheral T-cell lymphoma, not otherwise specified

Angio-immunoblastic T-cell lymphoma

Anaplastic large cell lymphoma, ALK positive

Anaplastic large cell lymphoma, ALK negative (provisional)

HODGKIN LYMPHOMA

Nodular lymphocyte-predominant Hodgkin lymphoma

Classic Hodgkin lymphoma

    Nodular sclerosis classic Hodgkin lymphoma

    Lymphocyte-rich classic Hodgkin lymphoma

    Mixed cellularity classic Hodgkin lymphoma

    Lymphocyte-depleted classic Hodgkin lymphoma

HISTIOCYTIC AND DENDRITIC CELL NEOPLASMS

Histiocytic sarcoma

Langerhans cell histiocytosis

Langerhans cell sarcoma

Interdigitating dendritic cell sarcoma

Follicular dendritic cell sarcoma

Fibroblastic reticular cell tumor

Indeterminate dendritic cell tumor

Disseminated juvenile xanthogranuloma

POST-TRANSPLANT LYMPHOPROLIFERATIVE DISORDERS (PTLD)

Early lesions

    Plasmacytic hyperplasia

    Infectious mononucleosis-like PTLD

Polymorphic PTLD

Monomorphic PTLD (B- and T/NK cell types)

Classic Hodgkin lymphoma type PTLD

---

manifestations of the disease at presentation" [1,9]. Primary cutaneous lymphomas should be separated from secondary skin manifestations of extracutaneous (usually nodal) lymphomas and leukemias, which represent metastatic disease characterized by a worse prognosis and require different treatment. Because the histopathology of primary and secondary cutaneous lymphomas may be similar or identical [3,10], in most cases complete staging investigations are needed to establish this distinction (early mycosis fungoides representing the most important exception) (see Chapter 2).

Classification of cutaneous lymphomas

As already mentioned, after the successful classification proposed by the EORTC in 1997 [2], a joint WHO-EORTC classification has been prepared and widely accepted (see Table 1.1) [1]. The new WHO classification of tumors of hematopoietic and lymphoid tissues includes most of the entities introduced in the WHO-EORTC classification of primary cutaneous lymphomas (see Table 1.3) [3].

Table 1.3 Comparison of the WHO-EORTC classification of 2005 and WHO classification of 2008 concerning primary cutaneous lymphomas

WHO-EORTC classification 2005	WHO classification 2008
Mycosis fungoides	Mycosis fungoides
Sézary syndrome	Sézary syndrome
Adult T-cell leukemia/lymphoma	Adult T-cell leukemia/lymphoma
Primary cutaneous CD30+ lymphoproliferative disorders	Primary cutaneous CD30+ lymphoproliferative disorders
Lymphomatoid papulosis	Lymphomatoid papulosis
Primary cutaneous anaplastic large cell lymphoma	Primary cutaneous anaplastic large cell lymphoma
Subcutaneous panniculitis-like T-cell lymphoma	Subcutaneous panniculitis-like T-cell lymphoma
Extranodal NK/T-cell lymphoma, nasal type	Extranodal NK/T-cell lymphoma, nasal type
Primary cutaneous CD8+ aggressive epidermotropic cytotoxic T-cell lymphoma	Primary cutaneous CD8+ aggressive epidermotropic cytotoxic T-cell lymphoma
Cutaneous γ/δ T-cell lymphoma	Primary cutaneous γ/δ T-cell lymphoma
Primary cutaneous CD4+ small/medium-sized pleomorphic T-cell lymphoma	Primary cutaneous CD4+ small/medium T-cell lymphoma
Primary cutaneous marginal zone B-cell lymphoma	Extranodal marginal zone lymphoma of mucosa-associated lymphoid tissue (MALT ly.)
Primary cutaneous follicle center lymphoma	Primary cutaneous follicle center lymphoma
Primary cutaneous diffuse large B-cell lymphoma, leg type	Primary cutaneous diffuse large B-cell lymphoma, leg type
Intravascular large B-cell lymphoma	Intravascular large B-cell lymphoma
CD4+/CD56+ hematodermic neoplasm (blastic NK cell lymphoma)	Blastic plasmacytoid dendritic cell neoplasm

In the following chapters we describe the clinicopathologic characteristics of lymphomas arising in the skin, with special emphasis on primary cutaneous lymphomas. A guideline for treatment is also included. In addition, a chapter on the inflammatory diseases that simulate lymphomas (cutaneous pseudolymphomas) and one on so-called "atypical lymphoid proliferations" are provided.

Examination of patients

Primary cutaneous lymphomas represent a heterogeneous group of diseases with different clinicopathologic presentations and prognostic features. In order to classify patients correctly, it is crucial that a complete clinical history is obtained and integrated with histopathologic, immunophenotypical and molecular data. To take one example, some lesions of lymphomatoid papulosis show histopathologic features that may be indistinguishable from those observed in mycosis fungoides or in anaplastic large cell lymphoma, and differentiation in these cases can only be achieved by correlation with the clinical picture.

As a general rule, complete staging investigations at presentation include physical examination, laboratory investigations, chest X-ray, ultrasound of lymph nodes and visceral organs, computed tomography (CT) scans and bone marrow biopsy. Positron emission tomography is also being increasingly used for staging of patients with cutaneous lymphoma [11]. Patients with patch-stage mycosis fungoides or lymphomatoid papulosis do not require extensive investigations. The necessity of bone

marrow biopsy in patients with primary cutaneous marginal zone lymphoma is questionable (see Chapter 11) [12].

Surgical techniques

Surgical specimens should be carefully removed, paying particular attention not to crush the tissue. Shave biopsies must be avoided. Punch biopsies, although sometimes insufficient for a definitive diagnosis, may be performed in special instances (i.e. early lesions of mycosis fungoides). It is a good rule to perform more than one biopsy on different lesions, in order to get as much information as possible, and to have enough material for further phenotypic and molecular studies. A common problem is the drying up of specimens immediately after the surgical procedures by putting them on a drying gauze; these specimens show artefacts that hinder a proper cytomorphologic evaluation; phenotypic stainings, too, cannot be judged properly.

Histopathology, immunophenotype and molecular genetics

Histopathology

Sections should be cut with a maximum thickness of 4 μm and subsequently stained with hematoxylin and eosin (H&E), periodic acid–Schiff (PAS) and, if possible, Giemsa. High-quality sections are necessary for a correct diagnosis. Morphologic examination of a biopsy specimen should assess the following criteria: architecture of the infiltrate (e.g. superficial, superficial and deep, subcutaneous, etc.), involvement of particular structures (e.g. epidermotropism, pilotropism, etc.), cell composition (e.g. monomorphous infiltrate, mixed cell infiltrate, etc.), cell morphology, and other specific clues and criteria (e.g. deposition of mucin within the hair follicles, angiocentricity/ angiodestruction, etc.). Much information can be gathered at low power by examination of the pattern of growth, and basic morphologic assessment is useful also for selection of appropriate panels of antibodies necessary for phenotypic analyses, and of other ancillary techniques useful in the study of the biopsy specimen.

Immunophenotype

Antigen retrieval-based techniques allow the study of phenotypical patterns on routinely fixed, paraffin-embedded tissue sections, and most antibodies are applied using methods such as microwave heating of sections [13–15]. In short, tissue sections are placed in a microwave heater and heated up to 100°C for 10–15 min, and then slowly cooled off before application of the first antibody. Microwave heating can be substituted by pressure cooking or by overnight incubation of sections at 80°C. A list of antibodies reactive with lymphocyte subsets and accessory cells (macrophages, dendritic reticulum cells and interdigitating cells) in routinely fixed, paraffin-embedded tissue sections is given in Table 1.4. It should be emphasized that immunohistochemical stainings are not necessary in each and every case of cutaneous lymphoma/pseudolymphoma: in early lesions of mycosis fungoides, for example, we don't use immunohistology as a routine investigation.

Gene rearrangement studies

Analysis of the T-cell receptor (TCR) and immunoglobulin heavy-chain (J_H) genes has provided a new and important technique for the study of cutaneous lymphomas. Early in their differentiation, T and B lymphocytes rearrange their TCR and J_H genes, respectively [16,17]. Analysis of the gene rearrangement by polymerase chain reaction (PCR) techniques provides clues to the clonality of a given infiltrate. Benign (reactive) lymphoid proliferations are characterized by a polyclonal pattern of TCR and/or J_H gene rearrangement. In contrast, malignant lymphomas reveal a monoclonal population of lymphocytes, identified as a single band with the PCR technique. Many variations of the original techniques have been introduced over the years, in an attempt to improve specificity and sensitivity of gene rearrangement analysis. In general, the different methods vary in the number and selection of the primers used to detect the TCR or J_H gene rearrangement. Capillary electrophoresis shows the monoclonal bands as peaks, allowing a better characterization and easier interpretation of the results. A standardized assay (BIOMED-2) has been introduced in an attempt to homogenize the different methods and to allow a better comparison of results of gene rearrangement studies [18,19]. Although these methods are effective and reliable, they have some limitations:

benign inflammatory dermatoses may rarely present a monoclonal pattern, and a "germline" or polyclonal pattern may be observed in clear-cut lymphomas. In addition, the presence of only a few neoplastic cells may give rise to negative results in cases of early cutaneous T- or B-cell lymphoma.

A common pitfall in molecular analysis of cutaneous lymphoproliferative disorders is the presence of "pseudomonoclonal" rearrangement of the J_H gene in cutaneous lymphoid infiltrates characterized by the presence of only a few B lymphocytes. In fact, it is not uncommon to observe this phenomenon in lesions of cutaneous T-cell lymphoma with reactive B lymphocytes. A good rule is to perform at least two (better three) separate extractions of DNA from different sections of the biopsy tissue, and to run one independent PCR assay for every extraction. In this way, different "pseudomonoclonal" bands will be observed, thus showing overall a polyclonal pattern. Comparing PCR results from different biopsies is also useful in confirming that the same clone is present in different lesions. Peak analyses allow a more reliable comparison than standard gel electrophoresis.

Other methods used in the study of cutaneous lymphoid infiltrates

Fluorescence *in situ* hybridization technique

Chromosomal abnormalities are becoming increasingly important in the study and classification of hematopoietic neoplasms. In recent years, new methods have been developed for evaluation of tissue specimens fixed in formalin and embedded in paraffin, allowing the investigation of routine biopsy samples and archive material. The fluorescence *in situ* hybridization (FISH) technique is based on the same principle as the Southern blot method, relying on the annealing of single-stranded DNA to complementary DNA.

Depending on the probes selected, the FISH method can be used to detect different types of chromosomal abnormalities, including monosomy, trisomy and other aneuploidies, as well as translocations and deletions. To give one example, the use of FISH applied to routinely processed tissue specimens identified a hitherto unknown t(14;18)(q32;q21) involving the *IGH* and *MALT1* genes in a subset of cases of primary cutaneous marginal zone lymphomas [20]. This method can be used routinely and can provide valuable information for a precise diagnosis and classification of controversial cases.

Microarrays

The development of techniques of comparative genomic hybridization, and the identification of over 19 000 human genes by the Human Genome Project, allows one to check copy numbers and expression profiles of thousands of genes in a single experiment (microarray technology), thus providing important new information on the genetic profiles of human cancers [21]. Microarrays can be used to detect copy

Table 1.4 Panel of antibodies for immunohistologic analysis of cutaneous lymphomas on routinely fixed, paraffin-embedded tissue sections

Antigen/antibody	Main immunostaining in cutaneous lymphomas/pseudolymphomas specificity
CD1a	Langerhans cells, precursor T cells
CD2	T cells
CD3	T cells
CD3ε	T cells (epsilon chain of CD3)
CD4	T-helper cells
CD5	T cells; B lymphocytes in some B-cell lymphoma/leukemia (e.g. B-CLL)
CD7	T cells
CD8	T-cytotoxic cells
CD10	CALLA; germinal center cells; angio-immunoblastic T-cell lymphoma
CD11c	Monocytes/macrophages, NK cells
CD13	Myeloid cells
CD14	Monocytes/macrophages
CD15	Hodgkin cells, granulocytes, monocytes
CD20	B cells
CD21	Follicular dendritic cells
CD23	B cells, B-CLL
CD25	IL-2 receptor, ATLL
CD30	Activated T and B cells, Hodgkin cells
CD31	Endothelial cells
CD33	Early myeloid cells, myelogenous leukemia
CD34	Precursor cells
CD35	Follicular dendritic cells
CD38	Plasma cells
CD43	T cells, myeloid cells
CD45	Leukocyte common antigen
CD45RA	Naive T cells
CD45RO	Memory T cells
CD52	Nature lymphocytes
CD56	NK cells, NCAM
CD57	NK cells
CD68	Histiocytes, macrophages
CD79a	B cells
CD99	Precursor cells
CD117	c-kit; mast cells, hematopoietic stem cells, myelogenous leukemia
CD123	Plasmacytoid dendritic cells II
CD138	Plasma cells
CD207	Langerin
CD246	ALK-1 (anaplastic large cell lymphoma kinase)
CD303	BDCA2 (plasmacytoid dendritic cells type II)
Ig heavy-chains	B cells (IgA, IgD, IgG, IgM)
Ig light-chains	B cells (κ, λ)
Ki-67	Proliferating cells
Cytokeratin	Epithelial cells
EMA	Epithelial membrane antigen
S100 protein	Langerhans cells, interdigitating reticulum cells
TdT	Precursor cells
TCR-β (βF1)	α/β T cells
TIA-1	Cytotoxic T cells
Granzyme-B	Cytotoxic T cells
Perforin	Cytotoxic T cells
Bcl-2	T and B cells
Bcl-6	B cells, germinal center
Anti-HLA-DR	HLA-DR
CXCL-13	Follicular T-helper lymphocytes, angio-immunoblastic T-cell lymphoma
Cyclin-D1	B cells, mantle cell lymphoma
FOX-P1	Forkhead box protein 1; large B-cell lymphoma
FOX-P3	Forkhead box protein 3; T-regulatory cells
ICOS	Inducible co-stimulator protein; angio-immunoblastic T-cell lymphoma
IRF8	Interferon regulatory factor 8
MUM-1	Multiple myeloma oncogene 1; large B-cell lymphoma
Myeloperoxidase	Myeloid cells
PAX-5	Paired box gene 5, B cells
PD-1	Immunoregulatory lymphoid cells
TCL-1	T cells, plasmacytoid dendritic cells type II

numbers of given genes (DNA microarrays), gene expression (RNA microarrays), RNA-inhibitor expression (RNAi micro-array) and proteins (proteomics).

Using these methods, different subgroups of patients with nodal diffuse large B-cell lymphoma have been identified, as well as prognostic categories of patients with diffuse large B-cell lymphoma after treatment [22,23]. In the skin, micro-array studies have been used mainly to characterize infiltrates of B-cell lymphomas and to elucidate their relationship to nodal counterparts, and to evaluate genetic features of myco-sis fungoides [21–27].

Comparative genomic hybridization

Changes in DNA copy number is one of many ways in which gene expression and function may be modified. Comparative genomic hybridization (CGH) is a powerful method of scan-ning the entire genome for copy number changes [28,29]. In chromosome CGH, genomic DNA is isolated from tumor and normal control cells, labeled with different fluorochromes, and hybridized to metaphase chromosomes. In array CGH, metaphase chromosomes are replaced by several thousand DNA spots, each representing a specific region of the human genome. The differentially labeled tumor and control DNA compete for the complementary binding sites on the micro-array and, therefore, the relative hybridization intensity at each spot is proportional to the relative copy number of the tumor and control DNA.

Laser-based microdissection

Microdissection of tissue specimens using a laser beam to isolate single cells or structures has been increasingly used in recent years in the study and characterization of cutaneous lymphoid infiltrates by PCR or other molecular techniques [30–35]. The main advantage over conventional microdis-section techniques lies in the more precise isolation of given structures, particularly of tiny ones that cannot be reliably isolated by manual microdissection techniques. This can be obtained either by selective destruction of tissue by laser beam energy, thus obtaining a contamination-free sample, with DNA from cells other than the target population totally destroyed, or by "shooting" the target structures out of the specimen (laser-catapulting). Most routine histologic or immunohisto-logic stains can be used. The laser is suitable for analysis of routinely fixed specimens, so there is no need for fresh-frozen tissue and archival material stored in paraffin blocks can be easily evaluated. As cutaneous lymphomas present commonly with mixed populations of neoplastic and reactive lympho-cytes, molecular techniques may be unable to detect specific abnormalities due to the dilution of neoplastic DNA by non-neoplastic cells (besides reactive lymphocytes, keratinocytes and other skin resident cells provide non-neoplastic DNA that hinders molecular studies). Thus, we use laser-based micro-dissection in connection with the CGH technique, in order to isolate DNA from pure populations of neoplastic cells.

Lymphoma microenvironment

The presence of accessory (non-neoplastic) cells within the infiltrate of cutaneous (and extracutaneous) lymphomas has been known for many years. In mycosis fungoides, for example, a population of S-100+ interdigitating reticulum cells has been observed in specific lesions, and several studies demonstrated that their number varies in different stages of the disease, decreasing in more advanced stages. In the last few years evidence has accumulated on the importance of non-neoplastic lymphoid and other accessory cells for the development and maintenance of malignant lymphomas, and a large number of such cells has been identified and better characterized ("lymphoma microenvironment"). Some lymphomas, such as angio-immunoblastic T-cell lymphoma, derive from specific subsets of follicular T-helper lymphocytes with a CD4+/CXCL13+ phenotype. T-regulatory cells (Treg) with a characteristic CD4+/CD25+/FOX-P3+ phenotype are present in variable numbers in many peripheral T-cell lymphomas, and may have a prognostic value. Rarely, some T-cell lym-phomas may show a Treg phenotype. Other regulatory cells involved in apoptosis and expressing the programmed cell death 1 (PD-1) antigen may also have prognostic value in some lymphomas.

This is a field of lymphoma research that is becoming increasingly important, and that in the future may provide crucial information on cutaneous and extracutaneous lym-phomas, as well as potential new therapeutic targets for these diseases.

References

1. Willemze R, Jaffe ES, Burg G et al. WHO-EORTC classification for cutaneous lymphomas. Blood 2005;**105**:3768–3785.
2. Willemze R, Kerl H, Sterry W et al. EORTC classification for primary cutaneous lymphomas: a proposal from the Cutaneous Lymphoma Study Group of the European Organization for Research and Treatment of Cancer. Blood 1997;**90**:354–371.
3. Swerdlow SH, Campo E, Harris NL et al, eds. WHO Classification of Tumours of Haematopoietic and Lymphoid Tissues. Lyon: IARC Press, 2008.
4. Kerl H, Kresbach H. Lymphoretikuläre Hyperplasien und Neoplasien der Haut. In: Schnyder UW, ed. Spezielle Pathologische Anatomie. Berlin: Springer Verlag, 1979: 351–480.
5. Burg G, Braun-Falco O. Cutaneous Lymphomas, Pseudolymphomas and Related Disorders. Berlin: Springer Verlag, 1983.
6. Kerl H, Cerroni L, Burg G. The morphologic spectrum of T-cell lymphomas in the skin: a proposal for a new classification. Semin Diagn Pathol 1991;**8**:55–61.
7. Edelson RL. Cutaneous T-cell lymphoma. J Dermatol Surg Oncol 1980;**6**:358–368.
8. Isaacson PG, Norton AJ. Cutaneous lymphoma. In: Isaacson PG, Norton AJ, eds. Extracutaneous Lymphomas. Edinburgh: Churchill Livingstone, 1994: 131–191.

9. Fink-Puches R, Zenahlik P, Bäck B *et al.* Primary cutaneous lymphomas: applicability of current classification schemes (European Organization for Research and Treatment of Cancer, World Health Organization) based on clinicopathologic features observed in a large group of patients. *Blood* 2002;**99**:800–805.

10. Lennert K, Feller AC. *Histopathology of Non-Hodgkin's Lymphomas*, 2nd edn. Berlin: Springer Verlag, 1992.

11. Kuo PH, McClennan BL, Carlson K *et al.* FDG-PET/CT in the evaluation of cutaneous T-cell lymphoma. *Molec Imag Biol* 2008; **10**:74–81.

12. Senff NJ, Kluin-Nelemans JC, Willemze R. Results of bone marrow examination in 275 patients with histological features that suggest an indolent type of cutaneous B-cell lymphoma. *Br J Haematol* 2008;**142**:52–56.

13. Cerroni L, Smolle J, Soyer HP, Martinez Aparicio A, Kerl H. Immunophenotyping of cutaneous lymphoid infiltrates in frozen and paraffin-embedded tissue sections: a comparative study. *J Am Acad Dermatol* 1990;**22**:405–413.

14. Cerroni L, Kerl H. Diagnostic immunohistology: cutaneous lymphomas and pseudolymphomas. *Semin Cutan Med Surg* 1999; **18**:64–70.

15. Gatter KC. Diagnostic immunocytochemistry: achievements and challenges. *J Pathol* 1989;**159**:183–190.

16. Van Dongen JJM, Wolvers-Tettero ILM. Analysis of immunoglobulin and T cell receptor genes. I. Basic and technical aspects. *Clin Chim Acta* 1991;**198**:1–91.

17. Van Dongen JJM, Wolvers-Tettero ILM. Analysis of immunoglobulin and T cell receptor genes. II. Possibilities and limitations in the diagnosis and management of lymphoproliferative diseases and related disorders. *Clin Chim Acta* 1991;**198**:93–174.

18. Van Dongen JJM, Langerak AW, Brüggemann M, et al. Design and standardization of PCR primers and protocols for detection of clonal immunoglobulin and T-cell receptor gene recombinations in suspect lymphoproliferations: Report of the BIOMED-2 Concerted Action BMH4-CT98-3936. *Leukemia* 2003;**17**:2257–2317.

19. Van Krieken JH, Langerak AW, Macintyre EA, et al. Improved reliability of lymphoma diagnostics via PCR-based clonality testing: report of the BIOMED-2 Concerted Action BHM4-CT98-3936. *Leukemia* 2007;**21**:201–206.

20. Streubel B, Lamprecht A, Dierlamm J *et al.* t(14;18)(q32;q21) involving *IGH* and *MALT1* is a frequent chromosomal aberration in MALT lymphoma. *Blood* 2003;**101**:2335–2339.

21. Pollack JR, Perou CM, Alizadeh AA *et al.* Genome-wide analysis of DNA copy-number changes using cDNA microarrays. *Nat Genet* 1999;**23**:41–46.

22. Alizadeh AA, Eisen MB, Davis RE *et al.* Distinct types of diffuse large B-cell lymphoma identified by gene expression profiling. *Nature* 2000;**403**:503–511.

23. Rosenwald A, Wright G, Chan WC *et al.* The use of molecular profiling to predict survival after chemotherapy for diffuse large-B-cell lymphoma. *N Engl J Med* 2002;**346**:1937–1947.

24. Storz MN, van de Rijn M, Kim YH *et al.* Gene expression profiles of cutaneous B cell lymphoma. *J Invest Dermatol* 2003;**120**:865–870.

25. Tracey L, Villuendas R, Dotor AM *et al.* Mycosis fungoides shows concurrent deregulation of multiple genes involved in the TNF signaling pathway: an expression profile study. *Blood* 2003;**102**:1042–1050.

26. Tracey L, Villuendas R, Ortiz P *et al.* Identification of genes involved in resistance to interferon-γ in cutaneous T-cell lymphoma. *Am J Pathol* 2002;**161**:1825–1837.

27. Hoefnagel JJ, Dijkman R, Basso K *et al.* Distinct types of primary cutaneous large B-cell lymphoma identified by gene expression profiling. *Blood* 2005;**105**:3671–3678.

28. Kallioniemi A. CGH microarrays and cancer. *Curr Opin Biotechnol* 2008;**19**:36–40.

29. Pinkel D, Albertson DG. Array comparative genomic hybridization and its applications in cancer. *Nat Genet* 2005;**37** (suppl): s11–17.

30. Cerroni L, Minkus G, Pütz B, Höfler H, Kerl H. Laser beam microdissection in the diagnosis of cutaneous B-cell lymphoma. *Br J Dermatol* 1997;**136**:743–746.

31. Cerroni L, Arzberger E, Pütz B *et al.* Primary cutaneous follicle center cell lymphoma with follicular growth pattern. *Blood* 2000; **95**:3922–3928.

32. Cerroni L, Arzberger E, Ardigó M, Pütz B, Kerl H. Monoclonality of intraepidermal T lymphocytes in early mycosis fungoides detected by molecular analysis after laser-beam-based microdissection. *J Invest Dermatol* 2000;**114**:1154–1157.

33. Gellrich S, Wilks A, Lukowsky A *et al.* T cell receptor-γ gene analysis of CD30 large atypical individual cells in CD30 large primary cutaneous T-cell lymphomas. *J Invest Dermatol* 2003; **120**:670–675.

34. Steinhoff M, Hummel M, Anagnostopoulos I *et al.* Single-cell analysis of CD30 cells in lymphomatoid papulosis demonstrates a common clonal T-cell origin. *Blood* 2002;**100**:578–584.

35. Gellrich S, Rutz S, Golembowski S *et al.* Primary cutaneous follicle center cell lymphomas and large B-cell lymphomas of the leg descend from germinal center cells: a single cell polymerase chain reaction analysis. *J Invest Dermatol* 2001;**117**:1512–1520.

Section 1: Cutaneous NK/T-cell lymphomas

In contrast to the situation in the lymph nodes, where B-cell lymphomas represent the majority of non-Hodgkin lymphomas, in the skin, T-cell lymphomas are the most frequent group of malignant lymphomas, and mycosis fungoides is by far the most frequent single entity, alone representing approximately half of all primary cutaneous lymphomas. The peculiar clinicopathologic and prognostic aspects of cutaneous T-cell lymphomas are well recognized, and prompted the inclusion in the new World Health Organization (WHO) classification of tumors of hematopoietic and lymphoid tissues of most entities recognized in the original European Organization for Research and Treatment of Cancer (EORTC) and subsequent WHO-EORTC classifications of primary cutaneous lymphomas [1–3].

In recent years, progress in immunohistochemistry and molecular genetics has allowed the reclassification of many of the cases diagnosed in the past as unusual variants of mycosis fungoides such as disseminated pagetoid reticulosis, mycosis fungoides "a tumeur d'emblee" and other cases of mycosis fungoides showing an aggressive course and short survival. It has been demonstrated that many of these cases belong to the recently described group of aggressive cytotoxic lymphomas, including mainly extranodal NK/T-cell lymphoma, nasal type, cutaneous γ/δ T-cell lymphoma, and primary cutaneous aggressive epidermotropic CD8 cytotoxic T-cell lymphoma. To this group of disorders belong also many of the cases classified in the past as "malignant histiocytosis." Many of the cytotoxic lymphomas are today well characterized, and the phenotype of cutaneous lesions can be evaluated on routinely fixed sections of tissue.

It should be noted that, with some exceptions, cytomorphologic features of neoplastic cells are of less importance in the classification of cutaneous T-cell lymphomas, and that a precise diagnosis can be achieved only by integration of clinical features with histopathologic, immunophenotypical and molecular ones. In fact, most cutaneous T-cell lymphomas (including mycosis fungoides) are characterized by a proliferation of small-, medium- or large-sized pleomorphic T lymphocytes. Thus, the distinction of rare entities of cutaneous T-cell lymphoma from mycosis fungoides can be achieved only by careful taking of the clinical history and clinical examination of the patients. In addition, although in mycosis fungoides the size of the neoplastic cells has a prognostic value and the onset of large cell transformation bears a worse prognosis (see Chapter 2), in many other entities of cutaneous T-cell lymphoma the size of the neoplastic cells is not a prognostic indicator, as the biologic behavior is independent of the cytomorphologic features. Thus, for example, an extranodal NK/T-cell lymphoma, nasal type, with predominance of small pleomorphic lymphocytes has a very aggressive behavior and bears a poor prognosis; in contrast, lymphomatoid papulosis and cutaneous CD30 anaplastic large cell lymphoma have an indolent behavior and an excellent prognosis in spite of the marked atypia and the large size of the neoplastic cells.

Although recent years have seen many advances in the field of malignant lymphomas in general and cutaneous lymphomas in particular, many controversies still exist that were mentioned in the second edition of this book. In spite of several studies and publications, for example, the definition of precise diagnostic criteria for Sézary syndrome is still a matter of discussion. Criteria for the early diagnosis of mycosis fungoides, as well as the exact nosologic classification of variants of it such as so-called small-plaque parapsoriasis, are also a matter of discussion. Exact definitions and diagnostic criteria for some subtypes of cytotoxic lymphomas are still lacking, and many overlaps exist among different entities. It is still unclear whether cutaneous small-medium pleomorphic T-cell lymphoma represents a specific entity, or not [4]. Until now, phenotypic and molecular data have not provided clear-cut answers to these questions.

References

1. Swerdlow SH, Campo E, Harris NL *et al* (eds). *WHO Classification of Tumors of Haematopoietic and Lymphoid Tissues*. Lyon: IARC Press, 2008.
2. Willemze R, Kerl H, Sterry W *et al*. EORTC classification for primary cutaneous lymphomas: a proposal from the Cutaneous Lymphoma Study Group of the European Organization for Research and Treatment of Cancer. *Blood* 1997;**90**:354–371.
3. Willemze R, Jaffe ES, Burg G *et al*. WHO-EORTC classification for cutaneous lymphomas. *Blood* 2005;**105**:3768–3785.
4. Kerl H, Cerroni L. Controversies in cutaneous lymphomas. *Semin Cutan Med Surg* 2000;**19**:157–160.

2 Mycosis fungoides

Mycosis fungoides represents the most common type of cutaneous T-cell lymphoma [1–5]. It is also a long-standing entity, having been described more than two centuries ago, in 1806, by the French dermatologist Alibert. Traditionally it is divided into three clinical phases: patch, plaque, and tumor stage. The clinical course can be protracted over years or decades. Indeed, in the World Health Organization (WHO)-European Organization for Research and Treatment of Cancer (EORTC) classification for cutaneous lymphomas the term "mycosis fungoides" is restricted to the classic (so-called "Alibert–Bazin") type of the disease, characterized by the typical slow evolution and protracted course [1]. The same definition has been adopted in the new classification of tumors of hematopoietic and lymphoid tissues published by the WHO in 2008 [5]. More aggressive entities (e.g. mycosis fungoides "a tumeur d'emblee"), characterized by onset with plaques and tumors, aggressive course and bad prognosis, are better classified among the group of aggressive cutaneous cytotoxic natural killer (NK)/ T-cell lymphomas (see Chapter 6).

In the past mycosis fungoides has been considered as an "incurable", albeit slowly progressive condition, that inevitably ended with the death of the patient. Recently an early form of mycosis fungoides has been recognized consisting of subtle patches of the disease [6–8]. These patients have relatively mild stable lesions which questions the traditional concept of the inevitability of disease progression till death. In fact, it is estimated that over 90% of patients with early mycosis fungoides neither progress to tumor stage nor show extracutaneous manifestations of the disease [3,9,10].

The incidence of the disease worldwide is probably around 6–7 cases/10^6, with many regional variations and with a regular increase in recent decades [11,12]. The increase is most likely due to better diagnosis (particularly of early lesions) rather than a true rise in the incidence.

In spite of decades of research, the etiology of mycosis fungoides remains unknown. A genetic predisposition may play a role in some cases, and a familial occurrence of the disease

has been reported in a few instances [13–15]. A study conducted among Israeli Jewish patients showed a significantly greater allele frequency of HLA DQBI*03, suggesting that genetic factors may play a role in the etiology of the disease [16]. On the other hand, mycosis fungoides has been rarely observed in unrelated married individuals, pointing at the existence of a possible environmental factor [17]. Association with long-term exposure to various allergens has also been advocated, as well as exposure to environmental agents and association with chronic skin disorders and viral infections [18–22]. Recently, exposure to halogenated hydrocarbons has been linked to a higher risk of developing the disease, but the number of affected individuals was very small [23]. Seropositivity for cytomegalovirus (CMV) has been observed at unusually high frequencies in patients with mycosis fungoides, suggesting a role for this virus in the pathogenesis of the disease [24], but these results have not been confirmed. Relationship to *Borrelia burgdorferi* infection or Epstein–Barr virus has also been suggested [25,26]. In some countries, disorders with mycosis fungoides-like clinicopathologic manifestations are clearly associated with viral infections (i.e. HTLV-I-associated adult T-cell leukemia/lymphoma – see Chapter 7), but the search for viral particles in patients with mycosis fungoides has so far been negative or controversial [27]. Recently, a possible prognostic role of HTLV *tax*-like sequences in lesions of mycosis fungoides has been hypothesized [28]. Interestingly, mycosis fungoides has been observed rarely in patients who received solid organ transplantation, suggesting that immunosuppression may contribute to the development of the disease [29]. In this context, herpes virus 8 has been detected in patients with mycosis fungoides [30], but an etiologic role seems unlikely. Genetic alterations have been identified mainly in late stages of the disease, and their importance for disease initiation is unclear [31–36].

Mycosis fungoides has been described in patients with other cutaneous or extracutaneous hematologic disorders, especially lymphomatoid papulosis and Hodgkin lymphoma. In occasional patients, the same clone has been detected in mycosis fungoides and associated lymphomas, raising questions about a common origin of the diseases [37–40]. In addition, patients with mycosis fungoides are at higher risk of developing a second (non-hematologic) malignancy [41].

Skin Lymphoma: The Illustrated Guide. By L. Cerroni, K. Gatter and H. Kerl.
Published 2009 Blackwell Publishing, ISBN: 978-1-4051-8554-7.

Table 2.1 TNMB staging of mycosis fungoides [41]

Skin

T_1	Patches, papules or plaques covering <10% of the skin surface
T_2	Patches, papules or plaques covering >10% of the skin surface
T_3	Tumors
T_4	Generalized erythroderma

Lymph nodes

N_0	No clinically abnormal lymph nodes; histology negative
N_1	Clinically abnormal peripheral lymph nodes
	N_{1o} Histology not performed
	N_{1n} Histology negative
	N_{1r} Histology reactive
	N_{1d} Dermopathic lymphadenitis
N_2	No clinically abnormal peripheral lymph nodes; histology positive
N_3	Clinically abnormal peripheral lymph nodes; histology positive

Visceral organs

M_0	No visceral involvement
M_1	Visceral involvement

Blood

B_0	<5% of atypical circulating cells
B_1	>5% of atypical circulating cells

Stage

Ia	$T_1N_0M_0$	Ib	$T_2N_0M_0$
IIa	$T_{1-2}N_1M_0$	IIb	$T_3N_{0-1}M_0$
III	$T_4N_{0-1}M_0$		
IVa	$T_{1-4}N_{2-3}M_0$	IVb	$T_{1-4}N_{0-3}M_1$

A staging classification system for mycosis fungoides was proposed in 1979 by the Mycosis Fungoides Cooperative Group (TNMB staging) (Table 2.1) [42]. This system takes into account the percentage of body area covered by lesions and the presence of lymph node or visceral involvement. Although the presence of malignant circulating cells in the blood should be recorded for each patient, these data are not used for staging. Modifications to the original schemes have been proposed [43]. More recently, a new staging classification for mycosis fungoides has been proposed by a joint working group of the International Society of Cutaneous Lymphoma (ISCL) and the EORTC (Table 2.2) [44]. Besides other changes, this system adds detection of a T-cell clone in the lymph nodes and/or blood to the traditional staging classification.

Although the traditional TNMB and ISCL-EORTC staging systems are useful for the evaluation of patients with advanced stages of mycosis fungoides, extensive staging investigations are usually not performed in patients presenting with patches of the disease only. Thus, some centers specializing in the study and management of skin lymphomas do not utilize exclusively the TNMB or ISCL-EORTC staging schemes, but classify mycosis fungoides according to the type of skin lesions (patches, plaques and tumors) and the presence or absence of large cell transformation and/or extracutaneous involvement. Table 2.3 summarizes a clinical staging system for patients with mycosis fungoides. In this scheme, stage I disease is confined to the skin and characterized morphologically by patches only. Survival is extremely long in these patients (usually decades), and non-aggressive treatments should be applied. Most patients in this stage, in fact, die of unrelated causes. Patients with stage II in this scheme also have disease limited to the skin, but characterized morphologically by the presence of plaques, tumors or erythroderma, or by large cell transformation histopathologically. The disease in these patients is inevitably progressive, and treatment should be more aggressive. Stage III patients have extracutaneous disease and should be managed with aggressive treatment options.

Staging investigations are not necessary in early mycosis fungoides (patch stage), and only clinical examination is performed (assessment of percentage of body involvement and of superficial lymph nodes). Patients with plaques, tumors or erythroderma should be screened for extracutaneous involvement (laboratory investigations, sonography of lymph nodes, CT scan of chest, abdomen and pelvis, bone marrow biopsy, examination of the peripheral blood). Although stages Ia and Ib are considered early stages in traditional systems, we perform staging investigations in patients who present with plaques of the disease in addition to patches. In this context, it should be underlined that clinicopathologic diagnosis of early mycosis fungoides is made differently in various countries, and that there may be discrepancies in the diagnostic threshold, particularly between the United States and European countries. The validity of magnetic resonance imaging (MRI) and ^{18}F-fluorodeoxyglucose positron emission tomography (FDG-PET) investigations in patients with mycosis fungoides has been reported only in a limited number of patients [45–47]. However, PET studies may be used in patients unable to safely undergo CT scans [44], and are commonly used in our centers. Suspect lymph nodes (lymph nodes that are either >1.5 cm in diameter and/or firm, irregular, clustered or fixed) should be biopsied. Although the presence of a monoclonal population of T lymphocytes within the peripheral blood has been observed by PCR technique in some patients with early mycosis fungoides, in many of these cases the clone was different from the one detected in the skin lesions [48–51]. In addition, the prognostic value of the detection of monoclonality in the peripheral blood is unclear.

Although many studies have addressed the identification of clinical markers of the disease, at present there is no investigation other than conventional physical examination and radiologic imaging that can allow reliable and repeatable monitoring of mycosis fungoides, particularly in early stages of the disease. Several markers have been the subject of recent investigations, including cancer antigen 27.29 (CA27.29) [52], transthyretin [53], peripheral blood mononuclear cell

Table 2.2 Staging of mycosis fungoides and Sézary syndrome according to the ISCL-EORTC [44]

Skin

T_1	Limited patches*, papules, and/or plaques[†] covering <10% of the skin surface. May further stratify into T_{1a} (patch only) vs T_{1b} (plaque ± patch)
T_2	Patches, papules or plaques covering >10% of the skin surface. May further stratify into T_{2a} (patch only) vs T_{2b} (plaque ± patch)
T_3	One or more tumors[‡] (≥1 cm diameter)
T_4	Confluence of erythema covering ≥80% body surface area

Lymph nodes

N_0	No clinically abnormal peripheral lymph nodes[§]; biopsy not required	
N_1	Clinically abnormal peripheral lymph nodes; histopathology Dutch grade 1 or NCI LN0-2	
	N_{1a}	Clone negative[#]
	N_{1b}	Clone positive[#]
N_2	Clinically abnormal peripheral lymph nodes; histopathology Dutch grade 2 or NCI LN3	
	N_{2a}	Clone negative[#]
	N_{2b}	Clone positive[#]
N_3	Clinically abnormal peripheral lymph nodes; histopathology Dutch grades 3–4 or NCI LN4; clone positive or negative	
N_x	Clinically abnormal peripheral lymph nodes; no histologic confirmation	

Visceral

M_0	No visceral organ involvement
M_1	Visceral involvement (must have pathology confirmation[¶] and organ involved should be specified)

Blood

B_0	Absence of significant blood involvement: ≤5% of peripheral blood lymphocytes are atypical (Sézary) cells[‖]	
	B_{0a}	Clone negative[#]
	B_{0b}	Clone positive[#]
B_1	Low blood tumor burden: >5% of peripheral blood lymphocytes are atypical (Sézary) cells but does not meet the criteria of B2	
	B_{1a}	Clone negative[#]
	B_{1b}	Clone positive[#]
B_2	High blood tumor burden: ≥1000/μL Sézary cells[‖] with positive clone[#]	

Stage

IA	$T_1N_0M_0B_{0,1}$	IB	$T_2N_0M_0B_{0,1}$			
II	$T_{1,2}N_{1,2}M_0B_{0,1}$	IIB	$T_3N_{0-2}M_0B_{0,1}$			
III	$T_4N_{0-2}M_0B_{0,1}$	IIIA	$T_4N_{0-2}M_0B_0$	IIIB	$T_4N_{0-2}M_0B_1$	
IVA1	$T_{1-4}N_{0-2}M_0B_2$	IVA2	$T_{1-4}N_3M_0B_{0-2}$	IVB	$T_{1-4}N_{0-3}M_1B_{0-2}$	

* For skin, patch indicates any size skin lesion without significant elevation or induration. Presence/absence of hypo- or hyperpigmentation, scale, crusting, and/or poikiloderma should be noted.

[†] For skin, plaque indicates any size skin lesion that is elevated or indurated. Presence or absence of scale, crusting, and/or poikiloderma should be noted. Histologic features such as folliculotropism or large-cell transformation (>25% large cells), CD30+ or CD30−, and clinical features such as ulceration are important to document.

[‡] For skin, tumor indicates at least one 1 cm diameter solid or nodular lesion with evidence of depth and/or vertical growth. Note total number of lesions, total volume of lesions, largest size lesion, and region of body involved. Also note if histologic evidence of large-cell transformation has occurred. Phenotyping for CD30 is encouraged.

[§] For node, abnormal peripheral lymph node(s) indicates any palpable peripheral node that on physical examination is firm, irregular, clustered, fixed or 1.5 cm or larger in diameter. Node groups examined on physical examination include cervical, supraclavicular, epitrochlear, axillary, and inguinal. Central nodes, which are not generally amenable to pathologic assessment, are not currently considered in the nodal classification unless used to establish N3 histopathologically.

[¶] For viscera, spleen and liver may be diagnosed by imaging criteria.

[‖] For blood, Sézary cells are defined as lymphocytes with hyperconvoluted cerebriform nuclei. If Sézary cells cannot be used to determine tumor burden for B2, then one of the following modified ISCL criteria along with a positive clonal rearrangement of the TCR may be used instead: (1) expanded CD4+ or CD3+ cells with CD4:CD8 ratio of 10 or more, (2) expanded CD4+ cells with abnormal immunophenotype including loss of CD7 or CD26.

[#] A T-cell clone is defined by PCR or Southern blot analysis of the T-cell receptor gene.

Table 2.3 Clinical staging for patients with mycosis fungoides (Department of Dermatology, Medical University of Graz)

Stage	
Ia	Patches <10% of body area
Ib	Patches >10% of body area
IIa	Plaques
IIb	Tumors
IIc	Erythroderma
IId	Large cell morphology
III	Lymph node involvement and/or visceral dissemination

cytokine expression [54], circulating CD8[+] lymphocytes [55], and testis-specific protein 10 (TSGA10) among others [56], but their value is yet to be confirmed. It has been suggested that flow cytometry analysis is highly effective in demonstrating and quantifying small numbers of circulating tumor cells in patients with mycosis fungoides [57,58].

Clinical features

Lesions of mycosis fungoides can be divided morphologically into patches, plaques, and tumors. Itching is often a prominent symptom. Erythroderma may develop in the course of the disease, rendering distinction from Sézary syndrome difficult without a proper clinical history (see also erythrodermic mycosis fungoides in this Chapter, and Chapter 3).

Patch stage

Patches of mycosis fungoides are characterized by variably large, erythematous, finely scaling lesions with a predilection for the buttocks and other sun-protected areas (Figs 2.1, 2.2). Loss of elastic fibers and atrophy of the epidermis may confer on the lesions a typical wrinkled appearance, and terms such as "parchment-like" or "cigarette paper-like" have been used to describe them (Fig. 2.3). Sometimes, these single patches have a yellowish hue, conferring a "xanthomatous"-like

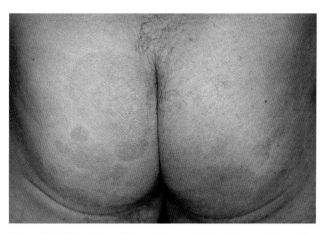

Figure 2.1 Mycosis fungoides, patch stage. Early patches on the buttocks.

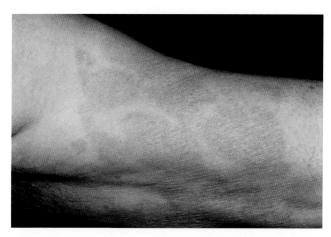

Figure 2.2 Mycosis fungoides, patch stage. Early patches on the arm.

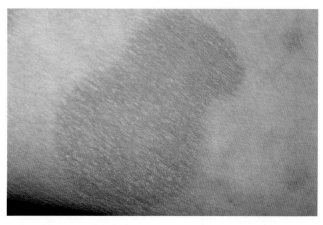

Figure 2.3 Mycosis fungoides, patch stage. Detail of a patch. Note finely wrinkled surface.

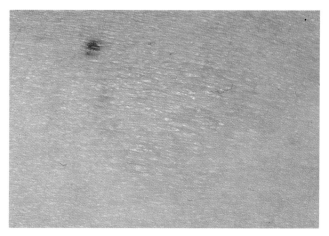

Figure 2.4 Mycosis fungoides, patch stage. Detail of a yellowish patch with clinical features of "xanthoerythroderma perstans."

aspect to the lesions (xanthoerythroderma perstans) (Fig. 2.4). In early phases, a "digitate" pattern can be observed (alone or in combination with larger patches) (see also section on small-plaque parapsoriasis) (Fig. 2.5).

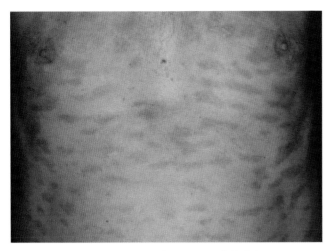

Figure 2.5 Mycosis fungoides, patch stage. So-called "digitate dermatosis." Histologic examination of two patches revealed in both a band-like infiltrate diagnostic of mycosis fungoides.

Plaque stage

Plaques of mycosis fungoides are characterized by infiltrated, variably scaling, reddish-brown lesions (Figs 2.6, 2.7). Typical patches are usually observed contiguous to plaques or at other sites on the body (Fig. 2.8). Plaques of mycosis fungoides should be distinguished from flat tumors of the disease (Figs 2.9, 2.10). Flat, infiltrated lesions should be biopsied in

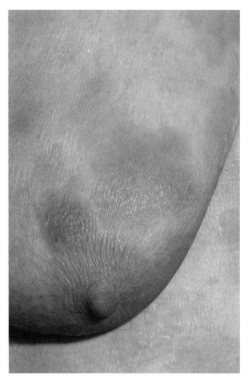

Figure 2.7 Mycosis fungoides, plaque stage. Small plaque near the nipple surrounded by infiltrated patches (detail of Fig. 2.6).

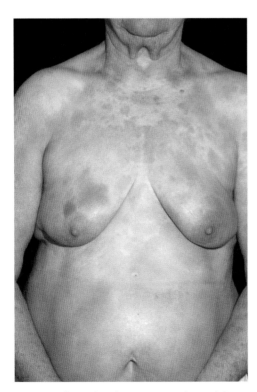

Figure 2.6 Mycosis fungoides, plaque stage. Patches and plaques on the trunk.

order to allow histopathologic examination and a precise classification of the lesions.

Tumor stage

In tumor-stage mycosis fungoides a combination of patches, plaques and tumors is usually found, but tumors may be observed in the absence of other lesions (Figs 2.11, 2.12). Tumors may be solitary or, more often, localized or generalized. Ulceration is common. Onychodystrophy may be prominent [59].

In tumor-stage mycosis fungoides unusual sites of involvement may be observed, such as the mucosal regions (Figs 2.13, 2.14). As oral and genital mucosa are frequently involved in cytotoxic NK/T-cell lymphomas, care should be taken to classify these cases correctly. Careful clinical history taking, re-evaluation of previous biopsies, and complete phenotypic and genotypic investigations are mandatory to make the diagnosis of mucosal involvement in mycosis fungoides.

It should be underlined that patients with tumor-stage mycosis fungoides who are in complete remission after successful treatment may relapse with patches, plaques or tumors. In fact, it is not uncommon that patches of the disease (clinically and histopathologically indistinguishable from early lesions of mycosis fungoides) are the first sign of relapse in these cases. The stage, of course, remains the highest reached by the patient and will not be downgraded; once recurrent

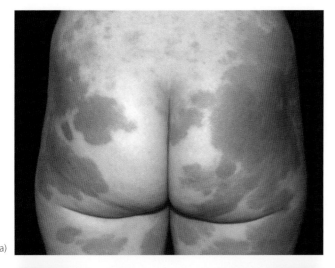

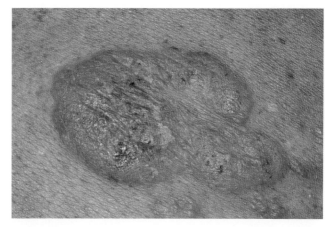

Figure 2.10 Mycosis fungoides, tumor stage. Detail of a flat tumor with small crusts and scales.

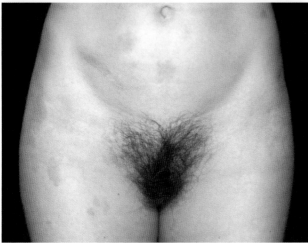

Figure 2.8 Mycosis fungoides, plaque stage. (a) Patches and early plaques on the buttocks. (b) Note concomitant small patches ("parapsoriasis en plaques") on the abdomen and upper legs.

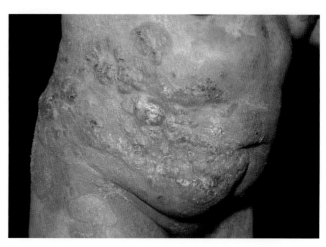

Figure 2.11 Mycosis fungoides, tumor stage. Patches, plaques and tumors.

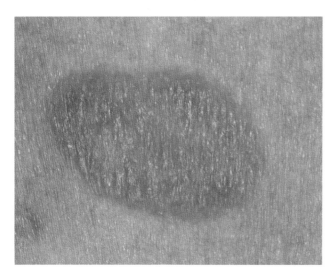

Figure 2.9 Mycosis fungoides, plaque stage. Detail of a plaque.

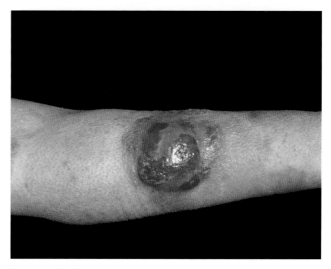

Figure 2.12 Mycosis fungoides, tumor stage. Large ulcerated tumor on the right arm. Note patches and plaques in the vicinity of the tumor.

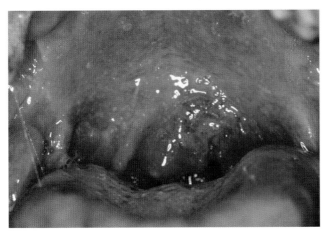

Figure 2.13 Mycosis fungoides, tumor stage. Involvement of the buccal mucosa.

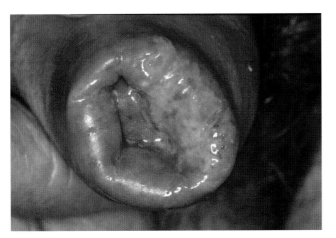

Figure 2.14 Mycosis fungoides, tumor stage. Involvement of the genital mucosa.

lesions arise, new tumors usually develop within short periods of time.

Extracutaneous involvement

Lymph nodes, lung, spleen and liver are the most frequent sites of extracutaneous involvement in mycosis fungoides, but specific lesions can arise in all organs [60,61]. The bone marrow is usually spared. Lymph node involvement may be difficult to differentiate histopathologically from so-called dermatopathic lymphadenopathy, and it has been suggested that, irrespective of the histopathologic features, enlarged lymph nodes represent a bad prognostic sign. A histopathologic staging system of lymph nodes in patients with mycosis fungoides or Sézary syndrome has been proposed recently by the ISCL-EORTC groups [44].

Because of the presence of ulcerated tumors and immune deficiency (due to both the lymphoma and the many treat-

ments typically administered to these patients during the course of the disease), septicemia and/or pneumonia are the major causes of death.

Association with other diseases

As mentioned before, mycosis fungoides can be observed in association with other hematologic disorders such as lymphomatoid papulosis, CD30+ anaplastic large cell lymphoma, and Hodgkin lymphoma. Onset of these disorders may precede, be concomitant with or occur later than the diagnosis of mycosis fungoides. In a few patients, molecular analyses revealed that the same neoplastic clone of T lymphocytes was present in mycosis fungoides and associated lymphomas [37–40]. It may be extremely difficult (if not impossible) to differentiate tumor-stage mycosis fungoides from lesions of lymphomatoid papulosis and CD30+ anaplastic large cell lymphoma (see also Chapter 4). It may be that at least some of the cases reported as lymphomatoid papulosis or cutaneous CD30+ anaplastic large cell lymphoma, arising after the onset of mycosis fungoides, in fact represent lesions of tumor-stage mycosis fungoides with expression of CD30 (see Chapter 2). In this context, it should be noted that spontaneous regression (usually partial regression) of single tumors of mycosis fungoides may be observed. Besides these disease entities, mycosis fungoides has been observed also in association with other non-Hodgkin lymphomas of T- or B-cell lineage [62–64].

An increased incidence of cancers other than lymphomas has been observed in patients with mycosis fungoides [62]. In these patients, mycosis fungoides may represent either the primary or the subsequent malignancy.

Specific infiltrates of mycosis fungoides can be observed in benign and malignant skin tumors such as melanocytic nevi, malignant melanoma and seborrheic keratoses, among others (Fig. 2.15) [65]. In these cases, the association of the two diseases represents an example of so-called "collision tumors".

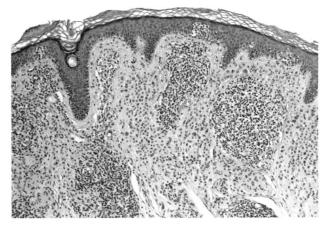

Figure 2.15 Mycosis fungoides. Specific infiltrate of the disease within a pre-existent melanocytic nevus. Note nests of intraepidermal lymphocytes.

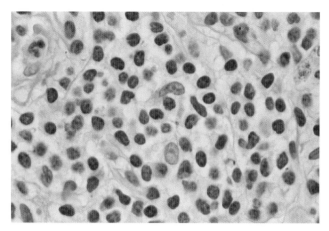

Figure 2.16 Cytomorphology of mycosis fungoides reveals predominance of small- and medium-sized pleomorphic ("cerebriform") lymphocytes.

Histopathology, immunophenotype and molecular genetics

Mycosis fungoides is a cutaneous T-cell lymphoma characterized cytomorphologically by the proliferation of small- to medium-sized pleomorphic ("cerebriform") lymphocytes (Fig. 2.16). Intraepidermal collections of lymphocytes (so-called "Pautrier's microabscesses"), considered for decades the hallmark of the disease, are present only in a minority of early patches of mycosis fungoides and can be absent from more advanced lesions as well. Parenthetically, the first description of the "microabscesses" was not by Pautrier but by Jean Ferdinand Darier several decades before [66]. Pautrier was puzzled by the attribution of this observation to himself and acknowledged that the intraepidermal collections of lymphocytes should have been termed "Darier's nests" (a term that was used in the 1920s) instead [66].

It should be emphasized that, although precise histopathologic criteria for the diagnosis of early mycosis fungoides have been identified (Table 2.4), in many cases a definitive diagnosis can only be made after a careful correlation with the clinical features of the disease [67]. Further problems can arise when biopsies are taken after different types of local treatment that alter the histopathologic features of the lesions. In unclear cases, a useful approach is to take multiple biopsies from morphologically different lesions, to repeat biopsies after a 2-week period without local treatment, and to perform repeat biopsies on recurrent lesions. Repeat biopsies on recurrent lesions should be performed also to check whether the features are stable or changing (i.e. occurrence of large cell transformation).

Scoring systems and algorithms for the diagnosis of mycosis fungoides have been proposed, combining the clinical aspect with the immunophenotypic and molecular features of the infiltrate [68–70]. However, in our view the diagnosis of mycosis fungoides can be achieved in most cases by accurate clinicopathologic correlation. In this context, we recently described several histopathologic patterns of early mycosis fungoides that were previously poorly characterized, showing the protean nature of the disease and the difficulties in histopathologic diagnosis [67].

Histopathology

Early lesions of mycosis fungoides reveal in the vast majority of cases a patchy lichenoid or band-like infiltrate in an expanded papillary dermis (Fig. 2.17). A psoriasiform hyperplasia of the epidermis can be seen (Figs 2.18, 2.19), but in many cases the epidermis is normal. Small lymphocytes predominate and atypical cells can be observed only in a minority of cases. Epidermotropism of solitary lymphocytes is usually found, but Darier's nests (Pautrier's microabscesses) are rare (Fig. 2.20). Useful diagnostic clues are the presence of epidermotropic lymphocytes with nuclei slightly larger than those of lymphocytes within the upper dermis and/or the presence of lymphocytes aligned along the basal layer of the epidermis (Figs 2.21, 2.22) [6–8,71–75]. Also useful is the presence of many intraepidermal lymphocytes in areas with scant spongiosis (Fig. 2.23). In this context, it should be emphasized

Table 2.4 Histopathologic criteria for the diagnosis of early mycosis fungoides

Epidermis
Intraepidermal collections of lymphocytes (Pautrier's microabscesses/ Darier's nests)
Lymphocytes aligned along the dermoepidermal junction
Intraepidermal lymphocytes larger than lymphocytes in the dermis
"Disproportionate" epidermotropism (epidermotropic lymphocytes with only scant spongiosis)
Intraepidermal lymphocytes with "haloed" nuclei

Dermis
Expanded papillary dermis with slight fibrosis and coarse bundles of collagen
Band-like or patchy-lichenoid infiltrate of lymphocytes

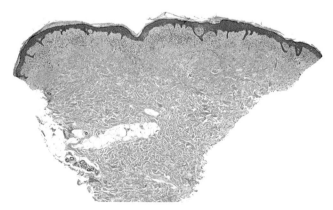

Figure 2.17 Mycosis fungoides, patch stage. Band-like infiltrate of lymphocytes within an expanded papillary dermis.

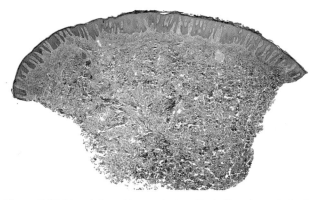

Figure 2.18 Mycosis fungoides, patch stage. Psoriasiform hyperplasia of the epidermis.

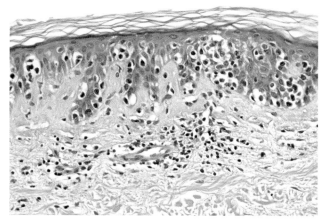

Figure 2.21 Mycosis fungoides, patch stage. Epidermotropic lymphocytes with nuclei larger than those of the lymphocytes within the superficial dermis. Note also lymphocytes with clear halo around the nuclei ("haloed lymphocytes").

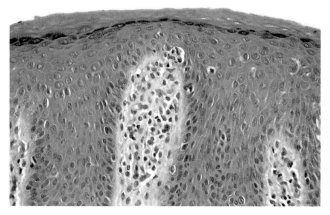

Figure 2.19 Mycosis fungoides, patch stage. Note a small intraepidermal collection of lymphocytes (detail of Fig. 2.18).

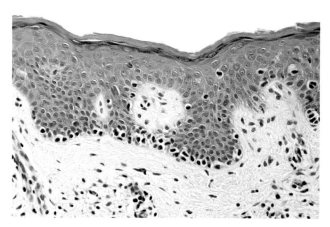

Figure 2.22 Mycosis fungoides, patch stage. Epidermotropism of solitary lymphocytes aligned along the basal layer of the epidermis.

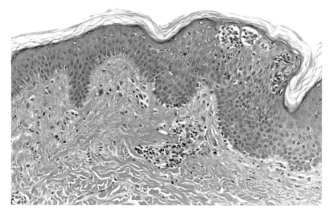

Figure 2.20 Mycosis fungoides, patch stage. Scant superficial perivascular infiltrate of lymphocytes and intraepidermal collections of lymphocytes ("Darier's nests," "Pautrier's microabscesses"). Note perivascular distribution of the infiltrate within the papillary dermis.

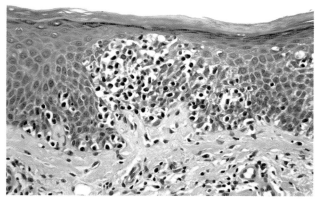

Figure 2.23 Mycosis fungoides, patch stage. "Disproportionate" epidermotropism (presence of many intraepidermal lymphocytes on the background of only scant spongiosis of the epidermis).

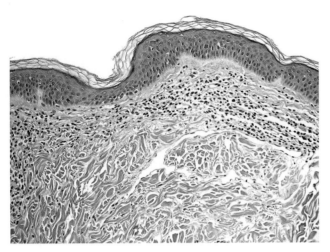

Figure 2.24 Mycosis fungoides, patch stage. Band-like infiltrate of lymphocytes within a thickened fibrotic papillary dermis. Note complete absence of epidermotropism.

that in a few cases (about 5% of the total) epidermotropism may be missing (Fig. 2.24). The papillary dermis shows a moderate to marked fibrosis with coarse bundles of collagen and a band-like or patchy-lichenoid infiltrate of lymphocytes. Dermal edema is usually not found.

Unusual histopathologic patterns of mycosis fungoides in early phases include the presence of a perivascular (as opposed to band-like) superficial infiltrate (Fig. 2.20), prominent spongiosis simulating the picture of acute contact dermatitis (Fig. 2.25), sometimes with Darier's nests (Pautrier's microabscesses) mimicking spongiotic vesicles (Fig. 2.26), an interface dermatitis, sometimes with several necrotic keratinocytes simulating a multiforme-like reaction (Figs 2.27, 2.28), marked pigment incontinence with melanophages in the

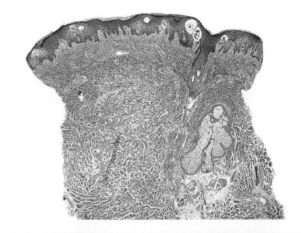

(a)

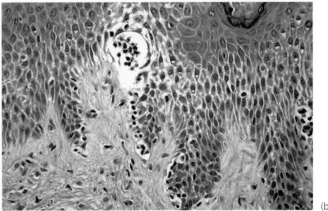

(b)

Figure 2.26 Mycosis fungoides, patch stage. (a) Psoriasiform hyperplasia of the epidermis with marked spongiosis and spongiform vesicles, some with lymphocytes. (b) Note prominent spongiosis and vesiculation with several lymphocytes within the vesicle.

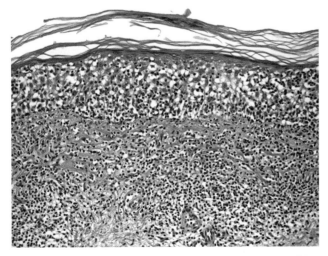

Figure 2.25 Mycosis fungoides, patch stage. Prominent spongiosis of the epidermis associated with several epidermotropic lymphocytes. Note also the presence of a band-like infiltrate of lymphocytes within an expanded fibrotic papillary dermis.

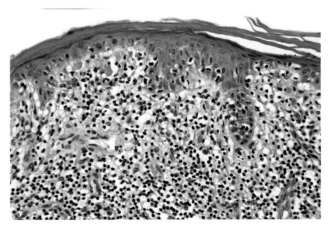

Figure 2.27 Mycosis fungoides, patch stage. Vacuolization of basal keratinocytes ("interface dermatitis") with several necrotic keratinocytes.

papillary dermis (Fig. 2.29), prominent epidermal hyperplasia simulating the picture of lichen simplex chronicus (Fig. 2.30), and prominent extravasation of erythrocytes simulating the picture of lichenoid purpura (Fig. 2.31). A pattern characterized

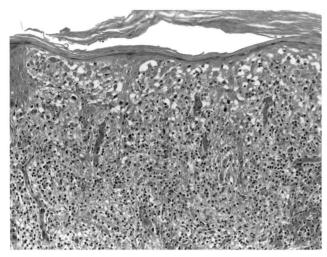

Figure 2.28 Mycosis fungoides, patch stage. Necrosis of clusters of keratinocytes simulating the picture of erythema multiforme. Note also many epidermotropic lymphocytes.

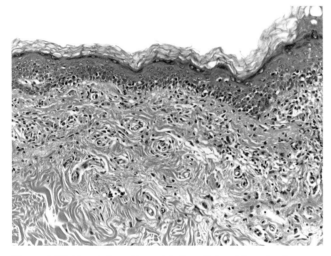

Figure 2.29 Mycosis fungoides, patch stage. Note epidermotropic lymphocytes and several melanophages within the papillary dermis.

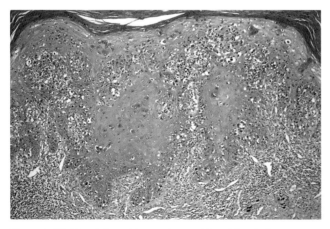

Figure 2.30 Mycosis fungoides, patch stage. The epidermis shows a prominent pseudocarcinomatous hyperplasia. Note epidermotropic lymphocytes with atypical nuclei.

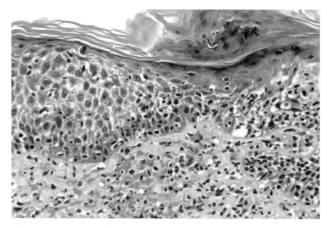

Figure 2.31 Mycosis fungoides, patch stage. Prominent extravasation of erythrocytes in "purpuric" mycosis fungoides. Note also spongiosis and epidermotropic lymphocytes.

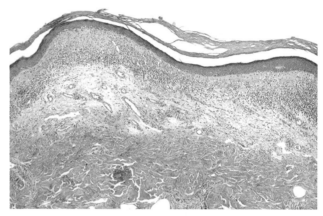

Figure 2.32 Mycosis fungoides, patch stage. Prominent atrophy of the epidermis with loss of rete ridges and epidermotropic lymphocytes within the lower layers (poikilodermatous mycosis fungoides). Note band-like infiltrate of lymphocytes within a fibrotic papillary dermis and increased number of telangiectatic vessels.

by a markedly flattened epidermis, a lichenoid infiltrate in the dermis, and increased, dilated vessels in the papillary dermis is the histopathologic counterpart of poikilodermatous mycosis fungoides (Fig. 2.32) (see Chapter 2). In rare cases the epidermal pattern may resemble that observed in lesions of pityriasis lichenoides et varioliformis acuta (PLEVA) (Fig. 2.33). This pattern can be observed more frequently in children (see corresponding section in this Chapter).

Plaques of mycosis fungoides are characterized by a dense, band-like infiltrate within the upper dermis (Fig. 2.34). Intraepidermal lymphocytes arranged in Darier's nests (Pautrier's microabscesses) are a common finding at this stage (Fig. 2.35). Cytomorphologically, small pleomorphic (cerebriform) cells predominate (Fig. 2.16). In some cases plaques or flat tumors of mycosis fungoides may present with a predominantly interstitial infiltrate (Fig. 2.36). This peculiar presentation can give rise to diagnostic problems and has been designated "interstitial

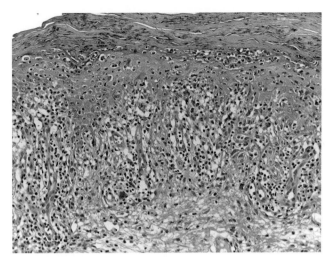

Figure 2.33 Mycosis fungoides, patch-stage. Scattered necrotic keratinocytes, prominent parakeratosis, and intraepidermal and intracorneal lymphocytes and neutrophils similar to the picture observed in pityriasis lichenoides et varioliformis acuta.

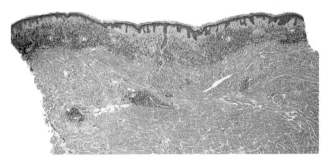

Figure 2.34 Mycosis fungoides, plaque stage. Dense band-like infiltrate of lymphocytes within the superficial dermis. Note small perivascular aggregates of lymphocytes in the mid-dermis.

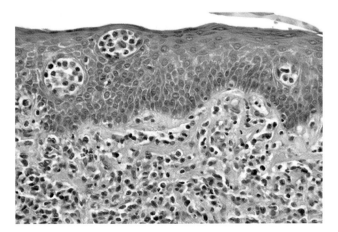

Figure 2.35 Mycosis fungoides, plaque stage. Intraepidermal collections of lymphocytes ("Darier's nests" or "Pautrier's microabscesses").

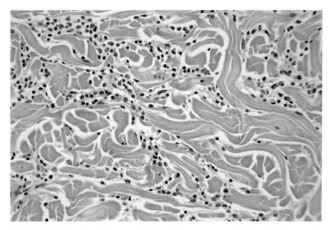

Figure 2.36 Interstitial mycosis fungoides. Note neoplastic cells arranged in intertwining cords within the collagen, simulating the histopathologic picture of the interstitial variant of granuloma annulare.

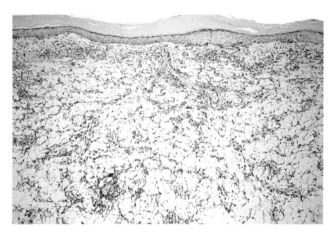

Figure 2.37 Interstitial mycosis fungoides. Staining for CD3 reveals that all interstitial cells are T lymphocytes.

mycosis fungoides" [76]. Immunohistology confirms that interstitial cells are T lymphocytes, which is a helpful clue for the differential diagnosis with the interstitial variant of granuloma annulare (Fig. 2.37). Interstitial mycosis fungoides is usually a manifestation of either plaque or tumor stage of the disease.

In tumors of mycosis fungoides a dense, nodular or diffuse infiltrate is found within the entire dermis, usually involving the subcutaneous fat (Fig. 2.38). Epidermotropism may be lost. Flat tumors are characterized histopathologically by dense infiltrates confined to the superficial and mid parts of the dermis (Fig. 2.39). Angiocentricity and/or angiodestruction may be observed in some cases [77].

Large cell transformation

In later stages, patients with mycosis fungoides usually develop lesions with many large cells (immunoblasts, large pleomorphic cells or large anaplastic cells) (Fig. 2.40) [78–81]. Large cell transformation in mycosis fungoides is defined as the presence

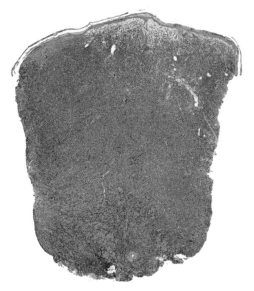

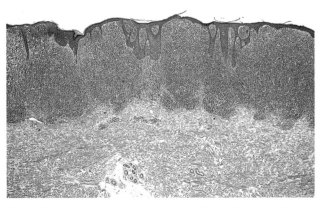

Figure 2.39 Mycosis fungoides, tumor stage. Histopathology of a flat tumor showing a dense diffuse infiltrate of lymphocytes within the superficial dermis involving the mid-dermis.

Figure 2.38 Mycosis fungoides, tumor stage. Dense nodular infiltrates of lymphocytes within the entire dermis involving the subcutaneous fat.

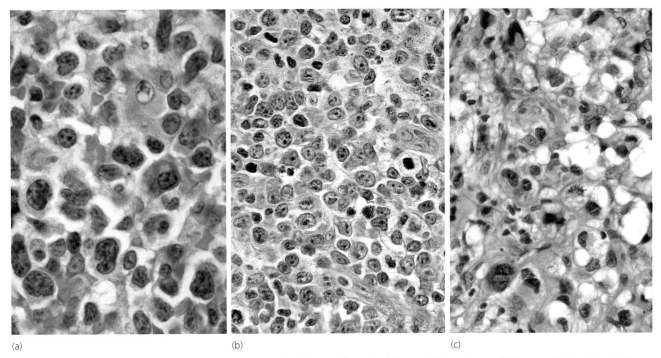

(a)   (b)   (c)

Figure 2.40 Mycosis fungoides with large cell transformation. (a) Medium- and large-sized pleomorphic lymphocytes. (b) T immunoblasts admixed with pleomorphic lymphocytes. (c) Large anaplastic cells predominate.

of large cells exceeding 25% of the infiltrate or large cells forming microscopic nodules, and has been detected in more than 50% of patients with tumor-stage mycosis fungoides [78]. Clusters of large cells may sometimes be observed in plaques of mycosis fungoides (usually in patients having tumors in other sites of the body), and rarely even in thin patches of the disease (these patients, too, usually also have plaques and tumors of mycosis fungoides at other sites of the body) (Fig. 2.41).

Tumors with a large cell morphology may or may not express CD30. Expression of the antigen does not have any prognostic significance in these patients. Spontaneous regression of some lesions and/or CD30 expression by neoplastic cells may suggest the diagnosis of anaplastic large cell lymphoma or lymphomatoid papulosis in these patients, but such a diagnosis should be made only upon compelling evidence in patients with known mycosis fungoides. Although lymphomatoid papulosis

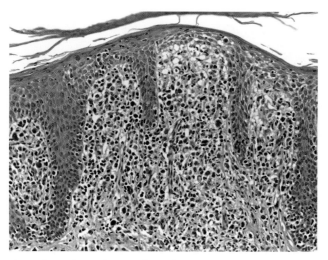

Figure 2.41 Plaque of mycosis fungoides with large cell transformation.

may be associated with mycosis fungoides, the highest degree of caution should be exercised in making this diagnosis when mycosis fungoides precedes the putative lymphomatoid papulosis. In fact, one patient with mycosis fungoides whom we published several years ago as "PUVA-induced lymphomatoid papulosis in mycosis fungoides" [82] turned out to have a CD30$^+$ large cell transformation with bad prognosis, and similar patients have been described recently [83,84]. Large cell transformation of mycosis fungoides bears a poor prognosis, and usually heralds the terminal stage of the disease.

Immunophenotype

Mycosis fungoides is characterized by an infiltrate of α/β T-helper memory lymphocytes (β F1$^+$, CD3$^+$, CD4$^+$, CD5$^+$, CD8$^-$, CD45Ro$^+$) (Fig. 2.42) [85,86]. Only a minority of cases exhibit a T-cytotoxic (β F1$^+$, CD3$^+$, CD4$^-$, CD5$^+$, CD8$^+$) or γ/δ (β F1$^-$, CD3$^+$, CD4$^-$, CD5$^+$, CD8$^+$ – the more specific δ1 staining is available only for frozen sections of tissue) lineage, which show no clinical and/or prognostic differences (Fig. 2.43) [87,88]. In these cases, correlation with the clinical features

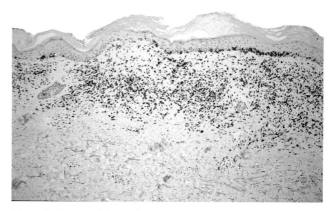

Figure 2.43 Mycosis fungoides, patch stage. Positive staining for CD8 in the CD8 variant of mycosis fungoides.

is crucial, in order to rule out skin involvement by aggressive cytotoxic lymphomas such as CD8$^+$ epidermotropic T-cell lymphoma or γ/δ T-cell lymphoma (see also Chapter 6). In late stages there may be a (partial) loss of pan-T-cell antigen expression. In plaque and tumor lesions (and rarely focally in patches, too) neoplastic T cells may express the CD30 antigen. Aberrant expression of the B-cell antigen CD20 has been observed exceptionally [89]. In these cases, negativity for other B-cell markers such as CD79a and positivity for T-cell markers helps in determining the exact lineage of the cells.

It has been suggested that a low CD8:CD3 ratio in skin infiltrates supports the histopathologic diagnosis of mycosis fungoides, but this finding should be confirmed in larger studies [90]. Loss of pan-T-cell markers (CD2, CD3, CD5) is a helpful sign for the diagnosis of mycosis fungoides [91], but in our experience it is very rare in early lesions of the disease. Rarely, early mycosis fungoides displays an aberrant CD4$^+$/CD8$^+$ or CD4$^-$/CD8$^-$ phenotype [88,92].

Particularly in tumor-stage disease, it may be important to assess the infiltrate for expression of molecules that may be potentially targeted for treatment. Campath, for example, is a monoclonal anti-CD52 antibody, and positivity for CD52 is a prerequisite for therapeutic effect. As more molecules are continuously characterized by genetic investigations, and some of them may be potentially targeted by specific therapies, it is likely that in the near future immunohistochemical investigations will be used not only for diagnostic purposes but also for predicting usefulness of given therapies.

Cytotoxic-associated markers such as T-cell intracellular antigen (TIA)-1, granzyme B and perforin are negative in mycosis fungoides, although occasionally in late stages of the disease positivity may be observed [93]. These cases should not be classified as cytotoxic lymphomas (see also Chapter 6), but as tumor-stage mycosis fungoides with cytotoxic phenotype. A similar phenotype may also be seen in early lesions of the rare γ/δ$^+$ mycosis fungoides, which besides cytotoxic proteins expresses also CD56 (Fig. 2.44), or in CD8$^+$ cytotoxic mycosis fungoides [88].

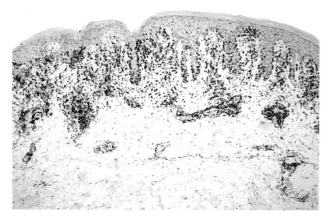

Figure 2.42 Mycosis fungoides, patch stage. Staining for CD3 helps to highlight intraepidermal T lymphocytes.

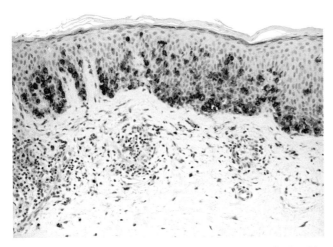

Figure 2.44 Mycosis fungoides, patch stage. Positive staining for CD56 in the γ/δ variant of mycosis fungoides.

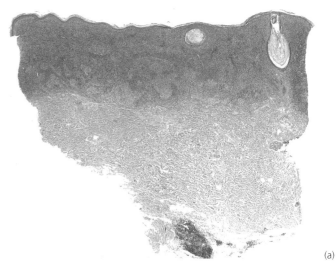

(a)

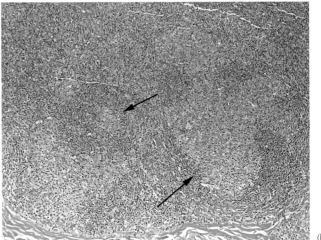

(b)

Figure 2.45 Mycosis fungoides, flat tumor (same case as Figs 2.46 and 2.47). (a) Prominent infiltrate of reactive cells. (b) Note reactive germinal centers (*arrows*).

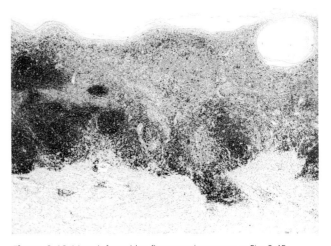

Figure 2.46 Mycosis fungoides, flat tumor (same case as Figs 2.45 and 2.47). Note prominent positivity for CD20 representing reactive B lymphocytes.

Multiple myeloma-1/interferon regulatory factor-4 (MUM1/IRF4), a member of the interferon regulatory factor (IRF) family of transcription factors, is positive in cutaneous CD30⁺ lymphoproliferative disorders and in CD30⁺ large cell transformation of mycosis fungoides, but it is otherwise negative in mycosis fungoides [94].

T-regulatory (Treg) cells comprise a T-cell population that can influence other cell types with suppression of the immune response, and that shows mostly a CD4⁺/CD25⁺/FOX-P3⁺ phenotype. They are present in the reactive infiltrate of lesions of early mycosis fungoides but tend to disappear in tumor stage, and are thought to be related to prognosis [95–98]. Convincing cases of mycosis fungoides with a true Treg phenotype have not been described. Dr Emilio Berti (Milan) recently showed to one of us (LC) one such case with positivity of most neoplastic cells.

An increased number of CD1a⁺ Langerhans cells as well as other dendritic cells can be observed in mycosis fungoides, particularly in early lesions, sometimes simulating the picture of a Langerhans cell histiocytosis [99]. We have come across cases that, besides the typical intraepidermal Darier's nests (Pautrier's microabscesses), revealed also small intraepidermal collections of Langerhans cells. Although these "Langerhans microabscesses" are considered a differential diagnostic tool for contact dermatitis (see Chapter 22), they can rarely be observed in mycosis fungoides as well. Besides CD1a⁺ cells, lesions of mycosis fungoides, particularly in advanced stages, may show a prominent amount of reactive CD20⁺ B lymphocytes, even forming germinal centers (Figs 2.45–2.47). The B lymphocytes may be prominent and mask the true T-cell nature of the neoplastic infiltrate. These cases should not be misinterpreted as B-cell lymphoma. As already mentioned, CD20 may also be expressed aberrantly by neoplastic T lymphocytes, thus underlining the need for complete phenotypic analyses of every case.

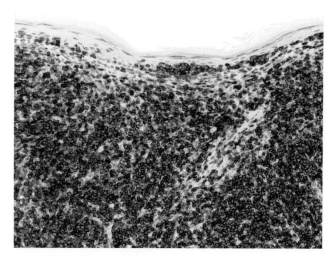

Figure 2.47 Mycosis fungoides, flat tumor (same case as Figs 2.45 and 2.46). Neoplastic cells express CD3. Note epidermotropism.

Molecular genetics

Studies on the genetic background of mycosis fungoides revealed a heterogenous picture, probably due to the differences in the study protocols and type of cases investigated so far, and to the inherent difficulties in analyzing early cases due to the small number of neoplastic cells. There are no specific abnormalities repeatedly associated with early mycosis fungoides, although more data are available for later stages of the disease. Using cDNA microarray analysis, a signature of 27 genes, including oncogenes and other genes involved in the control of apoptosis, has been identified in cases of early- and late-stage mycosis fungoides [100], but these results have not yet been confirmed. In a similar study, consensus clustering revealed the presence of two clusters that tended to include mostly patients with mycosis fungoides in early stages (Ia and Ib), and of a third cluster limited mostly to patients with more advanced disease [101]. However, the number of cases included was relatively small, and overlapping data were observed, thus necessitating confirmation of the results in larger series. Oncogenes such as p16 and p53 do not show alterations in early lesions, but are often mutated in late (tumor) phases of the disease [102]. Dysregulated expression of *JUNB* and *JUND* has been found in some cases [55,103,104], and FAS mutations in others [105]. Chromosomal aberrations observed in large cell transformation of mycosis fungoides include alterations of chromosomes 1, 2, 7, 9, 17, and 19, the most common imbalances being gain of chromosome regions 1p36, 7, 9q34, 17q24-qter, 19, and loss of 2q36-qter, 9p21, and 17p [106]. Loss of heterozygosity analysis allowed identification of specific loci associated with disease progression in one study, located particularly on chromosome 10 [107,108], whereas analysis of microsatellite instability failed to prove useful in determining the pathogenesis of the disease and/or the mechanisms of disease progression [109].

Recurrent deletions of tumor suppressor genes *BCL7A*, *SMAC/DIABLO*, and *RHOF* have been detected by comparative genome hybridization in cases of early mycosis fungoides [110]. Other gene alterations that have been detected in mycosis fungoides involve p15, p14, *PTEN*, HLA-G, Fas, and Fas ligand. In general, however, results of different studies did not reveal repeatable, reliable genetic alterations, even in tumor stages of the disease.

Only a few studies have addressed early genetic events in mycosis fungoides [111,112], and results have sometimes been contradictory [113,114]. In this context, it should be underlined that molecular analysis of early lesions of mycosis fungoides is hindered by the intrinsic difficulties in the identification of neoplastic cells, which are a small minority and look morphologically and phenotypically identical to reactive lymphocytes. As genetic techniques, especially on routinely fixed specimens, require a certain threshold of tumor DNA, it may be difficult to analyze early lesions of mycosis fungoides where only a few neoplastic cells can be observed.

Rearrangement of the T-cell receptor (TCR) gene is commonly found in plaques and tumors, but is present only in approximately 50–60% of early (patch) lesions analyzed by standard techniques [67,115,116]. More complicated systems for detection of TCR gene rearrangements bear a better sensitivity, but are time-consuming and not available routinely in all laboratories [117,118]. Moreover, dominant clones may be found in common inflammatory dermatoses (e.g. lichen planus), thus posing a problem of specificity as well. Development of "patient-specific" DNA probes can identify the neoplastic clone also in lesions that were not specific histopathologically [119–121], and may be a useful method (though not routinely available) for detection of residual disease. Recently, it has been shown that demonstration of T-cell clonality by standard polymerase chain reaction (PCR) assays at first diagnostic biopsy does not affect the prognosis of patients with early mycosis fungoides [88].

The presence of a monoclonal population of T lymphocytes has been detected in the peripheral blood in patients with early-stage mycosis fungoides [48–50]. In many of these patients the clone was different from that detected within the skin, but in some cases the same clone was present both in the peripheral blood and in the cutaneous lesions of mycosis fungoides, even after successful treatment and complete clinical remission [48,50,51]. The exact diagnostic and prognostic value of molecular genetic analysis of the TCR gene rearrangement within the peripheral blood in patients with early mycosis fungoides is still unclear [122]. Similarly, it is currently unclear what is the prognostic value (if any) of the detection of monoclonality within lymph nodes that are not affected clinically and/or histopathologically, but a prognostic implication has been suggested for lymph nodes that harbor a monoclonal population of T lymphocytes [123,124]. At present we do not advocate the routine performance of PCR assays from the peripheral blood or from clinically uninvolved lymph nodes in patients with early mycosis fungoides, but the determination of clonality may be of importance in lymph nodes showing dermopathic lymphadenopathy.

Recently, serum proteomic analyses have been used for identification of patients with tumor-stage mycosis fungoides [125]; however, these are currently useful mainly for scientific research and for identification of new therapeutic targets, as in this stage of the disease diagnosis is almost never a problem.

Histopathologic differential diagnosis

The histopathologic diagnosis of early mycosis fungoides may be extremely difficult, and in some cases classification of given histopathologic features as specific is simply not possible. In fact, in some instances differentiation from inflammatory skin conditions (i.e. psoriasis, chronic contact dermatitis, etc.) may be impossible on histopathologic grounds alone. In these cases clinical correlation is crucial to make a definitive diagnosis. It should be underlined that in many cases "non-specific" histopathologic features do not allow us to rule out a diagnosis of mycosis fungoides if the clinical presentation is suggestive of the disease. In such cases we describe the histopathologic aspects as "consistent with" the clinical diagnosis, rather than simply issuing a report of "non-specific chronic dermatitis." If only cases with marked epidermotropism and/or presence of Darier's nests (Pautrier's microabscesses) are reported as diagnostic, then the majority of early lesions of mycosis fungoides will be missed on histopathologic grounds. The ISCL proposed a scoring system for diagnosis of early patches of mycosis fungoides [69], but the crucial value of clinicopathologic correlation, integration of all available data, and especially repeated biopsies has been underlined again recently [70].

Immunohistologic features of mycosis fungoides are not distinctive, and are similar to those observed in many inflammatory skin conditions [85,86]. Staining for CD3 or CD4 may help by highlighting epidermotropic T lymphocytes (see Fig. 2.40). It has been suggested that in early stages of mycosis fungoides, in contrast to benign (inflammatory) cutaneous infiltrates of T lymphocytes, there is a loss of expression of the T-cell-associated antigen CD7 [126,127]. This finding has not been confirmed by other studies showing normal CD7$^+$ populations in early mycosis fungoides [85,115]. In addition, T lymphocytes in some cases of benign inflammatory dermatosis can also show partial loss of CD7 [128,129]. In our opinion, CD7 staining has very limited value in the differential diagnosis of cutaneous T-cell infiltrates [130].

Immunohistochemical analysis of the TCRs has also been advocated for differentiation of early mycosis fungoides from chronic benign inflammatory conditions [131,132], but at present this is not considered a useful method for differential diagnosis of mycosis fungoides from reactive conditions in routine settings. It has been suggested that the frequent expression of the same variable region of the TCRs in different cases of mycosis fungoides may reflect similarities in the etiology and/or pathogenesis (i.e. a distinct population of virus-infected cells) of this condition [132].

Molecular analysis of TCR gene rearrangement is a further method helpful in the differentiation of mycosis fungoides from benign skin conditions [115,116,133]. In particular, detection of clonality in lesions from different skin sites seems to be highly specific for mycosis fungoides [134]. It must be underlined, however, that using standard methods for detection of clonality in early lesions of mycosis fungoides a monoclonal rearrangement can be demonstrated only in about 50–60% of the cases, and that several benign dermatoses have been shown to harbor a monoclonal population of T lymphocytes (e.g. lichen planus and lichen sclerosus, among others) [88,135–137]. Thus, absence of clonality should not be considered as a criterion to rule out mycosis fungoides, particularly in cases that show suspicious clinical and/or histopathologic features. The reason for the low sensitivity of gene rearrangement analysis in mycosis fungoides may reside in the very low number of neoplastic lymphocytes in early phases of the disease, and it has been shown that sensitivity can be increased upon microdissection of the specimen [138]. Attempts to increase sensitivity of PCR techniques by refining the detection methods have been described as well [117,139, 140], but they are often too complex for routine examination of biopsy specimens. Moreover, increasing sensitivity has an adverse effect on the specificity of PCR techniques, as some inflammatory conditions may harbor a monoclonal population of T lymphocytes. At present, therefore, the presence or absence of a monoclonal pattern of TCR gene rearrangement cannot be considered as a crucial criterion in the early diagnosis of mycosis fungoides.

Besides the differential diagnosis with inflammatory (reactive) conditions, mycosis fungoides should be differentiated from other cutaneous lymphomas, particularly cytotoxic NK/T-cell lymphomas. Differential diagnostic criteria are discussed in Chapter 6.

Clinical and histopathologic variants

Mycosis fungoides has been recently defined as a "dermatologic masquerader" [141], and several clinical and/or histopathologic variants have been described (Table 2.5) [142,143]. It must be underlined that some of these "variants" are peculiar clinical or histopathologic presentations observed only in a few patients, but others are more frequent and represent a true pitfall in the diagnosis of the disease. Patients with these variants often also show features of "classic" mycosis fungoides at other sites of the body or develop more conventional lesions during follow-up.

Many of the clinicopathologic variants listed in Table 2.5 are quite rare. Some of them in the past were separated from mycosis fungoides and considered as distinct entities (e.g.

Table 2.5 Clinicopathologic variants of mycosis fungoides

Acanthosis nigricans-like mycosis fungoides
Anetodermic mycosis fungoides (mycosis fungoides with secondary anetoderma)
Angiocentric/angiodestructive mycosis fungoides
Bullous (vesiculobullous) mycosis fungoides
Dyshidrotic mycosis fungoides
Erythrodermic mycosis fungoides
Follicular (pilotropic) mycosis fungoides
Granulomatous mycosis fungoides
Granulomatous slack skin
Hyperpigmented mycosis fungoides
Hypopigmented mycosis fungoides
Ichthyosis-like mycosis fungoides
Interstitial mycosis fungoides
"Invisible" mycosis fungoides
Mucinous mycosis fungoides
Mycosis fungoides palmaris et plantaris
Mycosis fungoides with eruptive infundibular cysts
Mycosis fungoides with follicular mucinosis
Mycosis fungoides with large cell transformation
Pagetoid reticulosis (Woringer–Kolopp type)
Papular mycosis fungoides
Papuloerythroderma Ofuji
Perioral dermatitis-like mycosis fungoides
Pigmented purpura-like mycosis fungoides
PLEVA-like mycosis fungoides
Poikilodermatous mycosis fungoides (poikiloderma vasculare atrophicans)
Pustular mycosis fungoides
Small-plaque parapsoriasis
Syringotropic mycosis fungoides
Unilesional (solitary) mycosis fungoides
Verrucous/hyperkeratotic mycosis fungoides
Zosteriform mycosis fungoides

Table 2.6 Historical terms used for mycosis fungoides*

Erythrodermie pityriasique en plaques disseminées
Parakeratosis variegata
Parapsoriasis en plaques
Parapsoriasis lichenoides
Parapsoriasis variegata
Poikiloderma vasculare atrophicans
Premycotic erythema
Prereticulotic poikiloderma
Retiform type of parapsoriasis
Xanthoerythroderma perstans

* Some of these terms are still used today in some centers.

small-plaque parapsoriasis, pagetoid reticulosis, granulomatous slack skin, papuloerythroderma Ofuji). In fact, they are now thought to be variants of mycosis fungoides, although the exact nosologic classification of some of them is still debated. In the following text the main characteristics of some of these forms are summarized.

In addition to these variants, a plethora of terms has been used in the past for mycosis fungoides (Table 2.6), and unfortunately, some of them are still in use today. The use of these terms has brought much confusion to this field, and should be strongly discouraged.

Small-plaque parapsoriasis

The exact nosology of small-plaque parapsoriasis represents the most controversial issue in the discussion on early manifestations of mycosis fungoides. It is well known that small patches of disease are common in patients with otherwise "conventional" mycosis fungoides. Some patients present only with small, sometimes "digitated" patches, typically located on the trunk and upper extremities (see Fig. 2.5). In the past cases characterized by small lesions alone were variously diagnosed as "digitate" dermatosis, chronic superficial scaly dermatitis or small-plaque parapsoriasis (the term is a misnomer as these patients never present with plaques). Molecular genetic techniques revealed that in some of these lesions a monoclonal population of T-lymphocytes can be found.

At present there is lack of agreement concerning the exact relationship of small-plaque parapsoriasis and mycosis fungoides: some think that they represent one and the same disease, whereas others maintain that they are completely unrelated [144–146]. In Graz we have encountered patients with small patches of "parapsoriasis en plaques" who decades later developed typical plaques and tumors of mycosis fungoides, leading us to conclude that small-plaque parapsoriasis represents an early manifestation of the disease. A similar observation has been published recently by Väkevä and co-workers, who observed that 10% of their patients with small-plaque parapsoriasis developed mycosis fungoides during the course of the disease [147], and by Belousova and co-workers [148]. Regardless of the academic discussion, it is important to underline that patients with small-plaque parapsoriasis should not be treated aggressively, as progression of the disease is rare and, when it happens, takes place only after very long periods of time.

It should be clearly stated that we (as well as most other authors) do not believe that "large-plaque parapsoriasis" is a peculiar variant of mycosis fungoides but rather represents one of the most typical presentations of the disease. In this sense, we have not listed large-plaque parapsoriasis among the clinicopathologic variants of mycosis fungoides.

Mycosis fungoides with follicular mucinosis/follicular (pilotropic) mycosis fungoides

Some patients with mycosis fungoides present with follicular papules and plaques characterized histopathologically by abundant deposits of mucin within hair follicles that are surrounded by a more or less dense infiltrate of T lymphocytes

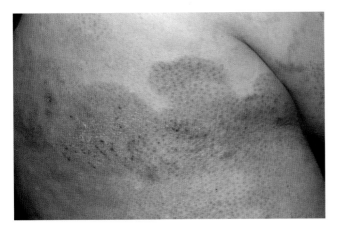

Figure 2.48 Mycosis fungoides with follicular mucinosis. Follicular erythematous papules and plaques on the thigh.

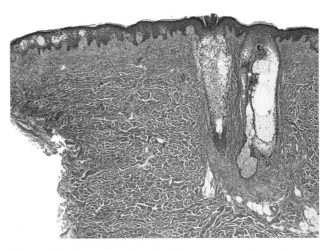

Figure 2.50 Mycosis fungoides with follicular mucinosis. Mucin deposits within two hair follicles as well as within the interfollicular epidermis ("epidermal mucinosis"). Note also patchy lichenoid infiltrate of lymphocytes with epidermotropism.

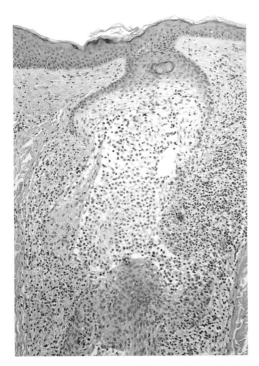

Figure 2.49 Mycosis fungoides with follicular mucinosis. Mucin deposits within a hair follicle with destruction of the follicle. Note lymphocytes infiltrating the hair follicle ("pilotropism").

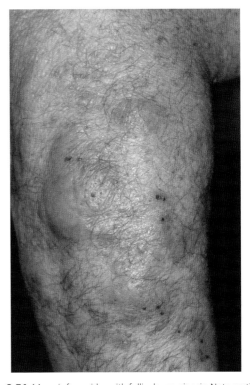

Figure 2.51 Mycosis fungoides with follicular mucinosis. Note partial loss of hairs within the affected skin ("alopecia mucinosa") and superficial erosions representing scratch artefacts resulting from intense itching.

(Figs 2.48, 2.49) [149]. The hair follicles are infiltrated by the lymphocytes ("pilotropism"). The epidermis between affected follicles may be spared or involved by the disease ("epidermal mucinosis") (Fig. 2.50). Alopecia due to destruction of the follicles is common (alopecia mucinosa), either generalized or localized (Fig. 2.51). Itching is severe and represents a major problem in this variant of mycosis fungoides, and may be non-responsive to standard treatments.

A variant of mycosis fungoides with marked involvement of the hair follicles but without deposition of mucin has also been described ("pilotropic mycosis fungoides") (Fig. 2.52); its relationship with follicular mucinosis-associated mycosis fungoides is unclear, but it seems that pilotropic mycosis fungoides with or without mucin deposition represents a spectrum of disease characterized by prominent involvement of the hair follicles [150,151].

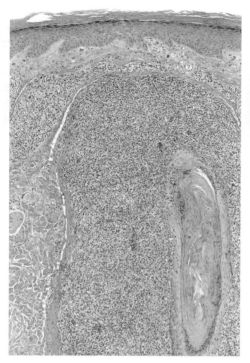

Figure 2.52 Pilotropic mycosis fungoides. Dense perifollicular infiltrate of lymphocytes without deposits of mucin within the hair follicle.

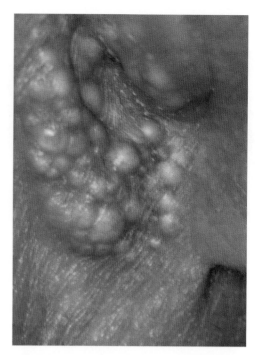

Figure 2.53 Mycosis fungoides with eruptive cysts and comedones. Retro-auricular eruption of small epidermal cysts (milia).

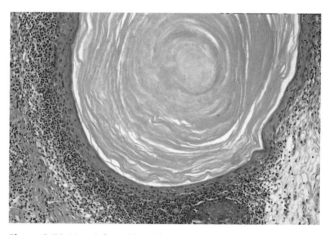

Figure 2.54 Mycosis fungoides with eruptive cysts and comedones. Dense infiltrate of lymphocytes involving the wall of a cyst.

In patients with marked involvement of the hair follicles, with or without deposition of mucin, a localized eruption of small infundibular cysts and comedones infiltrated by neoplastic T lymphocytes can be observed ("mycosis fungoides with eruptive cysts and comedones") (Figs 2.53, 2.54). The clinical picture is similar to that observed in so-called "milia en plaques."

We believe that so-called "idiopathic generalized follicular mucinosis" in fact represents a variant of mycosis fungoides with marked deposition of mucin within hair follicles, and cases of progression to late-stage mycosis fungoides and death have been well documented [149]. We have also observed patients with clear-cut mycosis fungoides-associated follicular mucinosis who entered clinical remission after conventional treatments, and who subsequently relapsed with skin lesions showing clinical and histopathologic features of "idiopathic" follicular mucinosis, again suggesting that this condition represents a variant of mycosis fungoides. Even "benign" localized follicular mucinosis may in fact represent a variant of mycosis fungoides, conceptually and biologically similar to localized pagetoid reticulosis and "unilesional" mycosis fungoides [149].

Prominent involvement of the hair follicles with follicular hyperplasia may lead to the formation of elevated lesions, clinically resembling tumors of the disease even in the absence of true neoplastic tumors ("pseudotumoral mycosis fungoides") [152,153]. Some authors report a worse prognosis in mycosis fungoides associated with follicular mucinosis in comparison to patients with "conventional" mycosis fungoides [154,155].

Syringotropic mycosis fungoides

Some patients present with unusual lesions consisting of dense lymphoid infiltrates located mainly around hyperplastic eccrine glands and coils, often with syringometaplasia (Figs 2.55, 2.56). Since the first observation of this peculiar variant of mycosis fungoides, its exact nosologic classification has been a matter of debate, as lesions are often solitary and there are no other signs of mycosis fungoides. The term "syringolymphoid hyperplasia with alopecia" has been used in the past to refer to these cases [156–160]. On the other hand, a relation to the cutaneous T-cell lymphomas was postulated in 1992 by Burg and Schmöckel [161] and has been con-

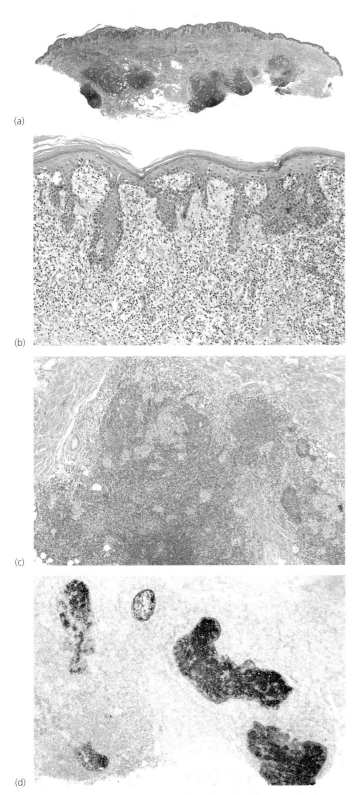

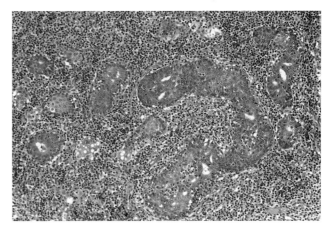

Figure 2.56 Syringotropic mycosis fungoides. Neoplastic lymphocytes arranged predominantly around and within sweat glands. Note syringometaplasia.

firmed by many other reports [162–166]. A specific relation to mycosis fungoides has also been suggested [167,168].

We have encountered several patients with similar lesions and believe that they represent a variant of mycosis fungoides with prominent involvement of the adnexal structures. In fact, in some cases there was a concomitant band-like infiltrate in the papillary dermis, and in others the hair follicles were involved as well, showing features indistinguishable from those of pilotropic mycosis fungoides. Sometimes these patients show clinically patchy areas of alopecia on affected parts, confirming the involvement of hair follicles with their destruction. Similar cases have been published in the literature [169].

Localized pagetoid reticulosis (Woringer–Kolopp type)/unilesional (solitary) mycosis fungoides

Localized pagetoid reticulosis is a variant of mycosis fungoides presenting with solitary, psoriasiform, scaly erythematous patches or plaques, usually located on the extremities (Fig. 2.57). The clinical picture can be deceptive, simulating that of benign conditions such as warts or eczematous dermatitis (Fig. 2.58) [170]. The histologic picture shows a markedly hyperplastic epidermis with striking epidermotropism of T lymphocytes (Figs 2.59, 2.60). Intraepidermal lymphocytes are characterized usually by medium-sized pleomorphic nuclei. Both T-helper and T-cytotoxic phenotypes have been described.

The term "pagetoid reticulosis" should be restricted to solitary lesions only (Woringer–Kolopp type) [1,2]. Patients presenting with the "generalized" form of pagetoid reticulosis (Ketron–Goodman type) probably have either classic mycosis fungoides, or, more frequently, one of the recently described primary cutaneous cytotoxic NK/T-cell lymphomas (cutaneous aggressive epidermotropic CD8+ cytotoxic T-cell lymphoma, cutaneous γ/δ T-cell lymphoma, extranodal NK/T-cell lymphoma, nasal type) (see also Chapter 6).

It should be emphasized that a histopathologic picture characterized by markedly hyperplastic epidermis with striking

Figure 2.55 Syringotropic mycosis fungoides. (a) At low power both a band-like infiltrate and prominent involvement of the eccrine glands are recognizable. (b) Note the superficial part with epidermotropism. (c) Detail of the eccrine glands with heavy lymphoid infiltrates, syringometaplasia, and small granulomas. (d) Staining for pancytokeratins highlights the syringometaplasia.

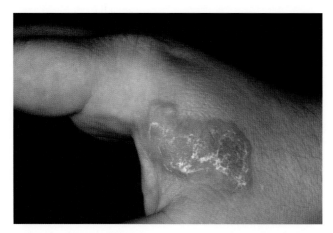

Figure 2.57 Localized pagetoid reticulosis. Erythematous plaque on the right hand. (Courtesy of Professor W. Sterry, Berlin.)

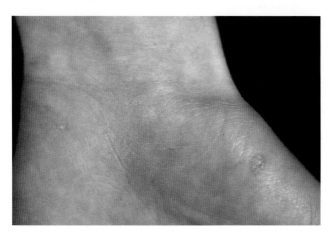

Figure 2.58 Localized pagetoid reticulosis. Two small erythematous papules on the left hand simulating clinically the picture of a wart.

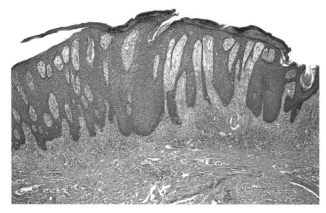

Figure 2.59 Localized pagetoid reticulosis. Hyperplastic epidermis with prominent epidermotropism of lymphocytes.

epidermotropism of innumerable T lymphocytes is not restricted to pagetoid reticulosis or aggressive cytotoxic NK/T-cell lymphomas: other lymphomas may rarely present with similar features, and a definitive diagnosis should be made only upon compeling clinicopathologic evidence and after complete

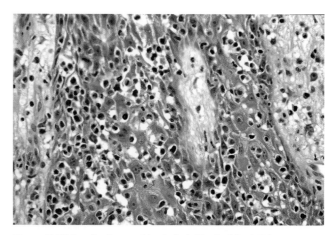

Figure 2.60 Localized pagetoid reticulosis (detail of Fig. 2.59).

phenotypic and genotypic studies [171]. We have observed a variant of lymphomatoid papulosis that is indistinguishable from pagetoid reticulosis histopathologically, but shows the typical waxing and waning course clinically (see Chapter 4). Presence of intraepidermal CD30+ neoplastic cells in "pagetoid reticulosis" should raise suspicion of such a variant of lymphomatoid papulosis; a precise classification of these cases can be achieved only upon clinicopathologic correlation.

The prognosis of patients with solitary pagetoid reticulosis is excellent, and involvement of internal organs has never been observed. In a few patients development of "classic" mycosis fungoides has been documented. The treatment of choice is surgical excision or local radiotherapy. Other skin-directed treatments may be used for more extensive lesions, including topical steroids, topical nitrogen mustard, PUVA, and narrow-band UV-B irradiation [172].

Besides localized pagetoid reticulosis, a solitary variant of mycosis fungoides with clinicopathologic features similar to "common" mycosis fungoides has been described (Fig. 2.61) [173–175]. It is as yet unclear whether the prognosis for these patients is better, but in some instances development of generalized lesions of mycosis fungoides has been observed over time.

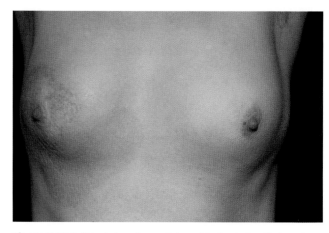

Figure 2.61 Solitary lesion of mycosis fungoides located on the breast.

Erythrodermic mycosis fungoides

Patients with mycosis fungoides may develop erythroderma during the course of their disease. Rarely, swelling of the lymph nodes and presence of circulating neoplastic cells ("Sézary cells") are observed as well, thus showing complete overlap of clinical features with Sézary syndrome (see Chapter 3). The histopathologic and phenotypic features are identical to those of conventional mycosis fungoides. After successful treatment patients may relapse with conventional patches, plaques or tumors of mycosis fungoides or with new flares of erythroderma. These cases probably should not be classified as Sézary syndrome but as erythrodermic mycosis fungoides, and the diagnosis of Sézary syndrome should be reserved to those patients presenting with the typical features of this disease from the onset [1]. In fact, a strong support to the distinction of mycosis fungoides from Sézary syndrome has been recently provided by oncogenomic analyses that showed major differences between the two diseases [176].

Poikilodermatous mycosis fungoides (poikiloderma vasculare atrophicans)

Poikilodermatous mycosis fungoides is characterized clinically by atrophic, red-brown macules and patches with prominent telangectasias (Fig. 2.62). Sites of predilection are the breast and buttocks. Histology reveals an atrophic epidermis with loss of rete ridges, an interface dermatitis with a superficial, band-like infiltrate of lymphocytes, and a thickened papillary dermis (see Fig. 2.32). Necrotic keratinocytes may be a prominent finding. Widely dilated capillaries are present within the superficial dermis. This variant of the disease has also been referred to as the "lichenoid" type of mycosis fungoides.

Hypopigmented/hyperpigmented mycosis fungoides

Patients with mycosis fungoides may develop hypopigmented patches and plaques (Fig. 2.63). These lesions may

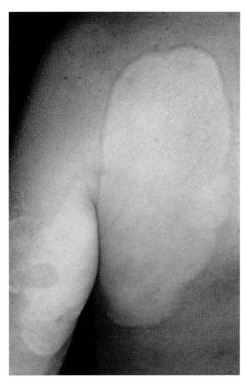

Figure 2.63 Hypopigmented patch of mycosis fungoides on the right shoulder. Note elevated, slightly erythematous margin.

be misinterpreted clinically as those of pityriasis versicolor, pityriasis alba or vitiligo. Histology reveals features typical of mycosis fungoides. Hypopigmented mycosis fungoides is observed more frequently in dark-skinned individuals and is one of the most frequent variants seen in children [177–178]. Repigmentation usually takes place after successful treatment of the lesions.

Although hypopigmented lesions may present as the sole manifestation of mycosis fungoides, in many cases, especially in Caucasians, careful examination of the patients will detect the presence of erythematous lesions as well (Fig. 2.64). Interestingly, patients with hypopigmented mycosis fungoides tend to develop more hypopigmented lesions during the course of the disease, suggesting that this is indeed an unusual variant of mycosis fungoides.

A predominant CD8+ phenotype has been described in patients with hypopigmented mycosis fungoides, possibly underlying some pathogenetic similarities to vitiligo [177]. However, a CD4+ phenotype can be observed as well. It should be underlined that differential diagnosis of hypopigmented mycosis fungoides from its simulators, including particularly atopic dermatitis and the inflammatory stages of vitiligo, may be extremely difficult, and it has been suggested that at least some of the cases published in the literature may not represent genuine examples of hypopigmented mycosis fungoides [179]. In our experience this problem is particularly evident in children, and sometimes only follow-up data provide a

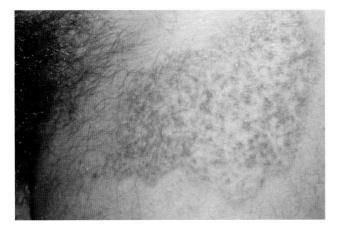

Figure 2.62 Poikilodermatous mycosis fungoides characterized by the presence of a reticulated atrophic plaque on the thigh.

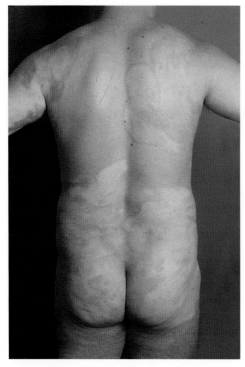

Figure 2.64 Hypopigmented mycosis fungoides covering large parts of the body. Note erythematous areas as well.

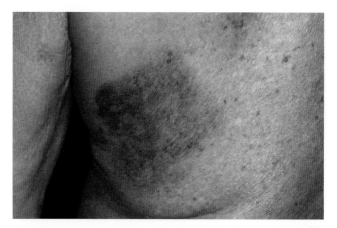

Figure 2.66 Purpuric mycosis fungoides. Same patient as Fig. 2.31. The patient also had "conventional" patches of mycosis fungoides elsewhere on the trunk.

precise diagnosis (see below) (see also the paragraph on vitiligo in Chapter 22). Another differential diagnosis of hypopigmented mycosis fungoides, particularly in children, is represented by pityriasis alba.

Rarely, the clinical picture of mycosis fungoides may be characterized by markedly hyperpigmented lesions, corresponding histopathologically to the presence of pigment incontinence and abundant melanophages in the papillary dermis (see Fig. 2.29; Fig. 2.65). Generalized hyperpigmented lesions have

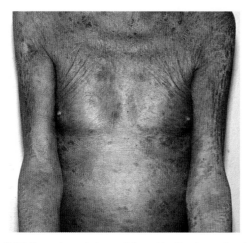

Figure 2.65 Hyperpigmented mycosis fungoides ("melanoerythroderma"). Note diffuse reddish brown color with multiple areas of marked hyperpigmentation.

been described as "melanoerythroderma" and are seen more frequently in patients with Sézary syndrome.

Pigmented purpura-like mycosis fungoides

In some patients, lesions of mycosis fungoides are characterized clinically by a purpuric hue, and histopathologically by the presence of many extravasated erythrocytes (see Fig. 2.31; Fig. 2.66). Differential diagnosis of these cases from lichenoid purpura and lichen aureus can be difficult on histopathologic grounds, and correlation with the clinical features is crucial (see also Chapter 22). The distinction of purpuric mycosis fungoides from purpuric dermatoses has been rendered more difficult in recent years by the introduction of the term "atypical pigmented purpura" and the concept of a possible relationship between some purpuric dermatoses and mycosis fungoides [180–183]. Patients with "pigmented purpura" progressing to mycosis fungoides probably had purpuric mycosis fungoides from the outset [183,184]. In this context, it should be emphasized that lichen aureus and lichenoid purpura are wholly benign disorders that should be clearly differentiated from mycosis fungoides.

Bullous (vesiculobullous) mycosis fungoides/ dyshidrotic mycosis fungoides

Some patients with mycosis fungoides present with vesiculous or bullous lesions, these last usually associated with large, superficial erosions (Fig. 2.67) [185]. Bullous lesions may be due to cleavage at the dermoepidermal junction or to confluence of intraepidermal vesicles (Fig. 2.68). A "dyshidrotic" variant of the disease located at the palms and soles has also been described (Figs 2.69, 2.70) [186,187]. Typical lesions of mycosis fungoides are commonly present near to the vesicular and bullous ones.

The reason(s) for the formation of vesicular and bullous lesions is unclear. Some patients may present with pre-existent dyshidrotic or vesicular dermatitis and subsequent colonization

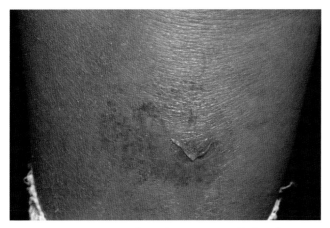

Figure 2.67 Bullous mycosis fungoides. Note ruptured bulla with superficial erosion.

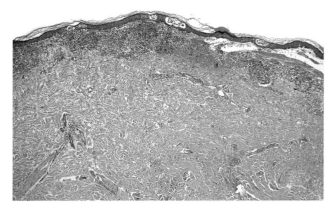

Figure 2.68 Bullous mycosis fungoides. Subepidermal bulla with dense band-like infiltrate of lymphocytes in the papillary dermis and epidermotropism.

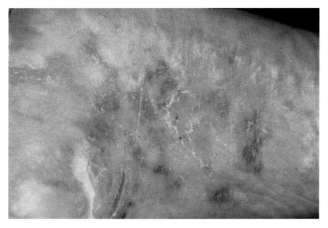

Figure 2.69 Dyshidrotic mycosis fungoides. Dyshidrotic vesicles and small erosions on the soles. (See histologic features depicted in Fig. 2.70.)

by neoplastic cells. In other patients a direct cytotoxic effect may be responsible for the detachment of the epidermis from the dermis, or pronounced spongiosis may lead to vesiculation, and eventually larger blisters may develop due to confluence

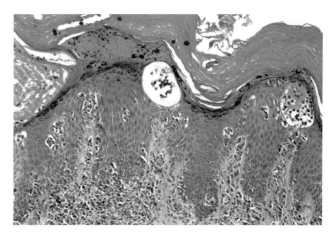

Figure 2.70 Dyshidrotic mycosis fungoides. Histology reveals epidermotropic lymphocytes, some within intraepidermal vesicles. (Same patient of Fig. 2.69.)

of vesicles. In some patients, onset of bullous lesions has been related to the use of interferon-α [188].

Granulomatous mycosis fungoides/granulomatous slack skin

Granulomatous mycosis fungoides is an unusual histologic variant of mycosis fungoides described first by Ackerman and Flaxman in 1970, who reported a patient with tumor-stage mycosis fungoides with huge giant cells scattered within the dermal infiltrate [189]. A granulomatous pattern can be observed in different lesions of mycosis fungoides including patches, plaques, and tumors, and in some cases even within affected lymph nodes (Figs 2.71, 2.72) [190]. Granulomatous lesions may either precede, be concomitant with or follow "classic" mycosis fungoides. Especially if the first manifestation of the disease shows prominent granulomatous features, the diagnosis of mycosis fungoides may be missed, and the histopathologic picture may be misinterpreted as that of a "granulomatous dermatitis." Histopathologically, granulomatous mycosis fungoides may also be difficult or even impossible to distinguish from other cutaneous T-cell lymphomas with granulomatous features (i.e. Sézary syndrome, small/medium pleomorphic T-cell lymphoma) [142,191], and clinicopathologic correlation is crucial for the diagnosis.

A rare variant of granulomatous mycosis fungoides is represented by so-called granulomatous slack skin, which is characterized clinically by the occurrence of bulky, pendulous skinfolds, usually located in flexural areas (Fig. 2.73) [142, 192–196]. Granulomatous slack skin is considered a specific manifestation of mycosis fungoides in most cases and is included as a variant of it in the WHO-EORTC classification [1], but association with other lymphomas has been reported [190]. It is difficult to state whether cases reported as "peripheral T-cell lymphoma" in patients with long-standing granulomatous slack skin represent mycosis fungoides or not [197]; irrespective of the precise classification of associated

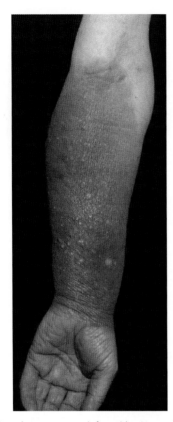

Figure 2.71 Granulomatous mycosis fungoides. Note reddish brown plaque with several papules and small nodules on the arm.

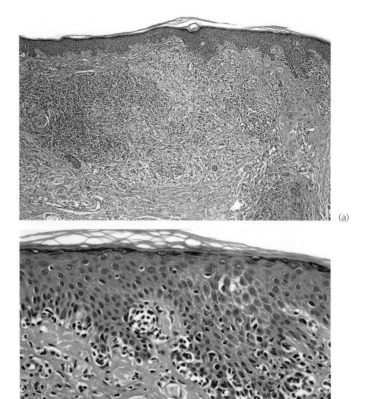

(a)

(b)

Figure 2.72 Granulomatous mycosis fungoides. (a) Dense lymphoid infiltrate admixed with large epithelioid granulomas in the dermis. (b) Note focal epidermotropism of lymphocytes.

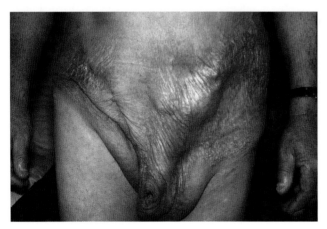

Figure 2.73 Granulomatous slack skin. Prominent atrophy of the skin with bulky pendulous skin folds in the lower abdomen and inguinal region. (Courtesy of Professor Giovanni Borroni, Pavia, Italy.)

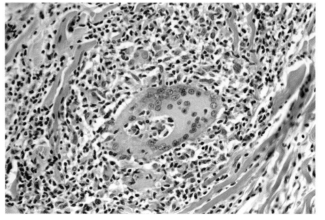

Figure 2.74 Granulomatous slack skin. Histiocytic giant cell with several intracellular leukocytes, surrounded by a dense infiltrate of lymphocytes.

lymphomas, however, it is clear that granulomatous slack skin has the potential for progression with involvement of internal organs and death of the patients. The granulomatous infiltrate in granulomatous slack skin is usually diffuse and involves the deep subcutaneous tissues, in contrast to the patchy, more superficial granulomas observed in "conventional" granulomatous mycosis fungoides. Giant cells with many nuclei are a common finding (Fig. 2.74). Elastophago-

cytosis is also typically present. The same rearrangement of T cells has been observed in skin and nodal lesions in one patient [198], and a t(3;9)(q12;p24) has been detected in another case [199].

Although it has been suggested that a granulomatous reaction is associated with a good prognosis in patients with mycosis fungoides [200], patients doing badly have been reported as well [142,201]. In addition, the amount of the granulomatous reaction is often variable in different biopsies from a single patient, suggesting that the term "granulomatous mycosis fungoides" should be used as a description of histopathologic specimens, and not for classifying the disease in a given patient [202]. Finally, it has recently been demonstrated that differentiation of "conventional" granulomatous mycosis fungoides from granulomatous slack skin cannot be achieved on histopathologic grounds only, and that correlation with the clinical picture is crucial for a precise classification [203].

Papular mycosis fungoides

In some patients with mycosis fungoides, small papules represent the predominant morphologic expression of the disease, and small and/or large patches are absent (Figs 2.75, 2.76) [204]. The absence of typical manifestations of the disease renders the clinical diagnosis very difficult. Moreover, differentiation from type B lymphomatoid papulosis can only be achieved by short-term follow-up of the patients, as the

histopathologic features may be indistinguishable (see also Chapter 4). In fact, papular lesions of mycosis fungoides do not show the spontaneous regression typical of type B lymphomatoid papulosis. Although we initially suggested that papular mycosis fungoides seemed to have the same prognosis as other variants of early mycosis fungoides [204], observation of cases who progressed to erythroderma or tumor stage within relative short periods of time should prompt great caution in the management of these patients.

"Invisible" mycosis fungoides

Normal-looking skin in patients with mycosis fungoides may show histopathologic, electron microscopic, immunophenotypic and/or molecular genetic evidence of neoplastic lymphocytes [205–207]. These cases have been termed "invisible" mycosis fungoides in the literature, because the lesions are clinically unapparent. The presence of such histologic features in normal-looking skin has been documented at the first diagnosis of mycosis fungoides, in patients with mycosis fungoides at sites distant from erythematous lesions, and in patients in complete clinical remission after treatment [205–207].

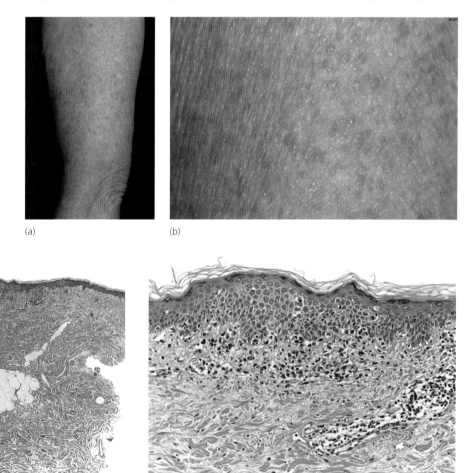

Figure 2.75 Papular mycosis fungoides. (a) Note small erythematous papules on the arm. (b) Detail of the papules.

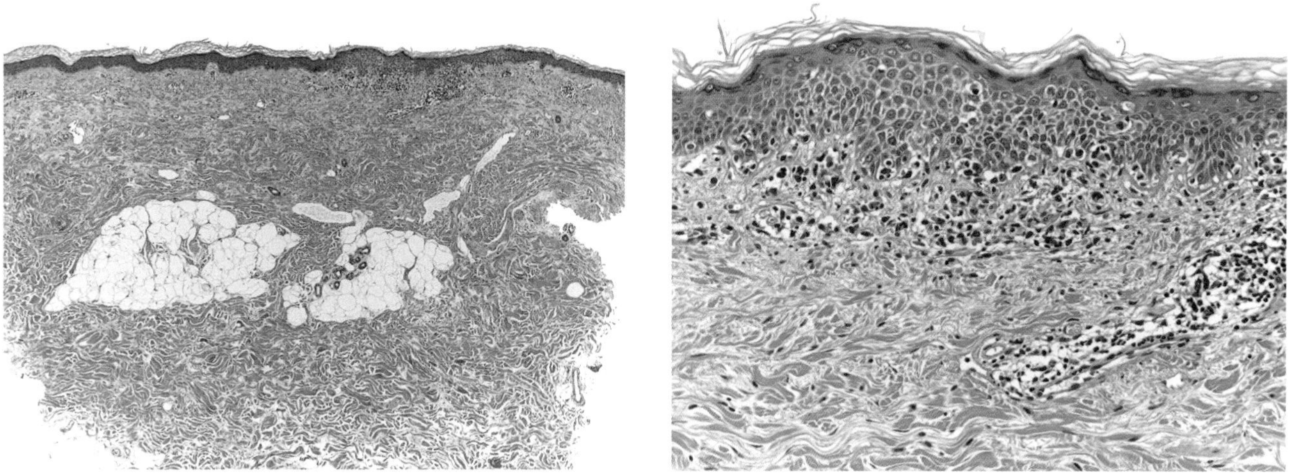

(a)   (b)

Figure 2.76 Papular mycosis fungoides. (a) Histology reveals an infiltrate confined to a small portion of the specimen. (b) Detail shows typical changes of mycosis fungoides (same patient of Fig. 2.75).

The finding of specific infiltrates of mycosis fungoides in skin that looks clinically normal poses two main questions: the first relates to the extent of the area treated by skin-targeted therapies, and the second concerns the proper monitoring of patients after treatment. At present it is difficult to answer either question, as the clinical implications (if any) of "invisible", persistent disease are not clear. In our experience, however, biopsies of normal-looking skin in cases of mycosis fungoides showing complete clinical remission do not add information relevant for further management of the patients.

Anetodermic mycosis fungoides

Two patients with secondary anetoderma developing on pre-existing lesions of mycosis fungoides have been described recently [208]. Some of the lesions depicted in this study resembled small tumors clinically, but represented probably just secondary anetodermic changes in flat lesions of mycosis fungoides, thus being a potential pitfall in clinical evaluation of the patients. Anetoderma secondary to mycosis fungoides has clinical and histopathologic features different from granulomatous slack skin.

Other unusual clinical presentations of mycosis fungoides

Besides those variants that have been described in the literature, and thus achieving a more or less "official" status, mycosis fungoides may present with clinical lesions different from the typical patches, plaques or tumors observed in most patients. We do not give special names to these variants, but it may be useful for readers to see some clinical pictures of cases that deviate from conventional presentation (Figs 2.77–2.82).

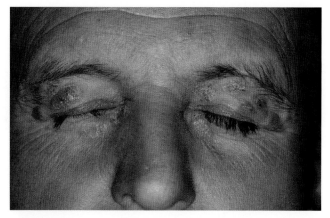

Figure 2.78 Mycosis fungoides, tumor stage. Bilateral papules and small tumors on the eyelids and periorbital regions. In this patient this was the first manifestation of recurrent disease after successful total-body electron beam therapy, possibly due to incorrect eye-shielding.

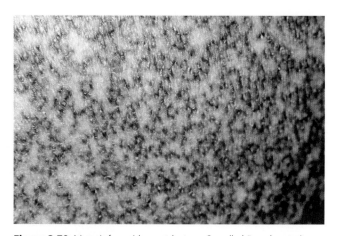

Figure 2.79 Mycosis fungoides, patch stage. So-called "parakeratosis variegata."

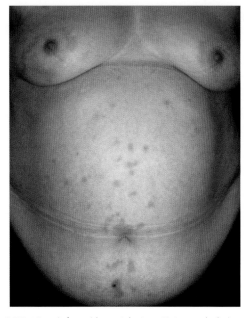

Figure 2.77 Mycosis fungoides, patch stage. Note annular lesion around both nipples and small patches on the abdomen.

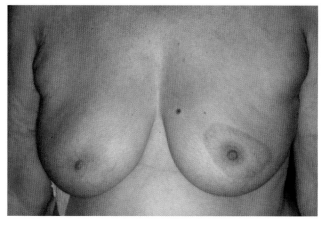

Figure 2.80 Mycosis fungoides, patch stage. Annular patch on the left breast. Note similarities with Fig. 2.77. We have frequently observed similar annular patches around the nipple, particularly in women (sun-protected area).

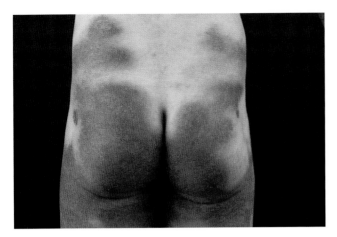

Figure 2.81 Mycosis fungoides, patch stage. Diffuse purpuric, hyperpigmented confluent patches.

Diagnosis in all of these patients was confirmed by histologic examination and/or follow-up data; in many of them more conventional lesions were present before or at the same time as the less typical ones.

Mycosis fungoides in children

Mycosis fungoides is the most common form of cutaneous lymphoma in childhood and adolescence (Fig. 2.83) [209]. In general, in patients younger than 20 years of age mycosis fungoides is rare, but the true incidence may be higher than generally assumed, because there is often a reluctance to perform biopsies in children, and the diagnosis can be delayed for several years [210,211]. The hypopigmented variant of mycosis fungoides appears with unusually high frequency in this age group, especially in children with dark skin [177, 210,212]. In addition, a distinct percentage of young patients with mycosis fungoides have localized pagetoid reticulosis (Woringer–Kolopp type), suggesting that this variant of mycosis fungoides may occur more frequently in childhood. The clinical presentation in these cases can be deceiving, and often lesions will be biopsied only after prolonged local treatment [170]. Other unusual variants observed in children include follicular mucinosis-associated mycosis fungoides, and CD8+ mycosis fungoides [149,213–216]. Cases reported in the literature as "annular lichenoid dermatitis of youth" [217] or "lymphomatoid annular erythema" [218] may represent another manifestation of mycosis fungoides in children (see also the paragraph on annular lichenoid dermatitis of youth in Chapter 22).

A peculiar type of mycosis fungoides in children simulates clinically and histopathologically the picture of pityriasis lichenoides et varioliformis acuta (PLEVA), and is particularly difficult to diagnose (see Fig. 2.33) [219]. Several young but

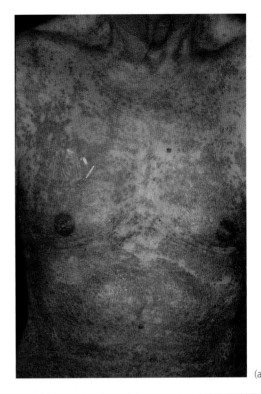

(a)

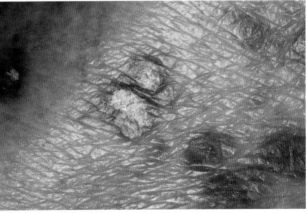

(b)

Figure 2.82 Mycosis fungoides, tumor stage. This patient had tumor-stage mycosis fungoides with tumors on the thighs and buttock. At the same time, he developed psoriasiform/lichenoid papules on the trunk and extremities (a). (b) Detail of the papules.

only one adult patient with this variant of mycosis fungoides have been reported, suggesting that this peculiar presentation is mostly restricted to children [220].

The overall outlook for children or adolescents with mycosis fungoides is difficult to predict, and it has been maintained that mycosis fungoides is more aggressive in childhood with a higher frequency of extracutaneous involvement [210,213]. Other reports suggested that the natural history of the disease is comparable with that seen in adults [214,221–223]. Indeed, it may be that at least some of the cases reported in the past as

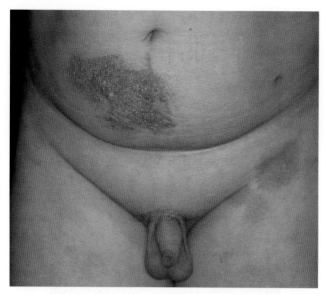

Figure 2.83 Mycosis fungoides in a 14-year-old boy. The patient also had lesions of hypopigmented mycosis fungoides on the back.

"atypical" or "aggressive" mycosis fungoides in children represent examples of cytotoxic NK/T-cell lymphomas, which usually show a more aggressive course with a poor prognosis. Overall it seems likely that the onset of lesions of mycosis fungoides in childhood will increase the probability of disease progression during the lifetime of the patient.

Treatment

Treatment of mycosis fungoides differs according to the stage of the disease, the extent of the cutaneous and/or extracutaneous manifestations, and the previous therapy (if any). It must be underlined that management of patients with advanced disease is extremely difficult, as can be inferred from the plethora of treatment modalities that are continually being proposed. In 1990 Jones wrote an editorial in the *Journal of the National Cancer Institute* titled "Enigma of therapy for cutaneous T-cell lymphoma" [224]: in spite of many improvements, the title would probably be similar today.

The standard treatment of early lesions of mycosis fungoides includes psoralens in association with UV-A irradiation (PUVA), interferon-α-2a, retinoids, or a combination of these three modalities [225–228]. PUVA treatment has also been administered in the form of so-called bath-PUVA [229]. Several other treatments have been used in the past (and are still in use at present), including UV-B irradiation (or narrow-band UV-B – 311 nm) and topical application of chemotherapeutic agents (nitrogen mustard, carmustine, methotrexate) [230–235]. In many cases, patients with localized patches of the disease can also be treated with local steroid ointments [236]. Localized variants of the disease have also been treated by laser vaporiza-

tion [237,238]. The administration of total body irradiation [239–241], proposed by some authors as a first-line treatment, should probably be restricted to patients with mycosis fungoides in the later stages. It should be noted that the administration of placebo as a topical vehicle devoid of active principle was found to produce an objective response in 24% of patients with early mycosis fungoides in a double-blind, randomized study [242]. The notion that a considerable proportion of patients with patch-stage mycosis fungoides shows complete clinical response upon local application of placebo suggests that in early phases the disease may be controlled also with a watchful waiting strategy.

Although interferon-α is well tolerated and shows good results in most patients with early mycosis fungoides, resistance to this drug has been observed, hindering its use in many patients. Analysis of these cases showed that multiple genes involved in signal transduction, apoptosis, transcription regulation, and cell growth are implicated in the mechanism of resistance [243]. Interferon treatment may be improved by the use of pegylated compounds but large studies are still lacking. Association with modalities other than PUVA or UV-B has been proven efficacious, too, even in advanced cases [244]. In our experience, interferon-α gives good results as monotherapy even in patients with tumor-stage disease, but the drug is used more commonly in the setting of combination treatments, particularly together with PUVA. In patients with early mycosis fungoides showing complete remissions after monotherapy or combination therapies including interferon-α, it is unclear whether the administration of the drug as a maintenance treatment carries any beneficial effect, and for how long it should be administered.

Among the retinoids, in recent years bexarotene (Targretin®, administered orally or topically) has been used commonly for the treatment of mycosis fungoides (in both early and late stages), either alone or, more often, in combination with other treatments [245–250]. The side effects can be minimized by proper management of the patients [251]. Tazarotene (Tazorac®) and alitretinoin (Panretin®) are other retinoids available for topical treatment in cream or gel formulas [252]. An inflammatory reaction on treated skin is the main side-effect of topical retinoids, being a limiting factor for their application to large areas of the body. Topical use of bexarotene gel is helpful in the adjuvant management of plaques or tumors that were unresponsive to the primary treatment [253].

Many other therapeutic protocols have been introduced for treatment of early mycosis fungoides during the years, including, among others, photodynamic therapy with 5-aminolaevulinic acid, new chemotherapeutic drugs for topical use, and immune response modifiers such as imiquimod [254–262]. At present there are not enough data to evaluate the efficacy of these new modalities in terms of remission and recurrence rates. Combinations of different protocols have not yet shown clear-cut advantages in terms of overall survival [263]. Some of the less aggressive modalities may be particularly suited for treatment of solitary patches of the disease [264,265].

A particular problem is represented by treatment of pilotropic or syringotropic mycosis fungoides, as skin-directed therapies may fail to reach a depth sufficient to achieve good results. In these patients, PUVA is usually combined with retinoids [266].

In the late stages, in addition to PUVA, retinoids and interferon-α, conventional systemic chemotherapy (CHOP), extracorporeal photopheresis and radiotherapy have been applied [239,267], including total skin electron beam irradiation [268]. Guidelines for the use of extracorporeal photopheresis have been published recently [269]. Autologous bone marrow transplantation showed good results with complete clinical responses, but recurrence within short periods of time is the rule [270]. Allogenic stem cell transplantation has been performed in a few patients and seems to be a promising treatment modality, perhaps with potential for cure due to a graft-versus-tumor response [271–274]. Although toxicity is still very high, at present this option seems to be the most promising for advanced-stage disease, particularly if patients are not heavily pretreated, and it is currently debated whether allogenic stem cell transplantation should be considered a main treatment option for early tumor-stage mycosis fungoides. A graft-versus-tumor response with prolonged remission has been observed also in a patient who failed a previous unrelated bone marrow transplantation and was subsequently treated with unrelated blood cord transplantation and discontinuation of immunosuppressive treatment [275].

Many other chemotherapeutic or immunologic agents have been tested in tumor-stage mycosis fungoides during the last years, including, among others, gemcitabine, fludarabine, temozolomide, pegylated liposomal doxorubicin (Caelyx), pentostatin, anti-CD52 antibody (alemtuzumab, Campath-IH), interleukin-12, DAB$_{389}$-IL-2 fusion protein (Ontak, denileukin diftitox), and trimetrexate [276–293]. Some patients have also been treated with different types of tumor vaccines [294–295], but results are not yet promising. Other treatment modalities for tumor stage mycosis fungoides, still in an experimental phase, include the anti-CD4 antibody zanolimumab [287], the inductor of cell death vorinostat [288,289], romidepsin (an inductor of cell cycle arrest and apoptosis), panobinostat (an histone deacetylase inhibitor) [292], belinostat (a pan-histone deacetylase inhibitor), bortezomib (a proteasome inhibitor) and forodesine (an inhibitor of purine nucleoside phosphorylase). Cancer-related genes may in the future be the target for immunotherapeutic strategies in mycosis fungoides [296]. It should be mentioned that treatment of advanced (tumor-stage) mycosis fungoides remains unsatisfactory, and that the disease usually progresses in spite of aggressive therapy. With the possible exception of allogenic stem cell or bone marrow transplantation, complete remissions are observed only in a small minority of patients, and are rarely durable.

An issue that only rarely has been properly addressed in controlled studies, but that should be carefully evaluated, concerns the quality of life in patients with late-stage mycosis fungoides [297–298]. In fact, patients may have tumor-stage disease for several years, underlying the need for proper palliation and alleviation of symptoms. In some patients, particularly those with pilotropic mycosis fungoides, pruritus may be intractable and so severe as to induce suicide, underlining the need for a proper, aggressive treatment of this symptom.

Onset of mycosis fungoides or exacerbation of undiagnosed disease under treatment with immunologic agents

In recent years, several cases of undiagnosed mycosis fungoides progressing to tumor-stage under treatment with different immunologic agents have been described (in the medical jargon often referred to as "biologicals") [299–301]. In some cases it may be that genuine association of two diseases (mycosis fungoides and an antecedent inflammatory disorder) may have occurred. In other cases, however, a wrong diagnosis of atopic dermatitis or psoriasis had been made initially, and a treatment with one of the many immunologic agents had been started, resulting in rapid progression of the disease. These cases underline the need for an accurate and precise diagnosis of inflammatory skin disorders that are to be treated with immunomodulatory agents, as a misdiagnosis can bear catastrophic consequences.

Prognosis

Mycosis fungoides is a malignant lymphoma of low-grade malignancy with prolonged survival, and progression from the clinical stage of patches to those characterized by plaques, tumors, and extracutaneous spread usually takes place over many years to decades [1,2]. Development of plaques and/or tumors, or of large cell transformation, heralds the terminal stages of the disease (patients may survive several years with tumor-stage mycosis fungoides, however). As the disease arises more commonly in the elderly, most patients never progress to plaque or tumor stage, and die of unrelated causes [302,303]. In fact, it has been estimated that only 15–20% of patients die of their disease [9]. However, a small subset of patients experience a more rapidly aggressive course with extracutaneous spread and death due to complications of the disease (usually sepsis or other severe infections). Moreover, a substantial subset of patients are middle-aged or young adults, and a few are children, thus having a higher risk of progression during their lifetime.

The most important prognostic parameters are stage at diagnosis, absence of complete remission after first treatment, age, and race (black patients have a worse prognosis, but this may be related to difficulties in gaining access to proper therapy) [9,10,302–304]. There are no significant differences in survival between stages Ia and Ib (TNM classification), or between patients with tumors and erythroderma [10,305]. Once extracutaneous spread takes place, initial prognostic parameters have no influence on survival and the prognosis is bad [61].

The exact implications of the detection of a clone in the blood or in the skin alone in the early phases of the disease remain unclear [305–309]. Recently, however, it has been demonstrated that presence of T-cell monoclonality in early lesions of mycosis fungoides, as detected by standard PCR assays, does not have any prognostic implications [88]. The finding of an identical clone in the blood and skin, on the other hand, seems to be an independent (bad) prognostic criterion [305,306,310]. Similarly, the finding of a monoclonal population of T lymphocytes in the lymph nodes of patients with mycosis fungoides has been linked to a worse prognosis compared to patients presenting with so-called "dermopathic lymphadenopathy" and no evidence of monoclonal rearrangement [311]. Although the influence of the presence of follicular mucinosis on survival is debated [149,154], it certainly complicates the treatment of these patients. Finally, analysis of histopathologic features of biopsy specimens of early mycosis fungoides has so far failed to detect parameters that might predict the course of the disease [312].

Although most treatments are efficacious in the early phases, and long-term remissions can be achieved, it is unlikely that cures will be obtained, with the possible exception of the solitary variants of the disease (though life-long follow-up is still needed in these patients). In a recent study with long-term follow-up data of patients with early mycosis fungoides treated with PUVA, 30–50% remained disease free for many years, but late relapses occurred [313]. The use of the PCR technique has been advocated for the detection of minimal residual disease after treatment, but the value of this method as a routine investigation needs to be confirmed by larger studies [314]. In addition, it has never been demonstrated that a more aggressive treatment of patch-stage disease (including treatment of recurrences) provides any survival advantages to the patients.

Résumé

Clinical	Adults. Patches, plaques and tumors can be found. Preferential location: buttocks, other sun-protected areas (early phases). Rarely observed in children (but the most common cutaneous lymphoma in this age group!).
Morphology	Small pleomorphic (cerebriform) cells. During the course of the disease large cell transformation may occur, indicating a worse prognosis (immunoblasts, large cell anaplastic, large cell pleomorphic). Epidermotropism is common but may be missing; Darier's nests (Pautrier's microabscesses) are rare in early lesions.
Immunology	CD2, 3, 4, 5, 45Ro + CD8 –(+) 45Ra – CD30 may be positive in tumors with large cell morphology; cytotoxic markers (e.g. TIA-1) may be positive in late stages and rarely in early lesions. Phenotypic variations occur!
Genetics	No specific abnormalities unequivocally identified in early phases. Some studies showed alterations of genes related to apoptosis and tumor suppression; frequent abnormalities of p53 and p16 in advanced disease. Monoclonal rearrangement of the TCR is not detected in about 40–50% of patients in early phases, depending on the technique used.
Treatment guidelines	*Early phases*: PUVA, interferon-α2a, new retinoids (bexarotene) (alone or in combination); topical chemotherapy; topical steroids; narrow-band UV-B (311 nm); photodynamic therapy. Watchful waiting if treatment can be postponed. *Advanced disease*: chemotherapy (single agent or multiagent); extracorporeal photopheresis; radiotherapy (including total body electron beam irradiation); allogenic stem cell transplantation may represent a curative option. *Experimental*: imiquimod; new chemotherapeutic drugs (many options, including gemcitabine, fludarabine, and pegylated doxorubicin among others); immunomodulatory agents; pentostatin.

TEACHING CASE

This 39-year-old man presented with a reddish tumor on the right forehead for the last few weeks (Fig. 2.84a). There was no relevant clinical history. A biopsy was taken showing a lymphoid tumor composed of pleomorphic and anaplastic cells admixed with some eosinophils (Fig. 2.84b, c) and strongly positive for CD30 (Fig. 2.84d). A diagnosis of cutaneous anaplastic CD30+ large cell lymphoma was made. The patient refused any further investigation. He was referred for local radiotherapy and subsequently lost to follow-up.

He presented again 3 years later showing several infiltrated erythematous patches and plaques that proved to be specific lesions of mycosis fungoides histopathologically. He admitted that he had suffered from "eczema" for many years. He subsequently developed clear-cut tumor-stage mycosis fungoides with follicular mucinosis (Fig. 2.84e), and finally succumbed to his lymphoma 14 years after first presentation.

Comment: Failure to perform complete investigations (in this particular case due to the patient's reluctance) led to an initial wrong diagnosis of cutaneous anaplastic CD30+ large cell lymphoma in this patient, who in truth had tumor-stage mycosis fungoides. In fact, this case was presented as an example of cutaneous anaplastic CD30+ large cell lymphoma in the first edition of this book, underlying the pitfalls in classification of cutaneous lymphomas when all clinical data (for whatever reason) are not available.

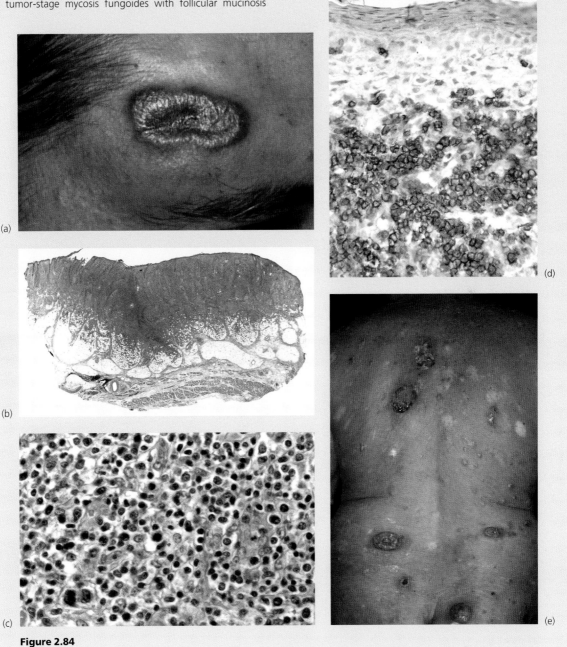

Figure 2.84

TEACHING CASE

This 67-year-old woman had a >20-year history of erythematous patches over the entire body. Clinical examination disclosed clear-cut features of mycosis fungoides (Fig. 2.85a). Two biopsies revealed only relatively mild infiltrates, particularly when compared with the clinical picture (taken at the same time as the two biopsies) (Fig. 2.85b–e).

Comment: This case illustrates the difficulties that may arise in the histopathologic diagnosis of mycosis fungoides. In spite of a clear-cut clinical presentation, the histopathologic changes were difficult to interpret and may have prompted a diagnosis of "non-specific chronic dermatitis" if the clinical picture had not been taken into account.

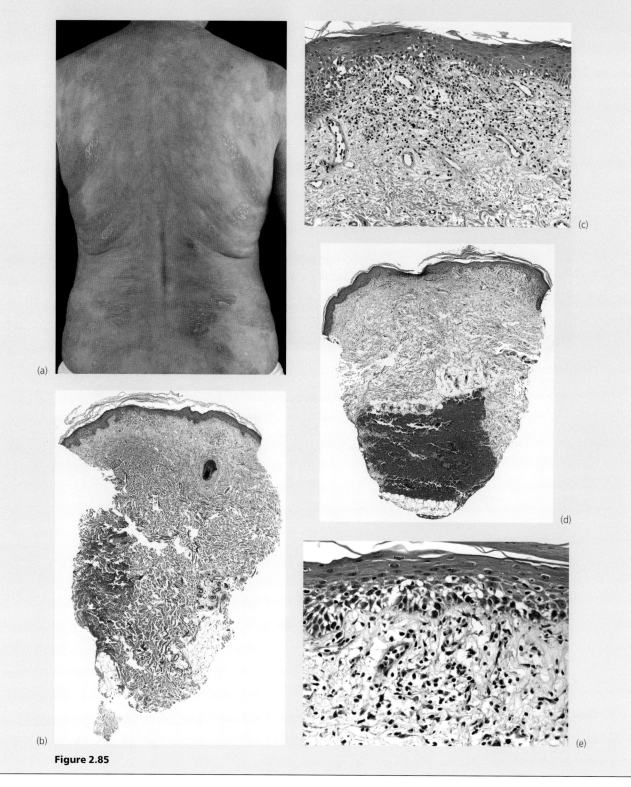

(a)

(b)

(c)

(d)

(e)

Figure 2.85

TEACHING CASE

This 64-year-old man had therapy-resistant, infiltrated lesions on the fifth finger of the right hand (Fig. 2.86a). The lesion had been treated previously for mycotic infection and eczema. A biopsy revealed a dense lymphoid infiltrate with peculiar accentuation around the eccrine glands and ducts and with syringometaplasia (Fig. 2.86b, c). At closer inspection there were also erythematous,

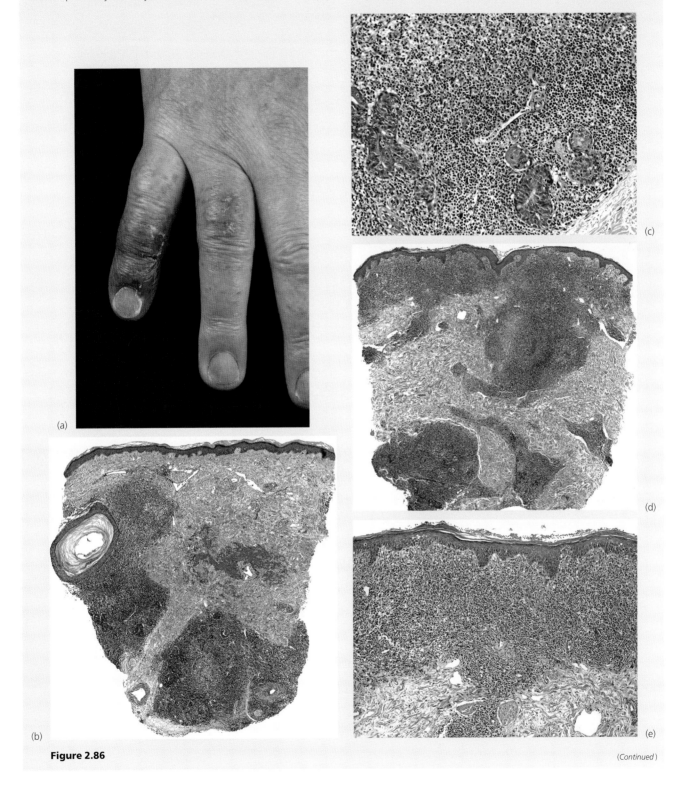

Figure 2.86

(Continued)

infiltrated lesions with follicular accentuation on the upper arms and one knee, which on biopsy revealed dense band-like infiltrates with small epidermal cysts surrounded by lymphocytes, as well as nodular lymphocytic infiltrates around the eccrine glands with syringometaplasia (Fig. 2.86d, e). A diagnosis of mycosis fungoides (syringomatous/pilotropic mycosis fungoides) was made.

Comment: This case exemplifies the difficulties (both clinically and histopathologically) in making a diagnosis of unusual variants of mycosis fungoides such as syringomatous mycosis fungoides. Syringometaplasia is constantly observed, and the infiltrate in this peculiar and rare type of mycosis fungoides often shows involvement of the hair follicles as well.

You can compare this case with the following one, occurring in an 84-year-old man with history of mycosis fungoides who, during the course of his disease, developed lesions on the chin (Fig. 2.87a). A biopsy revealed an infiltrate of lymphocytes arranged almost exclusively around the eccrine structures (Fig. 2.87b, c). A subsequent biopsy also showed features of conventional mycosis fungoides with infiltration of a hair follicle (Fig. 2.87d).

Syringotropic mycosis fungoides is one of the most difficult variants of the disease to diagnose on both clinical and histopathologic grounds. The finding of dense infiltrates of lymphocytes around the eccrine glands with syringometaplasia should always raise suspicion and prompt accurate clinicopathologic correlation.

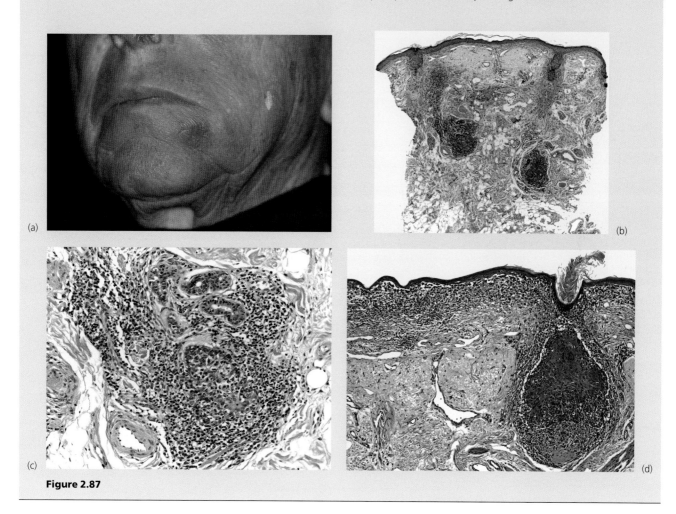

(a)　(b)　(c)　(d)

Figure 2.87

References

1. Willemze R, Jaffe ES, Burg G *et al.* WHO-EORTC classification for cutaneous lymphomas. *Blood* 2005;**105**:3768–3785.

2. Fink-Puches R, Zenahlik P, Bäck B *et al.* Primary cutaneous lymphomas: applicability of current classification schemes (European Organization for Research and Treatment of Cancer, World Health Organization) based on clinicopathologic features observed in a large group of patients. *Blood* 2002;**99**:800–805.

3. Hwang ST, Janik JE, Jaffe ES, Wilson WH. Mycosis fungoides and Sézary syndrome. *Lancet* 2008;**371**:945–957.

4. Zinzani PL, Ferreri AJM, Cerroni L. Mycosis fungoides. *Crit Rev Oncol/Hematol* 2008;**65**:172–182.

5. Ralfkiaer E, Cerroni L, Sander CA, Smoller BR, Willemze R. Mycosis fungoides. In: Swerdlow SH, Campo E, Harris NL *et al.*, eds. *WHO Classification of Tumours of Haematopoietic and Lymphoid Tissues.* Lyon: IARC Press, 2008: 296–298.

6. Sanchez JL, Ackerman AB. The patch stage of mycosis fungoides: criteria for histologic diagnosis. *Am J Dermatopathol* 1979;**1**:5–26.

7. Shapiro PE, Pinto FJ. The histologic spectrum of mycosis fungoides/Sezary syndrome (cutaneous T-cell lymphoma): a review of 222 biopsies, including newly described patterns and the earliest pathologic changes. *Am J Surg Pathol* 1994;**18**:645–667.

8. Santucci M, Biggeri A, Feller AC, Massi D, Burg G. Efficacy of histologic criteria for diagnosing early mycosis fungoides: an EORTC Cutaneous Lymphoma Study Group investigation. *Am J Surg Pathol* 2000;**24**:40–50.

9. Zackheim HS, Amin S, Kashani-Sabet M, McMillan A. Prognosis in cutaneous T-cell lymphoma by skin stage: long-term survival in 489 patients. *J Am Acad Dermatol* 1999;**40**:418–425.

10. Kim YH, Liu HL, Mraz-Gernhard S, Varghese A, Hoppe RT. Long-term outcome of 525 patients with mycosis fungoides and Sézary syndrome. *Arch Dermatol* 2003;**139**:857–866.

11. Criscione VD, Weinstock MA. Incidence of cutaneous T-cell lymphoma in the United States, 1973–2002. *Arch Dermatol* 2007;**143**:854–859.

12. Saunes M, Lund Nilsen TI, Johannesen TB. Incidence of primary cutaneous T-cell lymphoma in Norway. *Br J Dermatol* 2009;**160**:376–379.

13. Baykal C, Büyülbabani N, Kaymaz R. Familial mycosis fungoides. *Br J Dermatol* 2002;**146**:1108–1110.

14. Naji AA, Waiz MM, Sharquie KE. Mycosis fungoides in identical twins. *J Am Acad Dermatol* 2001;**44**:532–533.

15. Vassallo C, Brazzelli V, Cestone E *et al.* Mycosis fungoides in childhood: description and study of two siblings. *Acta Derm Venereol* 2007;**87**:529–532.

16. Hodak E, Klein T, Gabay B *et al.* Familial mycosis fungoides: report of 6 kindreds and a study of the HLA system. *J Am Acad Dermatol* 2005;**52**:393–402.

17. Schmidt AN, Robbins JB, Greer JP, Zic JA. Conjugal transformed mycosis fungoides: the unknown role of viral infection and environmental exposures in the development of cutaneous T-cell lymphoma. *J Am Acad Dermatol* 2006;**54**:s202–s205.

18. Morales MM, Olsen J, Johansen P *et al.* Viral infection, atopy and mycosis fungoides: a European multicentre case-control study. *Eur J Cancer* 2003;**39**:511–516.

19. Whittemore AS, Holly EA, Lee IM *et al.* Mycosis fungoides in relation to environmental exposures and immune response: a case-control study. *J Natl Cancer Inst* 1989;**81**:1560–1567.

20. Fransway AF, Winkelmann RK. Chronic dermatitis evolving to mycosis fungoides: report of four cases and review of the literature. *Cutis* 1988;**41**:330–335.

21. Tuyp E, Burgoyne A, Aitchison T, MacKie R. A case-control study of possible causative factors in mycosis fungoides. *Arch Dermatol* 1987;**123**:196–200.

22. Tan RSH, Butterworth CM, McLaughlin H, Malka S, Samman PD. Mycosis fungoides: a disease of antigen persistence. *Br J Dermatol* 1974; **91**: 607–16.

23. Morales Suarez-Varela MM, Olsen J, Johansen P *et al.* Occupational exposures and mycosis fungoides. A European multicentre case-control study (Europe). *Cancer Causes Control* 2005;**16**:1253–1259.

24. Herne KL, Talpur R, Breuer-McHam J, Champlin R, Duvic M. Cytomegalovirus seropositivity is significantly associated with mycosis fungoides and Sezary syndrome. *Blood* 2003;**101**:2132–2135.

25. Tothova SM, Bonin S, Trevisan G, Stanta G. Mycosis fungoides: is it a Borrelia burgdorferi-associated disease? *Br J Cancer* 2006; **94**:879–883.

26. Knol AC, Quereux G, Pandolfino MC, Khammari A, Dreno B. Presence of Epstein–Barr virus in Langerhans cells of CTCL lesions. *J Invest Dermatol* 2005;**124**:280–282.

27. Bazarbachi A, Soriano V, Pawson R *et al.* Mycosis fungoides and Sezary syndrome are not associated with HTLV-I infection: an international study. *Br J Haematol* 1997;**98**:927–933.

28. Zendri E, Pilotti E, Perez M *et al.* The HTLV tax-like sequences in cutaneous T-cell lymphoma patients. *J Invest Dermatol* 2008; **128**:489–492.

29. Rodriguez-Gil Y, Palencia SI, Lopez-Rios F, Ortiz PL, Rodriguez-Peralto JL. Mycosis fungoides after solid organ transplantation: report of 2 new cases. *Am J Dermatopathol* 2008;**30**:150–155.

30. Kreuter A, Bischoff S, Skrygan M *et al.* High association of human herpesvirus 8 in large-plaque parapsoriasis and mycosis fungoides. *Arch Dermatol* 2008;**144**:1011–1016.

31. Karenko L, Sarna S, Kähkönen M, Ranki A. Chromosomal abnormalities in relation to clinical disease in patients with cutaneous T-cell lymphoma: a 5-year follow-up study. *Br J Dermatol* 2003;**148**:55–64.

32. Dereure O, Levi E, Vonderheid EC, Kadin ME. Infrequent Fas mutations but no bax or p53 mutations in early mycosis fungoides: a possible mechanism for the accumulation of malignant T lymphocytes in the skin. *J Invest Dermatol* 2002; **118**:949–956.

33. Mao X, Lillington D, Scarisbrick JJ *et al.* Molecular cytogenetic analysis of cutaneous T-cell lymphomas: identification of common genetic alterations in Sézary syndrome and mycosis fungoides. *Br J Dermatol* 2002;**147**:464–475.

34. Scarisbrick JJ, Woolford AJ, Calonje E *et al.* Frequent abnormalities of the p15 and p16 genes in mycosis fungoides and Sezary syndrome. *J Invest Dermatol* 2002;**118**:493–499.

35. Scarisbrick JJ, Woolford AJ, Russell-Jones R, Whittaker SJ. Allelotyping in mycosis fungoides and Sézary syndrome: common regions of allelic loss identified on 9p, 10q, and 17p. *J Invest Dermatol* 2001;**117**:663–670.

36. Navas IC, Ortiz-Romero PL, Villuendas R *et al.* p16INK4a gene alterations are frequent in lesions of mycosis fungoides. *Am J Pathol* 2000;**156**:1565–1572.

37. Davis TH, Morton CC, Miller-Cassman R, Balk SP, Kadin ME. Hodgkin's disease, lymphomatoid papulosis, and cutaneous T-cell lymphoma derived from a common T-cell clone. *N Engl J Med* 1992;**326**:1115–1122.

38. Wood GS, Crooks CF, Uluer AZ. Lymphomatoid papulosis and associated cutaneous lymphoproliferative disorders exhibit a common clonal origin. *J Invest Dermatol* 1995;**105**:51–55.

39. Joly P, Lenormand B, Bagot M *et al.* Sequential analysis of T-cell receptor gene rearrangement in skin biopsy specimens from 6 patients with Hodgkin disease, lymphomatoid papulosis, mycosis fungoides and CD30 large cell lymphoma. *J Invest Dermatol* 1997;**109**:485.

40. Zackheim HS, Jones C, LeBoit PE *et al.* Lymphomatoid papulosis associated with mycosis fungoides: a study of 21 patients including analyses for clonality. *J Am Acad Dermatol* 2003;**49**:620–623.

41. Väkevä L, Pukkala E, Ranki A. Increased risk of secondary cancers in patients with primary cutaneous T cell lymphoma. *J Invest Dermatol* 2000;**115**:62–65.

42. Bunn P, Lamberg S. Report of the committee on staging and classification of cutaneous T-cell lymphoma. *Cancer Treat Rep* 1979;**63**:725–728.

43. Kashani-Sabet M, McMillan A, Zackheim HS. A modified staging classification for cutaneous T-cell lymphoma. *J Am Acad Dermatol* 2001;**45**:700–706.

44. Olsen E, Vonderheid E, Pimpinelli N *et al.* Revisions to the staging and classification of mycosis fungoides and Sezary syndrome: a proposal of the International Society for Cutaneous Lymphomas (ISCL) and the cutaneous lymphoma task force of the European Organization of Research and Treatment of Cancer (EORTC). *Blood* 2007;**110**:1713–1722.

45. Tsai EY, Taur A, Espinosa L *et al.* Staging accuracy in mycosis fungoides and Sézary syndrome using integrated positron emission tomography and computer tomography. *Arch Dermatol* 2006;**142**:577–584.

46. Valenvak J, Becherer A, Der-Petrossian M, Trautinger F, Raderer M, Hoffmann M. Positron emission tomography with [18F] 2–fluoro-D-2–deoxyglucose in primary cutaneous T-cell lymphomas. *Haematologica* 2005;**89**:115–116.

47. Kuo PH, McClennan BL, Carlson K *et al.* FDG-PET/CT in the evaluation of cutaneous T-cell lymphoma. *Molec Imag Biol* 2008;**10**:74–81.

48. Dereure O, Balavoine M, Salles MT *et al.* Correlations between clinical, histologic, blood, and skin polymerase chain reaction outcome in patients treated for mycosis fungoides. *J Invest Dermatol* 2003;**121**:614–617.

49. Muche JM, Lukowsky A, Asadullah K, Gellrich S, Sterry W. Demonstration of frequent occurrence of clonal T cells in the peripheral blood of patients with primary cutaneous T-cell lymphoma. *Blood* 1997;**90**:1636–1642.

50. Muche JM, Lukowsky A, Heim J *et al.* Demonstration of frequent occurrence of clonal T cells in the peripheral blood but not in the skin of patients with small plaque parapsoriasis. *Blood* 1999;**94**:1409–1417.

51. Delfau-Larue MH, Laroche L, Wechsler J *et al.* Diagnostic value of dominant T-cell clones in peripheral blood in 363 patients presenting consecutively with a suspicion of cutaneous lymphoma. *Blood* 2000;**96**:2987–2992.

52. Cen P, Duvic M, Cohen PR, Kurzrock R. Increased cancer antigen 27.29 (CA27.29) level in patients with mycosis fungoides. *J Am Acad Dermatol* 2008;**58**:382–386.

53. Escher N, Kaatz M, Melle C *et al.* Posttranslational modifications of transthyretin are serum markers in patients with mycosis fungoides. *Neoplasia* 2007;**9**:254–259.

54. Chong BF, Wilson AJ, Gibson HM *et al.* Immune function abnormalities in peripheral blood mononuclear cell cytokine expression differentiates stages of cutaneous T-cell lymphoma/mycosis fungoides. *Clin Cancer Res* 2008;**14**:646–653.

55. Abeni D, Frontani M, Sampogna F *et al.* Circulating CD8+ lymphocytes, white blood cells, and survival in patients with mycosis fungoides. *Br J Dermatol* 2005;**153**:324–330.

56. Theinert SM, Pronest MM, Peris K, Sterry W, Walden P. Identification of the testis-specific protein 10 (TSGA10) as serologically defined tumor-associated antigen in primary cutaneous T-cell lymphoma. *Br J Dermatol* 2005;**153**:639–641.

57. Washington LT, Huh YO, Powers LC, Duvic M, Jones D. A stable aberrant immunophenotype characterizes nearly all cases of cutaneous T-cell lymphoma in blood and can be used to monitor response to therapy. *BMC Clin Pathol* 2002;**2**:5.

58. Oshtory S, Apisarnthanarax N, Gilliam AC, Cooper KD, Meyerson HJ. Usefulness of flow cytometry in the diagnosis of mycosis fungoides. *J Am Acad Dermatol* 2007;**57**:454–462.

59. Grande-Sarpa H, Callis Duffin KP, Florell SR. Onychodystrophy and tumor-stage mycosis fungoides confined to a single digit: report of a case and review of nail findings in cutaneous T-cell lymphoma. *J Am Acad Dermatol* 2008;**59**:154–157.

60. Rappaport H, Thomas LB. Mycosis fungoides: the pathology of extracutaneous involvement. *Cancer* 1974;**34**:1198–1229.

61. de Coninck EC, Kim YH, Varghese A, Hoppe RT. Clinical characteristics and outcome of patients with extracutaneous mycosis fungoides. *J Clin Oncol* 2001;**19**:779–784.

62. Huang KP, Weinstock MA, Clarke CA, McMillan A, Hoppe RT, Kim YH. Second lymphomas and other malignant neoplasms in patients with mycosis fungoides and Sézary syndrome. Evidence from population-based and clinical cohorts. *Arch Dermatol* 2007;**143**:45–50.

63. Barzilai A, Trau H, David M *et al.* Mycosis fungoides associated with B-cell malignancies. *Br J Dermatol* 2006;**155**:179–186.

64. Hallermann C, Kaune MK, Tiemann M *et al.* High frequency of primary cutaneous lymphomas associated with lymphoproliferative disorders of different lineage. *Ann Hematol* 2007;**86**:509–515.

65. Kerl H, Cerroni L. Compare your diagnosis: seborrheic keratosis associated with mycosis fungoides. *Am J Dermatopathol* 1999;**21**:94–95.

66. Cribier BJ. The myth of Pautrier's microabscesses. *J Am Acad Dermatol* 2003;**48**:796–797.

67. Massone C, Kodama K, Kerl H, Cerroni L. Histopathologic features of early (patch) lesions of mycosis fungoides. A morphologic study on 745 biopsy specimens from 427 patients. *Am J Surg Pathol* 2005;**29**:550–560.

68. Stevens SR, Ke MS, Birol A *et al.* A simple clinical scoring system to improve the sensitivity and standardization of the diagnosis of mycosis fungoides type cutaneous T-cell lymphoma: logistic regression of clinical and laboratory data. *Br J Dermatol* 2003;**149**:513–522.

69. Pimpinelli N, Olsen EA, Santucci M *et al.* Defining early mycosis fungoides. *J Am Acad Dermatol* 2005;**53**:1053–1063.

70. Ferrara G, Di Blasi A, Zalaudek I, Argenziano G, Cerroni L. Regarding the algorithm for the diagnosis of early mycosis fungoides proposed by the International Society for Cutaneous Lymphomas: suggestions from routine histopathology practice. *J Cutan Pathol* 2008;**35**:549–553.

71. Smoller BR, Bishop K, Glusac E, Kim YH, Hendrickson M. Reassessment of histologic parameters in the diagnosis of mycosis fungoides. *Am J Surg Pathol* 1995;**19**:1423–1430.

72. Guitart J, Kennedy J, Ronan S *et al.* Histologic criteria for the diagnosis of mycosis fungoides: proposal for a grading system to standardize pathology reporting. *J Cutan Pathol* 2001;**28**:174–183.

73. Yeh YA, Hudson AR, Prieto VG, Shea CR, Smoller BR. Reassessment of lymphocytic atypia in the diagnosis of mycosis fungoides. *Mod Pathol* 2001;**14**:285–288.

74. Ming M, LeBoit PE. Can dermatopathologists reliably make the diagnosis of mycosis fungoides? If not, who can? *Arch Dermatol* 2000;**136**:543–546.

75. Kamarashev J, Burg G, Kempf W, Hess Schmid M, Dummer R. Comparative analysis of histological and immunohistological features in mycosis fungoides and Sézary syndrome. *J Cutan Pathol* 1998;**25**:407–412.

76. Su LD, Kim YH, LeBoit PE, Swetter SM, Kohler S. Interstitial mycosis fungoides, a variant of mycosis fungoides resembling granuloma annulare and inflammatory morphoea. *J Cutan Pathol* 2002;**29**:135–141.

77. Fujiwara Y, Abe Y, Kuyama M *et al.* CD8 cutaneous T-cell lymphoma with pagetoid epidermotropism and angiocentric and angiodestructive infiltration. *Arch Dermatol* 1990;**126**:801–804.

78. Cerroni L, Rieger E, Hödl S, Kerl H. Clinicopathologic and immunologic features associated with transformation of mycosis fungoides to large-cell lymphoma. *Am J Surg Pathol* 1992;**16**:543–552.

79. Vergier B, De Muret A, Beylot-Barry M *et al.* Transformation of mycosis fungoides: clinicopathologic and prognostic features of 45 cases. *Blood* 2000;**95**:2212–2218.

80. Diamandidou E, Colome-Grimmer MI, Fayad L, Duvic M, Kurzrock R. Transformation of mycosis fungoides/Sézary syndrome: clinical characteristics and prognosis. *Blood* 1998;**92**:1150–1159.

81. Arulogun SO, Prince HM, Ng J *et al.* Long-term outcomes of patients with advanced-stage cutaneous T-cell lymphoma and large cell transformation. *Blood* 2008;**112**:3082–3087.

82. Wolf P, Cerroni L, Smolle J, Kerl H. PUVA-induced lymphomatoid papulosis in a patient with mycosis fungoides. *J Am Acad Dermatol* 1991;**25**:422–426.

83. Ogino J, Saga K, Kagaya M *et al.* CD30+ large cell transformation of mycosis fungoides after psoralen plus ultraviolet A photochemotherapy. *Br J Dermatol* 2006;**156**:148–151.

84. Nakahigashi K, Ishida Y, Matsumura Y *et al.* Large cell transformation mimicking regional lymphomatoid papulosis in a patient with mycosis fungoides. *J Dermatol* 2008;**35**:283–288.

85. Willemze R, de Graaff-Reitsma CB, Cnossen J, van Vloten WA, Meijer CJLM. Characterization of T-cell subpopulations in skin and peripheral blood of patients with cutaneous T-cell lymphomas and benign inflammatory dermatoses. *J Invest Dermatol* 1983;**80**:60–66.

86. Ralfkiaer E, Lange Wantzin G, Mason DY *et al.* Phenotypic characterization of lymphocyte subsets in mycosis fungoides: comparison with large plaque parapsoriasis and benign chronic dermatoses. *Am J Clin Pathol* 1985;**84**:610–619.

87. Tosca AD, Varelzidis AG, Economidou J, Stratigos JD. Mycosis fungoides: evaluation of immunohistochemical criteria for the early diagnosis of the disease and differentiation between stages. *J Am Acad Dermatol* 1986;**15**:237–245.

88. Massone C, Crisman G, Kerl H, Cerroni L. The prognosis of early mycosis fungoides is not influenced by phenotype and T-cell clonality. *Br J Dermatol* 2008;**159**:881–886.

89. Sen F, Kang S, Cangiarella J, Kamino H, Hymes K. CD20 positive mycosis fungoides: a case report. *J Cutan Pathol* 2008;**35**:398–403.

90. Ortonne N, Buyukbabani N, Delfau-Larue MH, Bagot M, Wechsler J. Value of the CD8-CD3 ratio for the diagnosis of mycosis fungoides. *Mod Pathol* 2003;**16**:857–862.

91. Florell SR, Cessna M, Lundell RB *et al.* Usefulness (or lack thereof) of immunophenotyping in atypical cutaneous T-cell infiltrates. *Am J Clin Pathol* 2006;**125**:727–736.

92. Hodak E, David M, Maron L, Aviram A, Kaganovsky E, Feinmesser M. CD4/CD8 double-negative epidermotropic cutaneous T-cell lymphoma: an immunohistochemical variant of mycosis fungoides. *J Am Acad Dermatol* 2006;**55**:276–284.

93. Vermeer MH, Geelen FAMJ, Kummer JA, Meijer CJLM, Willemze R. Expression of cytotoxic proteins by neoplastic T cells in mycosis fungoides increases with progression from plaque stage to tumor stage disease. *Am J Pathol* 1999;**154**:1203–1210.

94. Wasco MJ, Fullen D, Su L, Ma L. The expression of MUM1 in cutaneous T-cell lymphoproliferative disorders. *Hum Pathol* 2008;**39**:557–563.

95. Gjerdrum LM, Woetmann A, Odum N *et al.* FOXP3+ regulatory T cells in cutaneous T-cell lymphomas: association with disease stage and survival. *Leukemia* 2007;**21**:2512–2518.

96. Tiemessen MM, Mitchell TJ, Hendry L, Whittaker SJ, Taams LS, John S. Lack of suppressive CD4+ CD25+ FOXP3+ T cells in advanced stages of primary cutaneous T-cell lymphoma. *J Invest Dermatol* 2006;**126**:2217–2223.

97. Hallermann C, Niermann C, Schulze HJ. Regulatory T-cell phenotype in association with large cell transformation of mycosis fungoides. *Eur J Haematol* 2007;**78**:260–263.

98. Fujimura T, Okuyama R, Ito Y, Aiba S. Profiles of Foxp3+ regulatory T cells in eczematous dermatitis, psoriasis vulgaris and mycosis fungoides. *Br J Dermatol* 2008;**158**:1256–1263.

99. Christie LJ, Evans AT, Bray SE *et al.* Lesions resembling Langerhans cell histiocytosis in association with other lymphoproliferative disorders: a reactive or neoplastic phenomenon? *Hum Pathol* 2006;**37**:32–39.

100. Tracey L, Villuendas R, Dotor AM *et al.* Mycosis fungoides shows concurrent deregulation of multiple genes involved in the TNF signaling pathway: an expression profile study. *Blood* 2003;**102**:1042–1050.

101. Shin J, Monti S, Aires DJ *et al.* Lesional gene expression profiling in cutaneous T-cell lymphoma reveals natural clusters associated with disease outcome. *Blood* 2007;**110**:3015–3027.

102. Navas IC, Ortiz-Romero PL, Villuendas R *et al.* p16(INK4a) gene alterations are frequent in lesions of mycosis fungoides. *Am J Pathol* 2000;**156**:1565–1572.

103. Mao X, Orchard G, Lillington DM *et al.* Amplification and over-expression of JUNB is associated with primary cutaneous T-cell lymphomas. *Blood* 2003;**101**:1513–1519.
104. Mao X, Orchard G, Mitchell TJ *et al.* A genomic and expression study of AP-1 in primary cutaneous T-cell lymphoma: evidence for dysregulated expression of JUNB and JUND in MF and SS. *J Cutan Pathol* 2008;**35**:899–910.
105. Dereure O, Levi E, Vonderheid EC, Kadin ME. Infrequent Fas mutations but no Bax or p53 mutations in early mycosis fungoides: a possible mechanism for the accumulation of malignant T lymphocytes in the skin. *J Invest Dermatol* 2002;**118**:949–956.
106. Prochazkova M, Chevret E, Mainhaguiet G *et al.* Common chromosomal abnormalities in mycosis fungoides transformation. *Genes Chrom Cancer* 2007;**46**:828–838.
107. Katona TM, O'Malley DPO, Cheng L *et al.* Loss of heterozygosity analysis identifies genetic abnormalities in mycosis fungoides and specific loci associated with disease progression. *Am J Surg Pathol* 2007;**31**:1552–1556.
108. Scarisbrick JJ, Woolford AJ, Russell-Jones R, Whittaker SJ. Loss of heterozygosity on 10q and microsatellite instability in advanced stages of primary cutaneous T-cell lymphoma and possible association with homozygous deletion of PTEN. *Blood* 2000;**95**:2937–2942.
109. Assaf C, Sanchez JAA, Lukowsky A *et al.* Absence of microsatellite instability and lack of evidence for subclone diversification in the pathogenesis and progression of mycosis fungoides. *J Invest Dermatol* 2007;**127**:1752–1761.
110. Carbone A, Bernardini L, Valenzano F *et al.* Array-based comparative genomic hybridization in early-stage mycosis fungoides: Recurrent deletion of tumor suppressor genes BCL7A, SMAC/DIABLO, and RHOF. *Genes Chromos Cancer* 2008;**47**:1067–1075.
111. Barba G, Matteucci C, Girolomoni G *et al.* Comparative genomic hybridization identifies 17q11.2~q12 duplication as an early event in cutaneous T-cell lymphomas. *Cancer Genetics Cytogen* 2008;**184**:48–51.
112. Wain EM, Mitchell TJ, Russell-Jones R, Whittaker SJ. Fine mapping of chromosome 10q deletions in mycosis fungoides and Sezary syndrome: identification of two discrete regions of deletion at 10q23.33–24.1 and 10q24.33–25.1. *Genes Chromos Cancer* 2005;**42**:184–192.
113. Karenko L, Hahtola S, Paivinen S *et al.* Primary cutaneous T-cell lymphomas show a deletion or translocation affecting NAV3, the human UNC-53 homologue. *Cancer Res* 2005;**65**:8101–8110.
114. Marty M, Prochazkova M, Laharanne E *et al.* Primary cutaneous T-cell lymphomas do not show specific NAV3 gene deletion or translocation. *J Invest Dermatol* 2008;**128**:2458–2466.
115. Böhncke WH, Krettek S, Parwaresch RM, Sterry W. Demonstration of clonal disease in early mycosis fungoides. *Am J Dermatopathol* 1992;**14**:95–99.
116. Wood GS, Tung RM, Haeffner AC *et al.* Detection of clonal T-cell receptor gamma gene rearrangements in early mycosis fungoides/Sezary syndrome by polymerase chain reaction and denaturing gradient gel electrophoresis (PCR/DGGE). *J Invest Dermatol* 1994;**103**:34–41.
117. Cozzio A, French LE. T-cell clonality assays: how do they compare? *J Invest Dermatol* 2008;**128**:771–773.
118. Nebozhyn M, Loboda A, Kari L *et al.* Quantitative PCR on 5 genes reliably identifies CTCL patients with 5% to 99% circulating tumor cells with 90% accuracy. *Blood* 2006;**107**:3189–3196.
119. Volkenandt M, Koch O, Wienecke R *et al.* Detection of monoclonal lymphoid subpopulations in clinical specimens by PCR and conformational polymorphism of cRNA molecules. *J Invest Dermatol* 1992;**98**:508.
120. Volkenandt M, Soyer HP, Cerroni L, Bertino JR, Kerl H. Molecular detection of clone-specific DNA in histopathologically unclassified lesions of a patient with mycosis fungoides. *Arch Dermatol Res* 1992;**284**:22–23.
121. Volkenandt M, Soyer HP, Cerroni L *et al.* Molecular detection of clone-specific DNA in hypopigmented lesions of a patient with early evolving mycosis fungoides. *Br J Dermatol* 1993;**128**:423–428.
122. Jones D, Duvic M. The current state and future of clonality studies in mycosis fungoides. *J Invest Dermatol* 2003;**121**:ix–xi.
123. Assaf C, Hummel M, Steinhoff M *et al.* Early TCR- and TCR-PCR detection of T-cell clonality indicates minimal tumor disease in lymph nodes of cutaneous T-cell lymphoma: diagnostic and prognostic implications. *Blood* 2005;**105**:503–510.
124. Fraser-Andrews EA, Mitchell T, Ferreira S, Seed PT, Russell-Jones R, Whittaker SJ. Molecular staging of lymph nodes from 60 patients with mycosis fungoides and Sezary syndrome: correlation with histopathology and outcome suggests prognostic relevance in mycosis fungoides. *Br J Dermatol* 2006;**155**:756–762.
125. Cowen EW, Liu CW, Steinberg SM *et al.* Differentiation of tumor-stage mycosis fungoides, psoriasis vulgaris and normal controls in a pilot study using serum proteomic analysis. *Br J Dermatol* 2007;**157**:946–953.
126. Wood GS, Abel EA, Hoppe RT, Warnke RA. Leu-8 and Leu-9 antigen phenotypes: immunological criteria for the distinction of mycosis fungoides from cutaneous inflammation. *J Am Acad Dermatol* 1986;**14**:1006–1013.
127. Ormsby A, Bergfeld WF, Tubbs RR, Hsi ED. Evaluation of a new paraffin-reactive CD7 T-cell deletion marker and a polymerase chain reaction-based T-cell receptor gene rearrangement assay: implications for diagnosis of mycosis fungoides in community clinical practice. *J Am Acad Dermatol* 2001;**45**:405–413.
128. Payne CM, Spier CM, Grogan TM *et al.* Nuclear contour irregularities correlate with Leu-9-, Leu-8-cells in benign lymphoid infiltrates of the skin. *Am J Dermatopathol* 1988;**10**:377–398.
129. Wood GS, Volterra AS, Abel EA, Nickoloff BJ, Adams RM. Allergic contact dermatitis: novel immunohistologic features. *J Invest Dermatol* 1986;**87**:688–693.
130. Cerroni L, Kerl H. Diagnostic immunohistology: cutaneous lymphomas and pseudolymphomas. *Semin Cutan Med Surg* 1999;**18**:64–70.
131. Michie SA, Abel EA, Hoppe RT, Warnke RA, Wood GS. Expression of T-cell receptor antigens in mycosis fungoides and inflammatory skin lesions. *J Invest Dermatol* 1989;**93**:116–120.
132. Jack AS, Boylston AW, Carrel S, Grigor I. Cutaneous T-cell lymphoma cells employ a restricted range of T-cell antigen receptor variable region genes. *Am J Pathol* 1990;**136**:17–21.
133. Alessi E, Coggi A, Venegoni L, Merlo V, Gianotti R. The usefulness of clonality for the detection of cases clinically and/or histopathologically not recognized as cutaneous T-cell lymphoma. *Br J Dermatol* 2005;**153**:368–371.

134. Thurber SE, Zhang B, Kim YH, Schrijver I, Zehnder J, Kohler S. T-cell clonality analysis in biopsy specimens from two different skin sites shows high specificity in the diagnosis of patients with suggested mycosis fungoides. *J Am Acad Dermatol* 2007;**57**:782–790.

135. Lukowsky A, Muche JM, Sterry W, Audring H. Detection of expanded T cell clones in skin biopsy samples of patients with lichen sclerosus et atrophicus by T cell receptor-γ polymerase chain reaction assays. *J Invest Dermatol* 2000;**115**:254–259.

136. Schiller PI, Flaig MJ, Puchta U, Kind P, Sander CA. Detection of clonal T cells in lichen planus. *Arch Dermatol Res* 2000;**292**:568–569.

137. Citarella L, Massone C, Kerl H, Cerroni L. Lichen sclerosus with histopathologic features simulating early mycosis fungoides. *Am J Dermatopathol* 2003;**25**:463–465.

138. Cerroni L, Arzberger E, Ardigó M, Pütz B, Kerl H. Monoclonality of intraepidermal T lymphocytes in early mycosis fungoides detected by molecular analysis after laser-beam-based microdissection. *J Invest Dermatol* 2000;**114**:1154–1157.

139. Scheller U, Muche JM, Sterry W, Lukowsky A. Detection of clonal T cells in cutaneous T cell lymphoma by polymerase chain reaction: comparison of mutation detection enhancement polyacrylamide gel electrophoresis, temperature gradient gel electrophoresis and fragment analysis of sequencing gels. *Electrophoresis* 1998;**19**:653–658.

140. Ponti R, Fierro MT, Quaglino P et al. TCR-g chain gene rearrangement by PCR-based GeneScan: diagnostic accuracy improvement and clonal heterogeneity analysis in multiple cutaneous T-cell lymphoma samples. *J Invest Dermatol* 2008;**128**:1030–1038.

141. Nashan D, Faulhaber D, Ständer S, Luger TA, Stadler R. Mycosis fungoides: a dermatological masquerader. *Br J Dermatol* 2007;**156**:1–10.

142. LeBoit PE. Variants of mycosis fungoides and related cutaneous T-cell lymphomas. *Semin Diagn Pathol* 1991;**8**:73–81.

143. Zackheim HS, McCalmont TH. Mycosis fungoides: the great imitator. *J Am Acad Dermatol* 2002;**47**:914–918.

144. Ackerman AB, Schiff TA. If small plaque (digitate) parapsoriasis is a cutaneous T-cell lymphoma, even an 'abortive' one, it must be mycosis fungoides! *Arch Dermatol* 1996;**132**:562–566.

145. Burg G, Dummer R, Nestle FO, Doebbeling U, Haeffner A. Cutaneous lymphomas consist of a spectrum of nosologically different entities including mycosis fungoides and small plaque parapsoriasis. *Arch Dermatol* 1996;**132**:567–572.

146. Ackerman AB, Denianke K, Sceppa J, Asgari M, Milette F, Sanchez J. *Mycosis Fungoides: Perspective Historical Allied with Critique Methodical for the Purpose of Illumination Maximal.* New York: Ardor Scribendi, 2008.

147. Väkevä L, Sarna S, Vaalasti A, Pukkala E, Kariniemi AL, Ranki A. A retrospective study of the probability of the evolution of parapsoriasis en plaques into mycosis fungoides. *Acta Derm Venereol (Stockh)* 2005;**85**:318–323.

148. Belousova IE, Vanecek T, Samtsov AV, Michal M, Kazakov DV. A patient with clinicopathologic features of small plaque parapsoriasis presenting later with plaque-stage mycosis fungoides: report of a case and comparative retrospective study of 27 cases of "nonprogressive" small plaque parapsoriasis. *J Am Acad Dermatol* 2008;**59**:474–482.

149. Cerroni L, Fink-Puches R, Bäck B, Kerl H. Follicular mucinosis: a critical reappraisal of clinicopathologic features and association with mycosis fungoides and Sézary syndrome. *Arch Dermatol* 2002;**138**:182–189.

150. Flaig MJ, Cerroni L, Schuhmann K et al. Follicular mycosis fungoides: a histopathologic analysis of nine cases. *J Cutan Pathol* 2001;**28**:525–530.

151. Gerami P, Guitart J. The spectrum of histopathologic and immunohistochemical findings in folliculotropic mycosis fungoides. *Am J Surg Pathol* 2007;**31**:1430–1438.

152. Kossard S, Weller P. Pseudotumorous folliculotropic mycosis fungoides. *Am J Dermatopathol* 2005;**27**:224–227.

153. Gerami P, Guitart, J. Basaloid folliculolymphoid hyperplasia: a distinctive finding in follicular mycosis fungoides. *J Cutan Pathol* 2007;**34** (suppl. 1):29–32.

154. van Doorn R, Scheffer E, Willemze R. Follicular mycosis fungoides, a distinct disease entity with or without associated follicular mucinosis. *Arch Dermatol* 2002;**138**:191–198.

155. Gerami P, Rosen S, Kuzel T, Boone SL, Guitart J. Folliculotropic mycosis fungoides. An aggressive variant of cutaneous T-cell lymphoma. *Archiv Dermatol* 2008;**144**:738–746.

156. Haller A, Elzubi E, Petzelbauer P. Localized syringolymphoid hyperplasia with alopecia and anhidrosis. *J Am Acad Dermatol* 2001;**45**:127–130.

157. Hobbs JL, Chaffins ML, Douglass MC. Syringolymphoid hyperplasia with alopecia: two case reports and review of the literature. *J Am Acad Dermatol* 2003;**49**:1177–1180.

158. Tomaszewski MM, Lupton GP, Krishnan J, Welch M, James WD. Syringolymphoid hyperplasia with alopecia. A case report. *J Cutan Pathol* 1994;**21**:520–526.

159. Tomaszewski MM, Lupton GP. Syringolymphoid hyperplasia with alopecia. Case report and review of the literature. *J Cutan Pathol* 1993;**30**:575.

160. Vakilzadeh F, Bröcker EB. Syringolymphoid hyperplasia with alopecia. *Br J Dermatol* 1984;**110**:95–101.

161. Burg G, Schmöckel C. Syringolymphoid hyperplasia with alopecia – a syringotropic cutaneous T-cell lymphoma? *Dermatology* 1992;**184**:306–307.

162. Garcovich A, Garcovich S, Massi G. An unusual variant of granulomatous adnexotropic cutaneous T-cell lymphoma. *Br J Dermatol* 2003;**148**:363–365.

163. Jacobs MA, Kocher W, Murphy GF. Combined folliculotropic/syringotropic cutaneous T-cell lymphoma without epidermal involvement: report of 2 cases and pathogenic implications. *Hum Pathol* 2003;**34**:1216–1220.

164. Thein M, Ravat F, Orchard G, Calonje E, Russell-Jones R. Syringotropic cutaneous T-cell lymphoma: an immunophenotypic and genotypic study of five cases. *Br J Dermatol* 2004;**151**:216–226.

165. Weng AA, Howatson SR, Goodlad JR, Patel MC, Gupta G. Erythrodermic syringotropic cutaneous T-cell lymphoma. *Br J Dermatol* 2003;**148**:349–352.

166. Tannous Z, Baldassano MF, Li VW, Kvedar J, Duncan LM. Syringolymphoid hyperplasia and follicular mucinosis in a patient with cutaneous T-cell lymphoma. *J Am Acad Dermatol* 1999;**41**:303–308.

167. Hitchcock MG, Burchette JL Jr, Olsen EA, Ratech H, Kamino H. Eccrine gland infiltration by mycosis fungoides. *Am J Dermatopathol* 1996;**18**:447–453.

168. Zelger B, Sepp N, Weyrer K, Grünewald K. Syringotropic cutaneous T-cell lymphoma: a variant of mycosis fungoides? *Br J Dermatol* 1994;**130**:765–769.

169. Hsiao PF, Hsiao CH, Tsai TF, Jee SH. Unilesional folliculotropic/ syringotropic cutaneous T-cell lymphoma presenting as an indurated plaque on the nape. *Int J Dermatol* 2006;**45**:1268–1270.

170. Scarabello A, Fantini F, Giannetti A, Cerroni L. Localized pagetoid reticulosis (Woringer–Kolopp disease). *Br J Dermatol* 2002;**147**:806.

171. Leinweber B, Chott A, Kerl H, Cerroni L. Epidermotropic precursor T-cell lymphoma with highly aggressive clinical behavior simulating localized pagetoid reticulosis. *Am J Dermatopathol* 2007;**29**:392–394.

172. Lee JL, Viakhireva N, Cesca C et al. Clinicopathologic features and treatment outcomes in Woringer-Kolopp disease. *J Am Acad Dermatol* 2008;**59**:706–712.

173. Cerroni L, Fink-Puches R, El-Shabrawi-Caelen L et al. Solitary skin lesions with histopathologic features of early mycosis fungoides. *Am J Dermatopathol* 1999;**21**:518–524.

174. Oliver GF, Winkelmann RK. Unilesional mycosis fungoides: a distinct entity. *J Am Acad Dermatol* 1989;**20**:63–70.

175. Heald PW, Glusac EJ. Unilesional cutaneous T-cell lymphoma: clinical features, therapy, and follow-up of 10 patients with a treatment-responsive mycosis fungoides variant. *J Am Acad Dermatol* 2000;**42**:283–285.

176. van Doorn R, van Kester MS, Dijkman R et al. Oncogenomic analysis of mycosis fungoides reveals major differences with Sézary syndrome. *Blood* 2009;**113**:127–136.

177. El Shabrawi-Caelen L, Cerroni L, Medeiros LJ, McCalmont TH. Hypopigmented mycosis fungoides: frequent expression of a CD8 T-cell phenotype. *Am J Surg Pathol* 2002;**26**:450–457.

178. Ardigó M, Borroni G, Muscardin L, Kerl H, Cerroni L. Hypopigmented mycosis fungoides in Caucasian patients: a clinicopathologic study of 7 cases. *J Am Acad Dermatol* 2003;**49**:264–270.

179. Werner B, Brown S, Ackerman AB. Hypopigmented mycosis fungoides is not always mycosis fungoides! *Am J Dermatopathol* 2005;**27**:56–67.

180. Toro JR, Sander CA, LeBoit PE. Persistent pigmented purpuric dermatitis and mycosis fungoides: simulant, precursor, or both? A study by light microscopy and molecular methods. *Am J Dermatopathol* 1997;**19**:108–118.

181. Crowson AN, Magro CM, Zahorchak R. Atypical pigmentary purpura: a clinical, histopathologic, and genotypic study. *Hum Pathol* 1999;**30**:1004–1012.

182. Boyd AS, Vnencak-Jones CL. T-cell clonality in lichenoid purpura: a clinical and molecular evaluation of seven patients. *Histopathology* 2003;**43**:302–303.

183. Barnhill RL, Braverman IM. Progression of pigmented purpura-like eruptions to mycosis fungoides: report of three cases. *J Am Acad Dermatol* 1988;**19**:25–31.

184. Viseux V, Schoenlaub P, Cnudde F, Le Roux P, Leroy JP, Plantin P. Pigmented purpuric dermatitis preceding the diagnosis of mycosis fungoides by 24 years. *Dermatology* 2003;**207**:331–332.

185. Bowman PH, Hogan DJ, Sanusi ID. Mycosis fungoides bullosa: report of a case and review of the literature. *J Am Acad Dermatol* 2001;**45**:934–939.

186. Jakob T, Tiemann M, Kuwert C et al. Dyshidrotic cutaneous T-cell lymphoma. *J Am Acad Dermatol* 1996;**34**:295–297.

187. Soyer HP, Smolle J, Kerl H. Dyshidrotic mycosis fungoides. *J Cutan Pathol* 1987;**14**:372.

188. Pföhler C, Ugurel S, Seiter S et al. Interferon-α-associated development of bullous lesions in mycosis fungoides. *Dermatology* 2000;**200**:51–53.

189. Ackerman AB, Flaxman BA. Granulomatous mycosis fungoides. *Br J Dermatol* 1970;**82**:397–401.

190. Scarabello A, Leinweber B, Ardigó M et al. Cutaneous lymphomas with prominent granulomatous reaction: a potential pitfall in the histopathologic diagnosis of cutaneous T- and B-cell lymphomas. *Am J Surg Pathol* 2002;**26**:1259–1268.

191. LeBoit PE, Zackheim HS, White CR Jr. Granulomatous variants of cutaneous T-cell lymphoma: the histopathology of granulomatous mycosis fungoides and granulomatous slack skin. *Am J Surg Pathol* 1988;**12**:83–95.

192. Ackerman AB. Granulomatous slack skin. In: Ackerman AB, ed. *Histologic Diagnosis of Inflammatory Skin Diseases*. Philadelphia: Lea and Febiger, 1978: 483–485.

193. Balus L, Manente L, Remotti D, Grammatico P, Bellocci M. Granulomatous slack skin: report of a case and review of the literature. *Am J Dermatopathol* 1996;**18**:199–206.

194. LeBoit PE. Granulomatous slack skin. *Dermatol Clin* 1994;**12**:375–89.

195. Clarijs M, Poot F, Laka A, Pirard C, Bourlond A. Granulomatous slack skin: treatment with extensive surgery and review of the literature. *Dermatology* 2003;**206**:393–397.

196. van Haselen CW, Toonstra J, van der Putte SCJ, van Dongen JJM, van Hees CLM, van Vloten WA. Granulomatous slack skin. Report of three patients with an updated review of the literature. *Dermatology* 1998;**196**:382–391.

197. Moreno-Gimenez JC, Jimenez-Puya R, Galan-Gutierrez M, Perez-Seoane C, Camacho FM. Granulomatous slack skin disease in a child: the outcome. *Ped Dermatol* 2007;**24**:640–645.

198. Belousova IE, Nikonova SM, Sima R, Kazakov DV. Granulomatous slack skin with clonal T-cell receptor-γ gene rearrangement in skin and lymph node. *Br J Dermatol* 2007;**157**:405–407.

199. Ikonomou IM, Aamot HV, Heim S, Fossa A, Delabie J. Granulomatous slack skin with a translocation t(3;9)(q12;p24). *Am J Surg Pathol* 2007;**31**:803–806.

200. Flaxmann BA, Koumans JAD, Ackerman AB. Granulomatous mycosis fungoides: a 14-year follow-up of a case. *Am J Dermatopathol* 1983;**5**:145–151.

201. Gomez de la Fuente E, Ortiz PL, Vanaclocha F, Rodriguez-Peralto JL, Iglesias L. Aggressive granulomatous mycosis fungoides with clinical pulmonary and thyroid involvement. *Br J Dermatol* 2000;**142**:1026–1029.

202. Cerroni L. Cutaneous granulomas and malignant lymphomas. *Derrmatology* 2003;**206**:78–80.

203. Kempf W, Ostheeren-Michaelis S, Paulli M et al. Granulomatous mycosis fungoides and granulomatous slack skin: a multicenter study of the Cutaneous Lymphoma Histopathology Task Force Group of the European Organization for Research and Treatment of Cancer (EORTC). *Arch Dermatol* 2008;**144**:1609–1617.

204. Kodama K, Fink-Puches R, Massone C, Kerl H, Cerroni L. Papular mycosis fungoides: a new clinical variant of early mycosis fungoides. *J Am Acad Dermatol* 2005;**52**:694–698.

205. Braverman JM, Klein S, Grant A. Electron microscopic and immunolabeling studies of the lesional and normal skin of patients with mycosis fungoides treated by total body electron beam irradiation. *J Am Acad Dermatol* 1987; **16**:61–74.

206. Bergman R, Cohen A, Harth Y *et al.* Histopathologic findings in the clinically uninvolved skin of patients with mycosis fungoides. *Am J Surg Pathol* 1995;**17**:452–456.

207. Pujol RM, Gallardo F, Llistosella E *et al.* Invisible mycosis fungoides: a diagnostic challenge. *J Am Acad Dermatol* 2000;**42**: 324–328.

208. Requena L, Gonzalez-Guerra E, Angulo J, DeVore AE, Sangueza OP. Anetodermic mycosis fungoides: a new clinico-pathological variant of mycosis fungoides. *Br J Dermatol* 2008; **158**:157–162.

209. Fink-Puches R, Chott A, Ardigo M *et al.* The spectrum of cutaneous lymphomas in patients under 20 years of age. *Pediatr Dermatol* 2004;**21**:525–533.

210. Hickham PR, McBurney EI, Fitzgerald RL. CTCL in patients under 20 years of age: a series of five cases. *Pediatr Dermatol* 1997;**14**:93–97.

211. Burns MK, Ellis CN, Cooper KD. Mycosis fungoides-type cutaneous T-cell lymphoma arising before 30 years of age. Immuno-phenotypic, immunogenotypic and clinicopathologic analysis of nine cases. *J Am Acad Dermatol* 1992;**27**:974–978.

212. Neuhaus IM, Ramos-Caro FA, Hassanein AM. Hypopigmented mycosis fungoides in childhood and adolescence. *Pediatr Dermatol* 2000;**17**:403–406.

213. Peters MS, Thibodeau SN, White JW Jr, Winkelmann RK. Mycosis fungoides in children and adolescents. *J Am Acad Dermatol* 1990;**22**:1011–1018.

214. Quaglino P, Zaccagna A, Verrone A, Dardano F, Bernengo MG. Mycosis fungoides in patients under 20 years of age: report of 7 cases, review of the literature and study of the clinical course. *Dermatology* 1999;**199**:8–14.

215. Ko JW, Seong JY, Suh KS, Kim ST. Pityriasis lichenoides-like mycosis fungoides in children. *Br J Dermatol* 2000;**142**:347–352.

216. Ben-Amitai D, David M, Feinmesser M, Hodak E. Juvenile mycosis fungoides diagnosed before 18 years of age. *Acta Derm Venereol (Stockh)* 2003;**83**:451–456.

217. Annessi G, Paradisi M, Angelo C *et al.* Annular lichenoid dermatitis of youth. *J Am Acad Dermatol* 2003;**49**:1029–1036.

218. Cogrel O, Boralevi F, Lepreux S *et al.* Lymphomatoid annular erythema: a new form of juvenile mycosis fungoides. *Br J Dermatol* 2005;**152**:565–566.

219. Whittam LR, Calonje E, Orchard G, Fraser-Andrews E, Woolford A, Russell-Jones R. CD-8-positive juvenile onset mycosis fungoides: an immunohistochemical and genotypic analysis of six cases. *Br J Dermatol* 2000;**143**:1199–1204.

220. Wang SH, Hsiao CH, Hsiao PH, Chu CY. Adult pityriasis lichenoides-like mycosis fungoides with high density of CD8-positive T-lymphocytic infiltration. *J Eur Acad Dermatol Venereol* 2007;**21**:401–402.

221. Zackheim HS, Mc Calmont TH, Deanovic FW, Odom RB. Mycosis fungoides with onset before 20 years of age. *J Am Acad Dermatol* 1997;**36**:557–562.

222. Crowley JJ, Nikko A, Varghese A, Hoppe RT, Kim YH. Mycosis fungoides in young patients: clinical characteristics and outcome. *J Am Acad Dermatol* 1998;**38**:696–701.

223. Wain EM, Orchard GE, Whittaker SJ, Spittle MF, Russell-Jones R. Outcome in 34 patients with juvenile-onset mycosis fungoides. A clinical, immunophenotypic, and molecular study. *Cancer* 2003;**98**:2282–2290.

224. Jones SE. Enigma of therapy for cutaneous T-cell lymphoma. *J Natl Cancer Inst* 1990;**82**:169–170.

225. Chiaron-Sileni V, Bononi A, Veller Fornasa C *et al.* Phase II trial of interferon-a-2a plus psoralen with ultraviolet light A in patients with cutaneous T-cell lymphoma. *Cancer* 2002;**95**: 569–575.

226. Stadler R, Otte HG, Luger T *et al.* Prospective randomized multi-center clinical trial on the use of interferon a-2a plus acitretin versus interferon a-2a plus PUVA in patients with cutaneous T-cell lymphoma stages I and II. *Blood* 1998;**92**:3578–3581.

227. Rupoli S, Goteri G, Pulini S *et al.* Long-term experience with low-dose interferon-α and PUVA in the management of early mycosis fungoides. *Eur J Haematol* 2005;**75**:136–145.

228. Trautinger F, Knobler R, Willemze R *et al.* EORTC consensus recommendations for the treatment of mycosis fungoides/ Sézary syndrome. *Eur J Cancer* 2006;**42**:1014–1030.

229. Weber F, Schmuth M, Sepp N, Fritsch P. Bath-water PUVA therapy with 8-methoxypsoralen in mycosis fungoides. *Acta Derm Venereol (Stockh)* 2005;**85**:329–332.

230. Diederen PVMM, van Weelden H, Sanders CJG, Toonstra J, van Vloten WA. Narrowband UVB and psoralen-UVA in the treatment of early-stage mycosis fungoides. A retrospective study. *J Am Acad Dermatol* 2003;**48**:215–219.

231. Kim YH, Martinez G, Varghese A, Hoppe RT. Topical nitrogen mustard in the management of mycosis fungoides. *Arch Dermatol* 2003;**139**:165–173.

232. Cochran Gathers R, Scherschun L, Malick F, Fivenson DP, Lim HW. Narrowband UVB phototherapy for early-stage mycosis fungoides. *J Am Acad Dermatol* 2002;**47**:191–197.

233. Hofer A, Cerroni L, Kerl H, Wolf P. Narrowband (311nm) UV-B therapy for small plaque parapsoriasis and early stage mycosis fungoides. *Arch Dermatol* 1999;**135**:1377–1380.

234. Boztepe G, Sahin S, Ayhan M, Erkin G, Kolemen F. Narrowband ultraviolet B phototherapy clear and maintain clearance in patients with mycosis fungoides. *J Am Acad Dermatol* 2005; **53**:242–246.

235. Brazzelli V, Antoninetti M, Palazzini S, Prestinari F, Borroni G. Narrow-band ultraviolet therapy in early-stage mycosis fungoides: study on 20 patients. *Photoderm Photoimmunol Photomed* 2007;**23**:229–233.

236. Zackheim HS, Kashani-Sabet M, Amin S. Topical corticosteroids for mycosis fungoides. Experience in 79 patients. *Arch Dermatol* 1998;**134**:949–954.

237. Goldberg DJ, Stampen TM, Schwartz RA. Mycosis fungoides palmaris et plantaris: successful treatment with the carbon dioxide laser. *Br J Dermatol* 1997;**136**:617–619.

238. Upjohn E, Foley P, Lane P *et al.* Long-term clearance of patch-stage mycosis fungoides with the 308-nm laser. *Clin Exp Dermatol* 2006;**32**:168–171.

239. Jones GW, Kacinski BM, Wilson LD *et al.* Total skin electron radiation in the management of mycosis fungoides: consensus of the European Organization for Research and Treatment of Cancer (EORTC) Cutaneous Lymphoma Project Group. *J Am Acad Dermatol* 2002;**47**:364–370.

240. Kaye FJ, Bunn PA Jr, Steinberg SM *et al.* A randomized trial comparing combination electron-beam radiation and chemotherapy with topical therapy in the initial treatment of mycosis fungoides. *N Engl J Med* 1989;**321**:1784–1790.

241. De Sanctis V, Osti MF, Berardi F *et al.* Primary cutaneous lymphoma: local control and survival in patients treated with radiotherapy. *Anticancer Res* 2007;**27**:601–605.

242. Duvic M, Olsen EA, Omura GA *et al.* A phase III, randomized, double-blind, placebo-controlled study of peldesine (BCX-34) cream as topical therapy for cutaneous T-cell lymphoma. *J Am Acad Dermatol* 2001;**44**:940–947.

243. Tracey L, Villuendas R, Ortiz P *et al.* Identification of genes involved in resistance to interferon-a in cutaneous T-cell lymphoma. *Am J Pathol* 2002;**161**:1825–1837.

244. Aviles A, Nambo MJ, Neri N *et al.* Interferon and low dose methotrexate improve outcome in refractory mycosis fungoides/sezary syndrome. *Cancer Biother Radiopharm* 2007;**22**:836–840.

245. Gniadecki R, Assaf C, Bagot M *et al.* The optimal use of bexarotene in cutaneous T-cell lymphoma. *Br J Dermatol* 2007;**157**:433–440.

246. Budgin JB, Richardson SK, Newton SB *et al.* Biological effects of bexarotene in cutaneous T-cell lymphoma. *Arch Dermatol* 2005;**141**:315–321.

247. Straus DJ, Duvic M, Kuzel T *et al.* Results of a phase II trial of oral bexarotene (Targretin) combined with interferon alfa-2b (Intron-A) for patients with cutaneous T-cell lymphoma. *Cancer* 2007;**109**:1799–1803.

248. Sepmeyer JA, Greer JP, Koyama T, Zic JA. Open-label pilot study of combination therapy with rosiglitazone and bexarotene in the treatment of cutaneous T-cell lymphoma. *J Am Acad Dermatol* 2007;**56**:584–587.

249. Lokitz ML, Wong HK. Bexarotene and narrowband ultraviolet B phototherapy combination treatment for mycosis fungoides. *Photoderm Photoimmunol Photomed* 2007;**23**:255–257.

250. Duvic M, Martin AG, Kim Y *et al.* Phase 2 and 3 clinical trial of oral bexarotene (targretin capsules) for the treatment of refractory or persistent early-stage cutaneous T-cell lymphoma. *Arch Dermatol* 2001;**137**:581–593.

251. Assaf C, Bagot M, Dummer R *et al.* Minimizing adverse side-effects of oral bexarotene in cutaneous T-cell lymphoma: an expert opinion. *Br J Dermatol* 2006;**155**:261–266.

252. Heald P, Mehlmauer M, Martin AG, Crowley CA, Yocum RC, Reich SD. Topical bexarotene therapy for patients with refractory or persistent early-stage cutaneous T-cell lymphoma: results of the phase III clinical trial. *J Am Acad Dermatol* 2003;**49**:801–805.

253. Berthelot C, Rivera A, Duvic M. Skin directed therapy for mycosis fungoides: a review. *J Drugs Dermatol* 2008;**7**:655–666.

254. Apisarnthanarax N, Talpur R, Duvic M. Treatment of cutaneous T cell lymphoma. Current status and future directions. *Am J Clin Dermatol* 2002;**3**:193–215.

255. Vonderheid EC. Treatment of cutaneous T cell lymphoma 2001. *Rec Res Cancer Res* 2002;**160**:309–320.

256. Dummer R, Urosevic M, Kempf W, Kazakov D, Burg G. Imiquimod induces complete clearance of a PUVA-resistant plaque in mycosis fungoides. *Dermatology* 2003;**207**:116–118.

257. Breneman D, Duvic M, Kuzel T, Yocum R, Truglia J, Stevens VJ. Phase 1 and 2 trial of bexarotene gel for skin-directed treatment of patients with cutaneous T-cell lymphoma. *Arch Dermatol* 2002;**138**:325–332.

258. Duvic M, Hymes K, Heald P *et al.* Bexarotene is effective and safe for treatment of refractory advanced-stage cutaneous T-cell lymphoma: multinational phase II–III trial results. *J Clin Oncol* 2001;**19**:2456–2471.

259. Demierre MF, Vachon L, Ho V, Sutton L, Cato A, Leyland-Jones B. Phase 1/2 pilot study of methotrexate-laurocapram topical gel for the treatment of patients with early-stage mycosis fungoides. *Arch Dermatol* 2003;**139**:624–628.

260. Wolf P, Fink-Puches R, Cerroni L, Kerl H. Photodynamic therapy for mycosis fungoides after topical photosensitization with 5-aminolevulinic acid. *J Am Acad Dermatol* 1994;**31**:678–680.

261. Martinez-Gonzalez MC, Verea-Hernando MM, Yebra-Pimentel MT, del Pozo J, Mazaira M, Fonseca E. Imiquimod in mycosis fungoides. *Eur J Dermatol* 2008;**18**:148–152.

262. Wiegleb Edström D, Hedblad MA. Long-term follow-up of photodynamic therapy for mycosis fungoides. *Acta Derm Venereol (Stockh)* 2008;**88**:288–290.

263. Duvic M, Apisarnthanarax N, Cohen DS, Smith TL, Ha CS, Kurzrock R. Analysis of long-term outcomes of combined modality therapy for cutaneous T-cell lymphoma. *J Am Acad Dermatol* 2003; **49**:35–49.

264. Chiam LYT, Chan YC. Solitary plaque mycosis fungoides on the penis responding to topical imiquimod therapy. *Br J Dermatol* 2007;**156**:560–562.

265. Zane C, Venturini M, Sala R, Calzavara Pinton P. Photodynamic therapy with methylaminolevulinate as a valuable treatment for unilesional cutaneous T-cell lymphoma. *Photoderm Photoimmun Photomed* 2006;**22**:254–258.

266. Leverkus M, Rose C, Bröcker EB, Goebeler M. Follicular cutaneous T-cell lymphoma: beneficial effect of isotretinoin for persisting cysts and comedones. *Br J Dermatol* 2005;**152**:193–194.

267. Rubegni P, De Aloe G, Fimiani M. Extracorporeal photochemotherapy in long-term treatment of early stage cutaneous T-cell lymphoma. *Br J Dermatol* 2000;**143**:894–896.

268. Kamstrup MR, Specht L, Skovgaard GL, Gniadecki R. A prospective, open-label study of low-dose total skin electron beam therapy in mycosis fungoides. *Int J Radiat Oncol Biol Phys* 2008;**71**:1204–1207.

269. Scarisbrick JJ, Taylor P, Holtick U *et al.* U.K. consensus statement on the use of extracorporeal photopheresis for treatment of cutaneous T-cell lymphoma and chronic graft-versus-host disease. *Br J Dermatol* 2008;**158**:659–678.

270. Olavarria E, Child F, Woolford A *et al.* T-cell depletion and autologous stem cell transplantation in the management of tumor stage mycosis fungoides with peripheral blood involvement. *Br J Haematol* 2001;**114**:624–631.

271. Soligo D, Ibatici A, Berti E *et al.* Treatment of advanced mycosis fungoides by allogeneic stem-cell transplantation with a non-myeloablative regimen. *Bone Marrow Trans* 2003;**31**:663–666.

272. Guitart J, Wickless SC, Oyama Y *et al.* Long-term remission after allogeneic hematopoietic stem cell transplantation for refractory cutaneous T-cell lymphoma. *Arch Dermatol* 2002;**138**:1359–1365.

273. Introcaso CE, Leber B, Greene K, Ubriani R, Rook AH, Kim EJ. Stem cell transplantation in advanced cutaneous T-cell lymphoma. *J Am Acad Dermatol* 2008;**58**:645–649.

274. Molina A, Zain J, Arber DA *et al.* Durable clinical, cytogenetic, and molecular remissions after allogeneic hematopoietic cell transplantation for refractory Sezary syndrome and mycosis fungoides. *J Clin Oncol* 2005;**23**:6163–6171.

275. Fukushima T, Horio K, Matsuo E, *et al.* Successful cord blood transplantation for mycosis fungoides. *Int J Hematol* 2008;**88**: 596–598.

276. Carretero-Margolis CD, Fivenson DP. A complete and durable response to denileukin diftitox in a patient with mycosis fungoides. *J Am Acad Dermatol* 2003;**48**:275–276.

277. Lundin J, Hagberg H, Repp R *et al.* Phase 2 study of alemtuzumab (anti-CD52 monoclonal antibody) in patients with advanced mycosis fungoides/Sézary syndrome. *Blood* 2003;**101**:4267–4272.

278. Pangalis GA, Dimopoulou MN, Angelopoulou MK *et al.* Campath-1H (anti-CD52) monoclonal antibody therapy in lymphoproliferative disorders. *Med Oncol* 2001;**18**:99–107.

279. Scarisbrick JJ, Child FJ, Clift A *et al.* A trial of fludarabine and cyclophosphamide combination chemotherapy in the treatment of advanced refractory primary cutaneous T-cell lymphoma. *Br J Dermatol* 2001;**144**:1010–1015.

280. Zinzani PL, Baliva G, Magagnoli M *et al.* Gemcitabine treatment in pretreated cutaneous T-cell lymphoma: experience in 44 patients. *J Clin Oncol* 2000;**18**:2603–2606.

281. Akpek G, Koh HK, Bogen S, O'Hara C, Foss FM. Chemotherapy with etoposide, vincristine, doxorubicin, bolus cyclophosphamide, and oral prednisone in patients with refractory cutaneous T-cell lymphoma. *Cancer* 1999;**86**:1368–1376.

282. Foss F, Demierre MF, DiVenuti G. A phase-1 trial of bexarotene and denileukin diftitox in patients with relapsed or refractory cutaneous T-cell lymphoma. *Blood* 2005;**106**:454–457.

283. Heinzerling L, Künzi V, Oberholzer PA, Kündig T, Naim H, Dummer R. Oncolytic measles virus in cutaneous T-cell lymphomas mounts antitumor immune responses in vivo and targets interferon-resistant tumor cells. *Blood* 2005;**106**: 2287–2294.

284. Marchi E, Almari L, Tani M *et al.* Gemcitabine as frontline treatment for cutaneous T-cell lymphoma. Phase II study of 32 patients. *Cancer* 2005;**104**:2437–2441.

285. Dumontet C, Thomas L, Berard F, Gimonet JF, Coiffier B. A phase II trial of miltefosine in patients with cutaneous T-cell lymphoma. *Bull Cancer* 2006;**93**:115–118.

286. Künzi V, Oberholzer PA, Heinzerling L, Dummer R, Naim HY. Recombinant measles virus induces cytolysis of cutaneous T-cell lymphoma *in vitro* and *in vivo*. *J Invest Dermatol* 2006;**126**: 2525–2532.

287. Kim YH, Duvic M, Obitz E *et al.* Clinical efficacy of zanolimumab (HuMax-CD4): two phase 2 studies in refractory cutaneous T-cell lymphoma. *Blood* 2007;**109**:4655–4662.

288. Duvic M, Talpur R, Ni X *et al.* Phase 2 trial of oral vorinostat (suberoylanilide hydroxamic acid, SAHA) for refractory cutaneous T-cell lymphoma (CTCL). *Blood* 2007;**109**:31–39.

289. Mann BS, Johnson JR, He K *et al.* Vorinostat for treatment of cutaneous manifestations of advanced primary cutaneous T-cell lymphoma. *Clin Cancer Res* 2007;**13**:2318–2322.

290. Yano H, Ishida T, Inagaki A *et al.* Defucosylated Anti-CC chemokine receptor 4 monoclonal antibody combined with immunomodulatory cytokines: A novel immunotherapy for aggressive/refractory mycosis fungoides and Sezary syndrome. *Clin Cancer Res* 2007;**13**:6494–6500.

291. Quereux G, Marques S, Nguyen JM *et al.* Prospective multi-center study of pegylated liposomal doxorubicin treatment in patients with advanced or refractory mycosis fungoides or Sezary syndrome. *Arch Dermatol* 2008;**144**:727–733.

292. Ellis L, Pan Y, Smyth GK *et al.* Histone deacetylase inhibitor pano-binostat induces clinical responses with associated alterations in gene expression profiles in cutaneous T-cell lymphoma. *Clin Cancer Res* 2008;**14**:4500–4510.

293. Tsimberidou AM, Giles F, Duvic M, Fayad L, Kurzrock R. Phase II study of pentostatin in advanced T-cell lymphoid malignancies. *Cancer* 2004;**100**:342–349.

294. Muche JM, Sterry W. Vaccination therapy for cutaneous T-cell lymphoma. *Clin Exp Dermatol* 2002; **27**:602–607.

295. Maier T, Tun-Kyi A, Tassis A *et al.* Vaccination of patients with cutaneous T-cell lymphoma using intranodal injection of autologous tumor-lysate-pulsed dendritic cells. *Blood* 2003; **102**:2338–2344.

296. Eichmüller S, Usener D, Thiel D, Schadendorf D. Tumor-specific antigens in cutaneous T-cell lymphoma: expression and sero-reactivity. *Int J Cancer* 2003;**104**:482–487.

297. LeBon B, Beynon TA, Whittaker SJ. Palliative care in patients with primary cutaneous lymphoma: symptom burden and characteristics of hospital palliative care team input. *Arch Dermatol* 2007;**143**:423–424.

298. Demierre MF, Tien A, Miller D. Health-related quality-of-life assessment in patients with cutaneous T-cell lymphoma. *Arch Dermatol* 2005;**141**:325–330.

299. Hernandez C, Worobec SM, Gaitonde S, Kiripolski ML, Aquino K. Progression of undiagnosed cutaneous T-cell lymphoma during efalizumab therapy. *Arch Dermatol* 2009;**145**: 92–94.

300. Lafaille P, Bouffard D, Provost N. Exacerbation of undiagnosed mycosis fungoides during treatment with etanercept. *Arch Dermatol* 2009;**145**:94–95.

301. Chuang GS, Wasserman DI, Byers HR, Demierre MF. Hypo-pigmented T-cell dyscrasia evolving to hypopigmented mycosis fungoides during etanercept therapy. *J Am Acad Dermatol* 2008;**59**:s121–s122.

302. Weinstock MA, Reynes JF. The changing survival of patients with mycosis fungoides. *Cancer* 1999; **85**:208–212.

303. van Doorn R, van Haselen CW, van Voorst Vader PC *et al.* Mycosis fungoides. Disease evaluation and prognosis of 309 Dutch patients. *Arch Dermatol* 2000;**136**:504–510.

304. Sun G, Berthelot C, Li Y, *et al.* Poor prognosis in non-Caucasian patients with early-onset mycosis fungoides. *J Am Acad Dermatol* 2009;**60**:231–235.

305. Fraser-Andrews E, Woolford AJ, Russell-Jones R, Seed PT, Whittaker SJ. Detection of a peripheral blood T cell clone is an independent prognostic marker in mycosis fungoides. *J Invest Dermatol* 2000;**114**:117–121.

306. Beylot-Barry M, Sibaud V, Thiebaut R *et al.* Evidence that an identical T cell clone in skin and peripheral blood lymphocytes is an independent prognostic factor in primary cutaneous T cell lymphoma. *J Invest Dermatol* 2001;**117**:920–926.

307. Delfau-Larue MH, Dalac S, Lepage E *et al.* Prognostic significance of a polymerase chain reaction-detectable dominant T-lymphocyte clone in cutaneous lesions of patients with mycosis fungoides. *Blood* 1998;**92**:3376–3380.

308. Guitart J, Camisa C, Ehrlich M, Bergfeld WF. Long-term implications of T-cell receptor gene rearrangement analysis by Southern blot in patients with cutaneous T-cell lymphoma. *J Am Acad Dermatol* 2003;**48**:775–779.

309. Vega F, Luthra R, Medeiros LJ *et al.* Clonal heterogeneity in mycosis fungoides and its relationship to clinical course. *Blood* 2002;**100**:3369–3373.

310. Sibaud V, Beylot-Barry M, Thiebaut R *et al.* Bone marrow histopathologic and molecular staging in epidermotropic T-cell lymphoma. *Am J Clin Pathol* 2003;**119**:414–423.

311. Bakels V, van Oostveen JW, Geerts ML *et al.* Diagnostic and prognostic significance of clonal T-cell receptor beta gene rearrangements in lymph nodes of patients with mycosis fungoides. *J Pathol* 1993;**170**:249–255.

312. Smoller BR, Detwiler SP, Kohler S, Hoppe RT, Kim YH. Role of histology in providing prognostic informations in mycosis fungoides. *J Cutan Pathol* 1998;**25**:311–315.

313. Querfeld C, Rosen ST, Kuzel TM *et al.* Long-term follow-up of patients with early-stage cutaneous T-cell lymphoma who achieved complete remission with psoralen plus UV-A monotherapy. *Arch Dermatol* 2005;**141**:305–311.

314. Poszepczynska-Guigne E, Bagot M, Wechsler J, Revuz J, Farcet JP, Delfau-Larue MH. Minimal residual disease in mycosis fungoides follow-up can be assessed by polymerase chain reaction. *Br J Dermatol* 2003;**148**:265–271.

3 Sézary syndrome

Sézary syndrome is characterized clinically by pruritic ery-throderma, generalized lymphadenopathy, and the presence of circulating malignant T lymphocytes (Sézary cells) [1–3]. Other typical cutaneous changes include palmoplantar hyper-keratosis, alopecia, and onychodystrophy [4]. Differentiation from non-neoplastic erythroderma may be extremely difficult. The main causes of erythroderma, besides cutaneous T-cell lymphoma, are atopic dermatitis, psoriasis, and drug reactions, but less frequently other cutaneous inflammatory disorders may show erythroderma as well [5]. In fact, the differential diagnosis of erythroderma is considered one of the most vexing problems in dermatology and dermatopathology, and in some cases only a descriptive diagnosis is used ("homme rouge," "red man syndrome"). Erythrodermic mycosis fun-goides should be distinguished from true Sézary syndrome (see Chapter 2) [1].

One of the major problems in Sézary syndrome is that vari-able diagnostic criteria have been used in different studies which hinders comparison of clinicopathologic and prog-nostic data. The demonstration of a monoclonal population of T lymphocytes within the peripheral blood by molecular or cytogenetic methods has been proposed by the European Organization for Research and Treatment of Cancer (EORTC)-Cutaneous Lymphoma Study Group, by the International Society for Cutaneous Lymphomas (ISCL) and by others as an important criterion for the diagnosis of Sézary syndrome [1,6–10], and is particularly important if the same T-cell clone is also detected in the skin[1]. Other useful criteria include the presence of at least 1000 circulating Sézary cells/mm^3, an expanded CD4$^+$ population in the peripheral blood, resulting in a markedly increased CD4$^+$:CD8$^+$ ratio (>10), an increased population of CD4$^+$/CD7$^-$ cells in the peripheral blood, Sézary cells larger than 14 μm in diameter, Sézary cells representing more than 20% of circulating lymphocytes, and the loss of T-cell antigens such as CD2, CD3, CD4, and CD5 [1,2,10,11].

Although Sézary syndrome is regarded as the leukemic variant of cutaneous T-cell lymphoma, involvement of the

bone marrow is rare in the early phases but may be found at a later stage [12]. The exact relation to mycosis fungoides is unclear although some authors consider the two diseases as variations of the same entity (see also Chapter 2). In fact, in 1975 the term "cutaneous T-cell lymphoma" was introduced to encompass mycosis fungoides, Sézary syndrome and related disorders [3]. The World Health Organization (WHO)-EORTC and WHO 2008 classifications list mycosis fungoides and Sézary syndrome as separate entities [1,13]. In this context, it should be mentioned that in many studies, particularly those con-ducted in the United States, mycosis fungoides and Sézary syndrome have been lumped together into a single group ("cutaneous T-cell lymphoma"), thus hindering precise ana-lysis of the data. This problem concerns diagnostic as well as therapeutic studies.

Patients with Sézary syndrome usually present with an abrupt onset of erythroderma or with erythroderma pre-ceded by itching and a non-specific skin rash. Rarely, a classic Sézary syndrome may develop in patients with preceding mycosis fungoides (see erythrodermic mycosis fungoides in Chapter 2). In the WHO-EORTC classification patients with a previous history of mycosis fungoides developing erythro-derma during the course of the disease are not classified as Sézary syndrome [1], but others have suggested classifica-tion of these cases as "Sézary syndrome preceded by mycosis fungoides" as it remains unclear whether the clinical features and prognosis are similar [10]. The presence of neoplastic T cells within the peripheral blood alone should not prompt a diagnosis of Sézary syndrome unless all other main diag-nostic criteria are met [10]; in fact, detection in the peripheral blood of a T-cell clone without clinical significance is not infrequent in elderly patients.

The etiology of Sézary syndrome is unknown. One case with a complex p53 gene mutation has been observed in a Chernobyl survivor, suggesting a possible relationship with environmental factors [14]. The association with viral infec-tions or previous long-standing dermatoses is unclear [15–17]. Much information on the neoplastic cells has been gathered by studies on tissue samples and cell lines. In most cases, so-called Sézary cells express a predominantly helper T cell type 2 (Th2) cytokine profile (characterized by expression of interleukin [IL]-4, IL-5 and IL-10). Several genetic aberrations as well as

Skin Lymphoma: The Illustrated Guide. By L. Cerroni, K. Gatter and H. Kerl.
Published 2009 Blackwell Publishing. ISBN: 978-1-4051-8554-7.

aberrant antigen, cytokine or molecular profiles have been documented in patients with Sézary syndrome, but the diagnostic and therapeutic implications of these findings are still unclear [18–32].

The TNM staging classification used for mycosis fungoides has also been adopted for Sézary syndrome. According to this system, Sézary syndrome is classified as stage III by definition (see Chapter 2). In the new ISCL staging system, depending on the tumor burden in the peripheral blood, cases are classified in stage III (B_1: low blood tumor burden, >5% of peripheral blood lymphocytes are atypical cells but do not meet the criteria of B_2; B_{1a}: clone negative; B_{1b}: clone positive;) or IV (B_2: high blood tumor burden, ≥1000/μL Sézary cells with positive clone) (see Chapter 2).

Similarly to mycosis fungoides, patients with Sézary syndrome have an increased risk of developing secondary malignancies [33,34].

Clinical features

Sézary syndrome is a rare malignant T-cell lymphoma affecting elderly adults of both sexes, with a predilection for males. "Non-specific" skin lesions (eczematous patches) may be present for some time before erythroderma develops. The erythroderma is characterized by intense pruritus and scaling (Fig. 3.1). Common clinical signs are the marked hyperker-

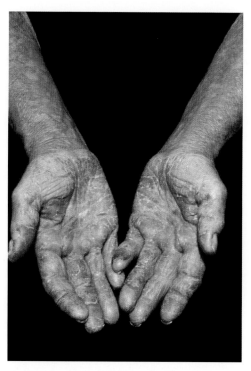

Figure 3.2 Sézary syndrome. Hyperkeratosis of the palms.

atosis of the palms and soles, alopecia, and onychodystrophy (Fig. 3.2). Large skin folds (groins, axillae) may be spared. Histopathologic analysis of peripheral lymph nodes usually shows evidence of involvement, but differentiation from

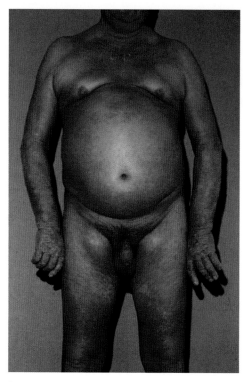

Figure 3.1 Sézary syndrome. Erythroderma. Note enlarged inguinal lymph nodes.

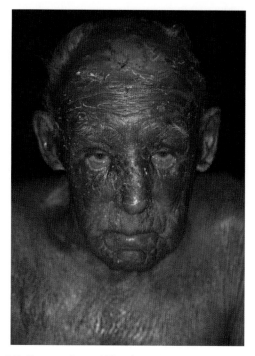

Figure 3.3 Sézary syndrome. Diffuse hyperpigmentation on the background of erythroderma ("melanoerythroderma"). Note ectropion.

so-called "dermatopathic lymphadenopathy" may be very difficult. As in mycosis fungoides, Sézary syndrome may be associated with follicular mucinosis [35,36]. Other clinical variants include the presence of diffuse hyperpigmentation as a consequence of melanosis or hemosiderosis (melanoerythroderma) (Fig. 3.3), and of vesiculobullous lesions. Analysis of peripheral blood may reveal features that have been considered helpful for the diagnosis of Sézary syndrome, such as the presence of a clonal population of CD4+/CD26− T lymphocytes [37–39], positivity for CD27 in the CD4+/CD26− T-cell population [40], presence of a CD158k+ clonal T-cell population [41], and paucity of forkhead box protein P3 (FOX-P3)+ circulating cells [42].

In some patients, prominent sensitivity may simulate the picture of actinic reticuloid and be the source of a giagnostic pitfall. In this context, as we mentioned before differential diagnosis of erythoderma is one of the most vexing fields of both dermatology and dermatopathology, and often only follow-up data allow a precise diagnosis to be made. Besides cutaneous and extracutaneous lymphomas (erythodermic mycosis fungoides, Sézary syndrome, other rare lymphomas), many inflammatory conditions may be responsible for the onset of erythoderma. The most frequent are psoriasis, atopic dermatitis, drug eruptions, and pityriasis rubra pilaris, but other diseases may be involved as well.

Histopathology, immunophenotype and molecular genetics

Histopathology

The histopathologic features of skin lesions in Sézary syndrome are indistinguishable from those of mycosis fungoides [43–45]. However, the features may be more subtle and difficult to interpret. Often there is a psoriasiform spongiotic pattern with a variably dense band-like infiltrate of lymphocytes (Fig. 3.4). Epidermotropism is usually less marked than in mycosis fungoides [46], but typical Darier's nests (Pautrier's

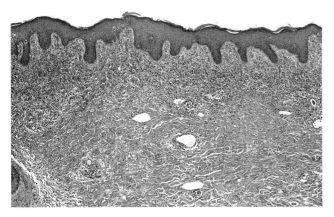

Figure 3.4 Sézary syndrome. Dense band-like infiltrate of lymphocytes within the superficial dermis. Note psoriasiform hyperplasia of the epidermis.

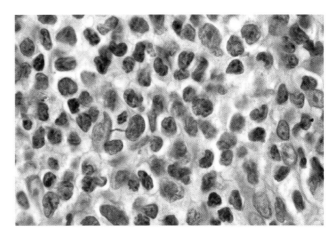

Figure 3.5 Sézary syndrome. Neoplastic cells are small- to medium-sized pleomorphic ("cerebriform") cells identical to those observed in mycosis fungoides.

microabscesses) may be observed. Cytomorphology reveals a predominance of small- to medium-sized pleomorphic (cerebriform) lymphocytes, often referred to as "Sézary cells" (Fig. 3.5). Differential diagnosis from mycosis fungoides can be achieved only by correlation of histopathologic features with clinical ones.

Histopathologic variants of Sézary syndrome include the presence of a prominent granulomatous reaction, deposition of mucin within hair follicles (follicular mucinosis), or large cell transformation [36,47–53]. Large cell transformation may be detected in skin lesions, lymph nodes or both, and is indistinguishable from that occurring in advanced mycosis fungoides (see Chapter 2).

In some cases the lymph nodes are characterized by monotonous infiltrates of neoplastic cells. Histopathologic differences from lymph nodes involved by cells of mycosis fungoides, suggesting a pathogenetic difference between the two diseases, have been described in one study [54].

Immunophenotype

Immunohistology reveals a predominance of T-helper lymphocytes (CD3+, CD4+, CD7−, CD8−). The findings are indistinguishable from those observed in mycosis fungoides. A recent study revealed a different expression of the multiple myeloma oncogene 1 (MUM-1) in neoplastic cells of Sézary syndrome (positive) and mycosis fungoides (negative), suggesting a potential value of this marker for differentiation between the two entities [55]. However, the number of cases included was very small, and these results should not be overemphasized.

Molecular genetics

Molecular genetic studies show clonal rearrangement of the T-cell receptor (TCR) genes in skin lesions in the majority of cases, but clonality may not be detected in the early stages. Amplification and overexpression of *JUNB* have been observed in some patients in two studies [56,57], and dysregulation of

JUNB and *JUND* in a third one [58]. A panel of eight genes that can distinguish Sézary syndrome in patients with low numbers of circulating cells has been detected by cDNA microarray technique [57]. In another study, copy number losses at 1p36p22, 6q24, and 15q11.2, as well as gains at 22q11.2q13.3, were capable of separating cases of Sézary syndrome from controls [59]. However, the number of cases studied was very limited.

Using quantitative polymerase chain reaction (PCR) analyses, gain of *cMYC* and loss of *cMYC* antagonists (*MXI1* and *MNT*) were observed in the majority of patients with Sézary syndrome, as well as alterations of the interleukin 2 (IL-2) pathway characterized by gain of STAT3/STAT5 and IL-2 (receptor) genes [60].

Although conventional immunohistochemical stainings for CD158k did not allow separation of neoplastic from reactive cases, mRNA expression of CD158k/KIR3DR2 detected by real-time reverse transcription PCR was significantly higher in lesional skin of Sézary syndrome than in reactive erythrodermic conditions, suggesting that detection of CD158k/KIR3DR2 transcripts may represent a molecular tool for the diagnosis of Sézary syndrome [61].

Support to the concept of biologic differences between mycosis fungoides and Sézary syndrome, and thus need for separate classification of the two entities, has been recently provided by oncogenomic analyses that showed major differences between the two diseases [62].

Treatment

The therapy of Sézary syndrome remains unsatisfactory. Patients may benefit from total body electron beam therapy, psoralen and UV-A (PUVA) (alone or associated with bexarotene, interferon-α or both) or chlorambucil combined with prednisone (Winkelmann scheme) [1,63–67]. Complete responses have been observed in several patients after extracorporeal photochemotherapy but recurrence is the rule, and the efficacy has been debated [68–72].

Guidelines for the use of extracorporeal photopheresis have been published recently [73]. Changes in the treatment protocols do not seem to alter the efficacy profile of this type of treatment [74]. An overall response rate of 62.5% (complete response 18.8%, partial response 43.7%) has been observed with pentostatin therapy in one study [75]. Total skin electron beam therapy was associated with improvement of tumor burden in the peripheral blood in a recent study [76].

Patients with cutaneous tumors and/or large cell transformation should be treated with systemic chemotherapy or other aggressive treatment modalities, similar to those used for advanced mycosis fungoides (see also Chapter 2).

As for mycosis fungoides, during the years many new compounds and new modalities have been introduced for the treatment of patients with Sézary syndrome, including IL-2, bone marrow transplantation, new retinoids such as bexarotene, and new immunomodulatory and chemotherapeutic agents as well as monoclonal antibodies, amongst others (see also Chapter 2) [77–86]. The association of extracorporeal photopheresis with other treatments has also been tested in a limited number of patients [87,88]. No single treatment modality revealed clear-cut benefits in comparison to the others, and the management of these patients is still extremely problematic. In addition, rapid progression of the disease and/or large cell transformation has been observed sometimes in patients treated with new therapeutic agents, particularly immunomodulatory drugs (see also Chapter 2). [89,90].

Prognosis

Overall survival of patients with Sézary syndrome depends on the criteria adopted for the diagnosis of the disease, and the 5-year survival varies between 11% and almost 50% in different studies, thus clearly showing that different criteria for diagnosis and classification are used in different centers. The disease-specific 5-year survival of 52 patients included in the Dutch and Austrian registries was 24% [1]. In this context, it should be underlined that patients with erythroderma, even if the cause is not Sézary syndrome or mycosis fungoides (non-neoplastic erythroderma), show a decreased survival [5]. If strict criteria are employed (i.e. presence of a neoplastic clone in the peripheral blood, CD4$^+$:CD8$^+$ ratio >10), the 5-year survival is poor [1]. The prognostic validity of B_1 and B_2 categories of peripheral blood involvement according to the ISCL staging system was confirmed in one study [91]. The presence of an identical clone in the skin and peripheral blood seems to be an independent prognostic criterion pointing to a worse prognosis [12,92]. Stage at diagnosis, failure to undergo remission after first treatment, age, and race also have prognostic value [93]. Other factors associated with reduced survival include elevated LDH and β_2-microglobulin serum levels, presence of an elevated tumor burden in the peripheral blood, advanced age at diagnosis, prior exposure to multiple systemic drugs, enlargement of peripheral lymph nodes (>3 cm), high blood tumor burden (CD4:CD8 ratio ≥10), chromosomally abnormal clone, and twofold increase in serum LDH level [94–96]. The number of circulating Sézary cells may predict the response to treatment, with higher counts showing better responses. The presence of Epstein–Barr virus (EBV) genome in keratinocytes was found to worsen the prognosis in one study [97].

A panel of 10 genes that can identify a group of patients with survival shorter than 6 months has been identified by cDNA microarray technique [46]. The expression of FOX-P3 by circulating Sézary cells has been related to a worse prognosis [98]. However, these results must be verified by larger studies.

Résumé	
Clinical	Elderly adults. Pruritic erythroderma, generalized lymphadenopathy and circulating Sézary cells. Strict diagnostic criteria include presence of a neoplastic clone and a CD4$^+$:CD8$^+$ ratio >10 in the peripheral blood.
	Usually aggressive course (5-year survival of about 25%).
Morphology	Small pleomorphic (cerebriform) cells. During the course of the disease there may be the appearance of tumors with large cell morphology (immunoblasts, large cell anaplastic, large cell pleomorphic).
Immunology	CD2, 3, 4, 5 +
	CD7, 8, 26 −
Genetics	Monoclonal rearrangement of the TCR gene may be absent in early phases. cDNA microarray studies revealed a class of genes that is altered in Sézary syndrome. Prominent aberrations involving genes encoding cMYC, cMYC regulating proteins, mediators of MYC-induced apoptosis, and IL-2 signaling pathway components.
Treatment guidelines	PUVA, interferon-α, retinoids (alone or in combination); extracorporeal photopheresis; radiotherapy; chlorambucil combined with prednisone (Winkelmann scheme); systemic chemotherapy. *Experimental:* new chemotherapeutic agents, pentostatin, bone marrow transplantation, new monoclonal antibodies.

TEACHING CASE

This 86-year-old man had erythroderma and marked pruritus for the last 6 years. Clinical examination revealed erythroderma and many erosions due to vigorous scratching (Fig. 3.6a). Three biopsy specimens revealed features consistent with a diagnosis of mycosis fungoides/Sézary syndrome. The patient had >10% circulating Sézary cells and a CD4:CD8 ratio of >10, and a diagnosis of Sézary syndrome was made. The bone marrow biopsy revealed infiltration by neoplastic T cells. A lesion diagnosed clinically as suspect tumor-stage Sézary syndrome was biopsied and revealed a well-differentiated, superficial squamous cell carcinoma (Fig. 3.6b, c) infiltrated by cells of the Sézary syndrome (Fig. 3.6d).

Comment: This case illustrates well the difficulties in distinguishing erythrodermic mycosis fungoides from Sézary syndrome, and the overlapping histopathologic features of these two variants of the cutaneous T-cell lymphomas. It also shows that in patients with leukemic stage of cutaneous (or extracutaneous) lymphoma, it is not uncommon to find specific cells of the hematologic neoplasm infiltrating epithelial tumors or at sites of cutaneous inflammation.

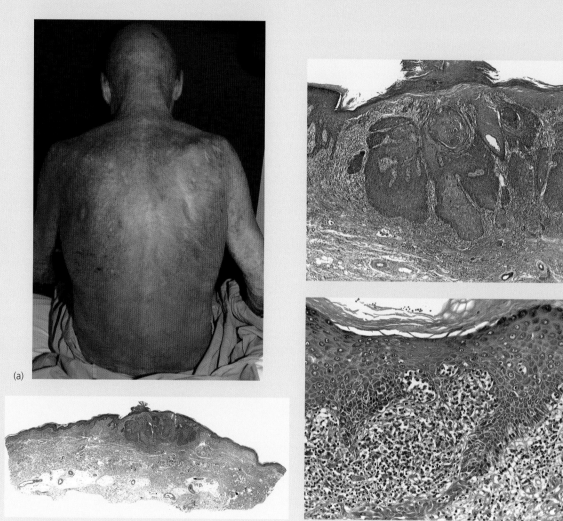

(a)

(b)

(c)

(d)

Figure 3.6

References

1. Willemze R, Jaffe ES, Burg G et al. WHO-EORTC classification for cutaneous lymphomas. *Blood* 2005;**105**:3768–3785.

2. Hwang ST, Janik JE, Jaffe ES, Wilson WH. Mycosis fungoides and Sézary syndrome. *Lancet* 2008;**371**:945–957.

3. Edelson RL. Cutaneous T cell lymphoma: the Sézary syndrome, mycosis fungoides, and related disorders (NIH Conference). *Ann Intern Med* 1975;**83**:534–552.

4. Kerl H. Das Sézary Syndrom. *Zbl Haut Geschl* 1981;**144**:359–380.

5. Sigurdsson V, Toonstra J, Hezemans-Boer M, van Vloten WA. Erythroderma: a clinical and follow-up study of 102 patients, with special emphasis on survival. *J Am Acad Dermatol* 1996;**35**:53–57.

6. Cherny S, Mraz S, Su L, Harvell J, Kohler S. Heteroduplex analysis of T-cell receptor γ gene rearrangement as an adjuvant diagnostic tool in skin biopsies for erythroderma. *J Cutan Pathol* 2001;**28**:351–355.

7. Delfau-Larue MH, Laroche L, Wechsler J et al. Diagnostic value of dominant T-cell clones in peripheral blood in 363 patients presenting consecutively with a suspicion of cutaneous lymphoma. *Blood* 2000;**96**:2987–2992.

8. Fraser-Andrews EA, Russell-Jones R, Woolford AJ et al. Diagnostic and prognostic importance of T-cell receptor gene analysis in patients with Sézary syndrome. *Cancer* 2001;**92**:1745–1752.

9. Russell-Jones R, Whittaker S. T-cell receptor gene analysis in the diagnosis of Sézary syndrome. *J Am Acad Dermatol* 1999;**41**:254–259.

10. Vonderheid EC, Bernengo MG, Burg G et al. Update on erythrodermic cutaneous T-cell lymphoma: report of the International Society for Cutaneous Lymphomas. *J Am Acad Dermatol* 2002;**46**:95–106.

11. Vonderheid EC, Bigler RD, Kotecha A et al. Variable CD7 expression on T cells in the leukemic phase of cutaneous T cell lymphoma (Sézary syndrome). *J Invest Dermatol* 2001;**117**:654–662.

12. Sibaud V, Beylot-Barry M, Thiebaut R et al. Bone marrow histopathologic and molecular staging in epidermotropic T-cell lymphoma. *Am J Clin Pathol* 2003;**119**:414–423.

13. Ralfkiaer E, Willemze R, Whittaker SJ. Sezary syndrome. In: Swerdlow SH, Campo E, Harris NL et al., eds. *WHO Classification of Tumours of Haematopoietic and Lymphoid Tissues.* Lyon: IARC Press, 2008: 299.

14. Fraser-Andrews E, McGregor JM, Crook T et al. Sézary syndrome with a complex, frameshift *p53* gene mutation in a Chernobyl survivor. *Clin Dermatol* 2001;**26**:683–685.

15. Herne KL, Talpur R, Breuer-McHam J, Champlin R, Duvic M. Cytomegalovirus seropositivity is significantly associated with mycosis fungoides and Sézary syndrome. *Blood* 2003;**101**:2132–2135.

16. Bazarbachi A, Soriano V, Pawson R et al. Mycosis fungoides and Sézary syndrome are not associated with HTLV-I infection: an international study. *Br J Haematol* 1997;**98**:927–933.

17. van Haselen CW, Toonstra J, Preesman AH et al. Sézary syndrome in a young man with severe atopic dermatitis. *Br J Dermatol* 1999;**140**:704–707.

18. Bernengo MG, Novelli M, Quaglino P et al. The relevance of the CD4 CD26 subset in the identification of circulating Sézary cells. *Br J Dermatol* 2001;**144**:125–135.

19. Ferenczi K, Fuhlbrigge RC, Pinkus JL, Pinkus GS, Kupper TS. Increased CCR4 expression in cutaneous T cell lymphoma. *J Invest Dermatol* 2002;**119**:1405–1410.

20. Hwang ST, Fitzhugh DJ. Aberrant expression of adhesion molecules by Sézary cells: functional consequences under physiologic shear stress conditions. *J Invest Dermatol* 2001;**116**:466–470.

21. Karenko L, Nevala H, Raatikainen M, Franssila K, Ranki A. Chromosomally clonal T cells in the skin, blood, or lymph nodes of two Sézary syndrome patients express CD45RA, CD45RO, CDw150, and interleukin-4, but no interleukin-2 or interferon-γ. *J Invest Dermatol* 2001;**116**:188–193.

22. Karenko L, Sarna S, Kähkönen M, Ranki A. Chromosomal abnormalities in relation to clinical disease in patients with cutaneous T-cell lymphoma: a 5-year follow-up study. *Br J Dermatol* 2003;**148**:55–64.

23. Leroy S, Dubois S, Tenaud I et al. Interleukin-15 expression in cutaneous T-cell lymphoma (mycosis fungoides and Sézary syndrome). *Br J Dermatol* 2001;**144**:1016–1021.

24. Mao X, Lillington D, Scarisbrick JJ et al. Molecular cytogenetic analysis of cutaneous T-cell lymphomas: identification of common genetic alterations in Sézary syndrome and mycosis fungoides. *Br J Dermatol* 2002;**147**:464–475.

25. Papadavid E, Economidou J, Psarra A et al. The relevance of peripheral blood T-helper 1 and 2 cytokine pattern in the evaluation of patients with mycosis fungoides and Sézary syndrome. *Br J Dermatol* 2003;**148**:709–718.

26. Qin JZ, Dummer R, Burg G, Döbbeling U. Constitutive and interleukin-7/interleukin-15 stimulated DNA binding of Myc, Jun, and novel Myc-like proteins in cutaneous T-cell lymphoma cells. *Blood* 1999;**93**:260–267.

27. Scarisbrick JJ, Woolford AJ, Calonje E et al. Frequent abnormalities of the *p15* and *p16* genes in mycosis fungoides and Sézary syndrome. *J Invest Dermatol* 2002;**118**:493–499.

28. Scarisbrick JJ, Woolford AJ, Russell-Jones R, Whittaker SJ. Allelotyping in mycosis fungoides and Sézary syndrome: common regions of allelic loss identified on 9p, 10q, and 17p. *J Invest Dermatol* 2001;**117**:663–670.

29. Wysocka M, Zaki MH, French LE et al. Sézary syndrome patients demonstrate a defect in dendritic cell populations: effects of CD40 ligand and treatment with GM-CSF on dendritic cell numbers and the production of cytokines. *Blood* 2002;**100**:3287–3294.

30. Zaki MH, Shane RB, Geng Y et al. Dysregulation of lymphocyte interleukin-12 receptor expression in Sézary syndrome. *J Invest Dermatol* 2001;**117**:119–127.

31. Brender C, Nielsen M, Kaltoft K et al. STAT3-mediated constitutive expression of SOCS-3 in cutaneous T-cell lymphoma. *Blood* 2001;**97**:1056–1062.

32. Magazin M, Poszepczynska-Guigne E, Bagot M et al. Sezary syndrome cells unlike normal circulating T lymphocytes fail to migrate following engagement of NT1 receptor. *J Invest Dermatol* 2004;**122**:111–118.

33. Väkevä L, Pukkala E, Ranki A. Increased risk of secondary cancers in patients with primary cutaneous T cell lymphoma. *J Invest Dermatol* 2000;**115**:62–65.

34. Scarisbrick JJ, Child FJ, Evans AV, Fraser-Andrews E, Spittle M, Russell-Jones R. Secondary malignant neoplasms in 71 patients with Sézary syndrome. *Arch Dermatol* 1999;**135**:1381–1385.

35. Cerroni L, Fink-Puches R, Bäck B, Kerl H. Follicular mucinosis. A critical reappraisal of clinicopathologic features and association with mycosis fungoides and Sézary syndrome. *Arch Dermatol* 2002;**138**:182–189.

36. Gerami P, Guitart J. Folliculotropic Sézary syndrome: a new variant of cutaneous T-cell lymphoma. *Br J Dermatol* 2007;**156**: 781–783.

37. Introcaso CE, Hess SD, Kamoun M, Ubriani R, Gelfand JM, Rook AH. Association of change in clinical status and change in the percentage of the CD4+ CD26– lymphocyte population in patients with Sézary syndrome. *J Am Acad Dermatol* 2005;**53**:428–434.

38. Kelemen K, Guitart J, Kuzel TM, Goolsby CL, Peterson LC. The usefulness of CD26 in flow cytometric analysis of peripheral blood in Sézary syndrome. *Am J Clin Pathol* 2008;**129**:146–156.

39. Sokolowska-Wojdylo M, Wenzel J, Gaffal E *et al.* Circulating clonal CLA+ and CD4+ T cells in Sezary syndrome express the skin-homing chemokine receptors CCR4 and CCR10 as well as the lymph node-homing chemokine receptor CCR7. *Br J Dermatol* 2005;**152**:258–264.

40. Fierro MT, Novelli M, Quaglino P *et al.* Heterogeneity of circulating CD4+ memory T-cell subsets in erythrodermic patients: CD27 analysis can help to distinguish cutaneous T-cell lymphomas from inflammatory erythrodermas. *Dermatology* 2008;**216**:213–221.

41. Ortonne N, Huet D, Gaudez C *et al.* Significance of circulating T-cell clones in Sézary syndrome. *Blood* 2006;**107**:4030–4038.

42. Klemke CD, Fritzsching B, Franz B *et al.* Paucity of FOXP3+ cells in skin and peripheral blood distinguishes Sezary syndrome from other cutaneous T-cell lymphomas. *Leukemia* 2006;**20**:1123–1129.

43. Kohler S, Kim YH, Smoller BR. Histologic criteria for the diagnosis of erythrodermic mycosis fungoides and Sézary syndrome: a critical reappraisal. *J Cutan Pathol* 1997;**24**:292–297.

44. Trotter MJ, Whittaker SJ, Orchard GE, Smith NP. Cutaneous histopathology of Sézary syndrome: a study of 41 cases with a proven circulating T-cell clone. *J Cutan Pathol* 1997;**24**:286–291.

45. Walsh NMG, Prokopetz R, Tron VA *et al.* Histopathology in erythroderma: review of a series of cases by multiple observers. *J Cutan Pathol* 1994;**21**:419–423.

46. Diwan AH, Prieto VG, Herling M, Duvic M, Jones D. Primary Sézary syndrome commonly shows low-grade cytologic atypia and an absence of epidermotropism. *Am J Clin Pathol* 2005;**123**: 510–515.

47. Cerroni L, Rieger E, Hödl S, Kerl H. Clinicopathologic and immunologic features associated with transformation of mycosis fungoides to large-cell lymphoma. *Am J Surg Pathol* 1992;**16**: 543–552.

48. Diamandidou E, Colome-Grimmer MI, Fayad L, Duvic M, Kurzrock R. Transformation of mycosis fungoides/Sézary syndrome: clinical characteristics and prognosis. *Blood* 1998;**92**: 1150–1159.

49. Carrozza PM, Kempf W, Kazakov DV, Dummer R, Burg G. A case of Sézary's syndrome associated with granulomatous lesions, myelodysplastic syndrome and transformation into CD30-positive large-cell pleomorphic lymphoma. *Br J Dermatol* 2002;**147**:582–586.

50. Diamandidou E, Colome-Grimmer MI, Fayad L, Duvic M, Kurzrock R. Transformation of mycosis fungoides/Sézary syndrome: clinical characteristics and prognosis. *Blood* 1998;**92**:1150–1159.

51. Gregg PJ, Kantor GR, Telang GH, Lessin SR, Nowell PC, Vonderheid EC. Sarcoidal tissue reaction in Sezary syndrome. *J Am Acad Dermatol* 2000;**43**:372–376.

52. So CC, Wong KF, Siu LL, Kwong YL. Large cell transformation of Sezary syndrome. A conventional and molecular cytogenetic study. *Am J Clin Pathol* 2000;**113**:792–797.

53. Scarabello A, Leinweber B, Ardigó M *et al.* Cutaneous lymphomas with prominent granulomatous reaction. A potential pitfall in the histopathologic diagnosis of cutaneous T- and B-cell lymphomas. *Am J Surg Pathol* 2002;**26**:1259–1268.

54. Scheffer E, Meijer CJLM, Willemze R, van Vloten WA. Lymph node histopathology in mycosis fungoides and Sezary's syndrome. In: van Vloten W, Willemze R, Lange Vejlsgaard G, Thomsen K, eds. *Cutaneous Lymphomas and Pseudolymphomas.* Basel: Karger, 1990: 105–113.

55. Wasco MJ, Fullen D, Su L, Ma L. The expression of MUM1 in cutaneous T-cell lymphoproliferative disorders. *Hum Pathol* 2008;**39**:557–563.

56. Mao X, Orchard G, Lillington DM, Russell-Jones R, Young BD, Whittaker SJ. Amplification and overexpression of JUNB is associated with primary cutaneous T-cell lymphomas. *Blood* 2003; **101**:1513–1519.

57. Kari L, Loboda A, Nebozhyn M *et al.* Classification and prediction of survival in patients with the leukemic phase of cutaneous T cell lymphoma. *J Exp Med* 2003;**197**:1477–1488.

58. Mao X, Orchard G, Mitchell TJ *et al.* A genomic and expression study of AP-1 in primary cutaneous T-cell lymphoma: evidence for dysregulated expression of JUNB and JUND in MF and SS. *J Cutan Pathol* 2008;**35**:899–910.

59. Mao X, McElwaine S. Functional copy number changes in Sezary syndrome: toward an integrated molecular cytogenetic map III. *Cancer Genet Cytogenet* 2008;**185**:86–94.

60. Vermeer MH, van Doorn R, Dijkman R *et al.* Novel and highly recurrent chromosomal alterations in Sézary syndrome. *Cancer Res* 2008;**68**:2689–2698.

61. Ortonne N, Le Gouvello S, Mansour H *et al.* CD158K/KIR3DL2 transcript detection in lesional skin of patients with erythroderma is a tool for the diagnosis of Sézary syndrome. *J Invest Dermatol* 2008;**128**:465–472.

62. van Doorn R, van Kester MS, Dijkman R *et al.* Oncogenomic analysis of mycosis fungoides reveals major differences with Sézary syndrome. *Blood* 2009;**113**:127–136.

63. Apisarnthanarax N, Talpur R, Duvic M. Treatment of cutaneous T cell lymphoma. Current status and future directions. *Am J Clin Dermatol* 2002;**3**:193–215.

64. Jones GW, Rosenthal D, Wilson LD. Total skin electron radiation for patients with erythrodermic cutaneous T-cell lymphoma (mycosis fungoides and the Sézary syndrome). *Cancer* 1999;**85**: 1985–1995.

65. Jumbou O, N'Guyen JM, Tessier MH, Legoux B, Dreno B. Long-term follow-up in 51 patients with mycosis fungoides and Sézary syndrome treated by interferon-alfa. *Br J Dermatol* 1999; **140**:427–431.

66. Wilson LD, Jones GW, Kim D *et al.* Experience with total skin electron beam therapy in combination with extracorporeal photopheresis in the management of patients with erythrodermic (T4) mycosis fungoides. *J Am Acad Dermatol* 2000;**43**:54–60.

67. Trautinger F, Knobler R, Willemze R *et al.* EORTC consensus recommendations for the treatment of mycosis fungoides/Sézary syndrome. *Eur J Cancer* 2006;**42**:1014–1030.

68. Heald P, Rook A, Perez M *et al.* Treatment of erythrodermic cutaneous T-cell lymphoma with extracorporeal photochemotherapy. *J Am Acad Dermatol* 1992;**27**:427–433

69. Edelson RL. Sézary syndrome, cutaneous T-cell lymphoma, and extracorporeal photopheresis. *Arch Dermatol* 1999;**135**:600–601.

70. Evans AV, Wood WP, Scarisbrick JJ *et al.* Extracorporeal photopheresis in Sézary syndrome: hematologic parameters as predictors of response. *Blood* 2001;**98**:1298–1301.

71. Fraser-Andrews E, Seed P, Whittaker S, Russell-Jones R. Extracorporeal photopheresis in Sézary syndrome. No significant effect in the survival of 44 patients with a peripheral blood T-cell clone. *Arch Dermatol* 1998;**134**:1001–1005.

72. Ferenczi K, Yawalkar N, Jones D, Kupper TS. Monitoring the decrease of circulating malignant T cells in cutaneous T-cell lymphoma during photopheresis and interferon therapy. *Arch Dermatol* 2003;**139**:909–913.

73. Scarisbrick JJ, Taylor P, Holtick U *et al.* U.K. consensus statement on the use of extracorporeal photopheresis for treatment of cutaneous T-cell lymphoma and chronic graft-versus-host disease. *Br J Dermatol* 2008;**158**:659–678.

74. Arulogun S, Prince HM, Gambell P *et al.* Extracorporeal photopheresis for the treatment of Sezary syndrome using a novel treatment protocol. *J Am Acad Dermatol* 2008;**59**:589–595.

75. Dearden C, Matutes E, Catovsky D. Pentostatin treatment of cutaneous T-cell lymphoma. *Oncology* 2000;**14**(suppl. 2):37–40.

76. Introcaso CE, Micaily B, Richardson SK *et al.* Total skin electron beam therapy may be associated with improvement of peripheral blood disease in Sézary syndrome. *J Am Acad Dermatol* 2008;**58**:592–595.

77. Foss FM. Activity of pentostatin (Nipent) in cutaneous T-cell lymphoma: single-agent and combination studies. *Sem Oncol* 2000;**27**(suppl 5):58–63.

78. Molina A, Nademanee A, Arber DA, Forman SJ. Remission of refractory Sezary syndrome after bone marrow tranplantation from a matched unrelated donor. *Biol Blood Marrow Transplant* 1999;**5**:400–404.

79. Sarris AH, Phan A, Duvic M *et al.* Trimetrexate in relapsed T-cell lymphoma with skin involvement. *J Clin Oncol* 2002;**20**:2876–2880.

80. Scarisbrick JJ, Child FJ, Clift A, Sabroe R, Whittaker SJ, Spittle M, Russell-Jones R. A trial of fludarabine and cyclophosphamide combination chemotherapy in the treatment of advanced refractory primary cutaneous T-cell lymphoma. *Br J Dermatol* 2001;**144**:1010–1015.

81. Shapiro M, Rook AH, Lehrer MS *et al.* Novel multimodality biologic response modifier therapy, including bexarotene and long-wave ultraviolet A for a patient with refractory stage IVa cutaneous T-cell lymphoma. *J Am Acad Dermatol* 2002;**47**:956–961.

82. Osborne GEN, Pagliuca A, Ho A, du Vivier AWP. Novel treatment of Sezary-like syndrome due to adult T-cell leukaemia/lymphoma with daclizumab (humanized anti-interleukin-2 receptor a antibody). *Br J Dermatol* 2006;**155**:617–620.

83. Bernengo MG, Quaglino P, Comessatti A *et al.* Low-dose intermittent alemtuzumab in the treatment of Sézary syndrome: clinical and immunologic findings in 14 patients. *Haematologica* 2007;**92**:784–794.

84. Querfeld C, Rosen ST, Guitart J *et al.* Phase II trial of subcutaneous injections of human recombinant interleukin-2 for the treatment of mycosis fungoides and Sézary syndrome. *J Am Acad Dermatol* 2007;**56**:580–583.

85. Rupoli S, Goteri G, Pimpinelli N *et al.* Pegylated liposomal doxorubicin in the treatment of primary cutaneous T-cell lymphomas. *Haematologica* 2007;**92**:686–689.

86. Kahata K, Hashino S, Takahata M, *et al.* Durable remission of Sézary syndrome after unrelated bone marrow transplantation by reduced-intensity conditioning. *Acta Haematol* 2008;**120**:14–18.

87. Fritz TM, Kleinhans M, Nestle FO, Burg G, Dummer R. Combination treatment with extracorporeal photopheresis, interferon alfa and interleukin-2 in a patient with the Sezary syndrome. *Br J Dermatol* 1999;**140**:1144–1147.

88. McGinnis KS, Ubriani R, Newton S, *et al.* The addition of interferon gamma to oral bexarotene therapy with photopheresis for Sézary syndrome. *Arch Dermatol* 2005;**141**:1176–1178.

89. Bouwhuis SA, Davis MDP, el-Azhary RA *et al.* Bexarotene treatment of late-stage mycosis fungoides and Sézary syndrome: development of extracutaneous lymphoma in 6 patients. *J Am Acad Dermatol* 2005;**52**:991–996.

90. Faguer S, Launay F, Ysebaert L *et al.* Acute cutaneous T-cell lymphoma transformation during treatment with alemtuzumab. *Br J Dermatol* 2007;**157**:841–842.

91. Vonderheid EC, Pena J, Nowell P. Sezary cell counts in erythrodermic cutaneous T-cell lymphoma: Implications for prognosis and staging. *Leukem Lymph* 2006;**47**:1841–1856.

92. Beylot-Barry M, Sibaud V, Thiebaut R *et al.* Evidence that an identical T cell clone in skin and peripheral blood lymphocytes is an independent prognostic factor in primary cutaneous T cell lymphoma. *J Invest Dermatol* 2001;**117**:920–926.

93. Kim YH, Liu HL, Mraz-Gernhard S, Varghese A, Hoppe RT. Long-term outcome of 525 patients with mycosis fungoides and Sézary syndrome. *Arch Dermatol* 2003;**139**:857–866.

94. Diamandidou E, Colome M, Fayad L, Duvic M, Kurzrock R. Prognostic factor analysis in mycosis fungoides/Sézary syndrome. *J Am Acad Dermatol* 1999;**40**:914–924.

95. Scarisbrick JJ, Whittaker S, Evans AV *et al.* Prognostic significance of tumor burden in the blood of patients with erythrodermic primary cutaneous T-cell lymphoma. *Blood* 2001;**97**:624–630.

96. Stevens SR, Baron ED, Masten S, Cooper KD. Circulating CD4+ CD7– lymphocyte burden and rapidity of response. Predictors of outcome in the treatment of Sézary syndrome and erythrodermic mycosis fungoides with extracorporeal photopheresis. *Arch Dermatol* 2002;**138**:1347–1350.

97. Foulc P, N'Guyen JM, Dreno B. Prognostic factors in Sézary syndrome: a study of 28 patients. *Br J Dermatol* 2003;**149**:1152–1158.

98. Capriotti E, Vonderheid EC, Thoburn CJ *et al.* Expression of T-plastin, FoxP3 and other tumor-associated markers by leukemic T-cells of cutaneous T-cell lymphoma. *Leuk Lymph* 2008;**49**:1190–1201.

4
Primary cutaneous CD30⁺ lymphoproliferative disorders

One of the changes made in the World Health Organization (WHO)-European Organization of Research and Treatment of Cancer (EORTC) classification of primary cutaneous lymphomas concerns lymphomatoid papulosis and cutaneous anaplastic CD30⁺ large cell lymphoma [1]. These two entities are now included in the group of the "CD30⁺ cutaneous lymphoproliferative disorders" as they represent two ends of a spectrum without clear-cut boundaries. This approach has been used in the new WHO classification of tumors of hematopoietic and lymphoid tissues as well [2].

The CD30 antigen is a cytokine receptor belonging to the tumor necrosis factor receptor superfamily. The antigen was initially described within Reed–Sternberg and Hodgkin cells of Hodgkin lymphoma, and subsequently identified within neoplastic cells of a new group of non-Hodgkin lymphomas (anaplastic large cell lymphoma) [3,4]. Soon after the first description, it become clear that anaplastic large cell lymphomas could occur as a primary skin tumor, where they were characterized by a good prognosis [5–10]. The term "cutaneous CD30⁺ lymphoproliferative disorders" has been subsequently proposed to denote a group of primary cutaneous T-cell lymphomas characterized by expression of the CD30 antigen phenotypically and a favorable prognosis biologically, including lymphomatoid papulosis and primary cutaneous anaplastic large cell lymphoma [11–16]. Cases described in the past as "regressing atypical histiocytosis" or "pseudo-Hodgkin disease" are part of the spectrum of primary cutaneous CD30⁺ lymphoproliferative disorders [17,18].

As already mentioned, it is important to emphasize that there is no clear-cut boundary between "classic" lymphomatoid papulosis and primary cutaneous anaplastic large cell lymphoma. The term "borderline lymphomatoid papulosis – anaplastic large cell lymphoma" has been used by some authors for cases where a definitive diagnosis is not possible based on clinicopathologic features. In this group are cases with the clinical aspect of lymphomatoid papulosis and the histopathology of primary cutaneous anaplastic large cell lymphoma and vice versa.

Skin Lymphoma: The Illustrated Guide. By L. Cerroni, K. Gatter and H. Kerl. Published 2009 Blackwell Publishing, ISBN: 978-1-4051-8554-7.

The typical features of cutaneous CD30⁺ lymphoproliferative disorders, including partial or complete spontaneous resolution of the lesions and good prognosis, have been the subject of several studies in an attempt to elucidate the reasons for this peculiar clinical behavior. It has been suggested that CD30 and CD30-ligand are involved in the control of apoptosis, and that activation of the CD30 signaling pathway plays a role in tumor regression [19–23]. Resistance to CD30-mediated growth inhibition provides a possible mechanism for escape from tumor regression in cases with more aggressive behavior. A higher expression of apoptotic-related proteins has been observed in lymphomatoid papulosis as compared to primary cutaneous anaplastic large cell lymphoma, suggesting that the apoptosis index may play a role in the spontaneous resolution of the lesions and better prognosis of lymphomatoid papulosis [24].

At this point, it should also be stressed that CD30 is a very important marker for diagnosis and classification of cutaneous lymphomas, but interpretation of the staining cannot be made without knowledge of full phenotypic features and complete clinical information. We have received in consultation cases of aggressive cytotoxic lymphomas or even B-cell lymphomas (not to mention the many pseudolymphomas) that were erroneously classified as cutaneous anaplastic large cell lymphoma because of CD30 positivity. These mistakes can have disastrous consequences for patients. Similar cases with incomplete phenotypic features and possibly erroneous diagnoses have been published in the literature [25]. In this context, we would like to stress that a diagnosis of lymphomatoid papulosis or cutaneous anaplastic large cell lymphoma should be made only upon compelling evidence, particularly in cases that present with clinical features not typical of these disorders.

LYMPHOMATOID PAPULOSIS

Lymphomatoid papulosis is defined as a chronic, recurrent, self-healing eruption of papules and small nodules with the histopathologic features of a cutaneous T-cell lymphoma ("rhythmic paradoxical eruption") [26].

Although in the past it has been classified among the cutaneous pseudolymphomas, lymphomatoid papulosis is considered today as a low-grade cutaneous T-cell lymphoma, and has been included as such in the WHO-EORTC classification of cutaneous lymphomas [1]. In the new WHO classification of tumors of hematopoietic and lymphoid tissues it is included in the spectrum of CD30⁺ cutaneous lymphoproliferative disorders; however, it is stated that "from a clinical perspective lymphomatoid papulosis is not considered a malignant disorder, despite demonstration of clonality in many cases" [2].

No specific genetic alterations, association with inflammatory skin disorders or viral infections have been consistently demonstrated in lymphomatoid papulosis, and the etiology of the disease is still unknown. No association with Epstein–Barr virus (EBV) infection has been found in a recent Korean study [27]. The interchromosomal (2;5) translocation is absent [28,29].

In 10–20% of patients lymphomatoid papulosis is preceded, concomitant with or followed by another type of lymphoma (usually mycosis fungoides, Hodgkin lymphoma and anaplastic large cell lymphoma, but other malignant hematologic disorders have also been observed) (see also Chapter 2) [30–40]. In some of these patients, the same clone of neoplastic T lymphocytes has been identified in lesions of lymphomatoid papulosis and those of the associated lymphomas, raising the question of a possible common origin of the diseases [41–44]. However, their response to treatment is different as the lesions of lymphomatoid papulosis may continue to appear while the second lymphoma is in complete remission [45]. In patients with mycosis fungoides, self-healing papules with CD30⁺ lymphoid infiltrates may develop during the course of the disease, suggesting a diagnosis of lymphomatoid papulosis associated with mycosis fungoides. In these patients it is of crucial importance to rule out large cell transformation of mycosis fungoides. In fact, one case that we published originally in 1991 as "PUVA-induced lymphomatoid papulosis in a patient with mycosis fungoides" [46] died with large cell transformation of mycosis fungoides 48 months after the onset of the "lymphomatoid papulosis." (See also Chapter 2).

In addition to these hematologic malignancies, patients with lymphomatoid papulosis are also at higher risk of developing non-lymphoid second malignancies [47].

In the absence of specific symptoms of other associated diseases, complete staging investigations are not necessary in patients with classic lymphomatoid papulosis. Some authors found T-cell clonality within the peripheral blood or the bone marrow in some patients, but the clinical and prognostic value of these findings is unclear [48,49]. However, a recent study revealed that in all cases of lymphomatoid papulosis and cutaneous anaplastic large cell lymphoma with a clonal T-cell population detected both in the blood and in the skin, the clones were different, thus demonstrating that they are not related [50].

Clinical features

Young adults are usually affected but the disease has been reported in children and in the elderly as well [32,33,51–56].

Clinically, lymphomatoid papulosis presents in most patients as a generalized eruption of reddish-brown papules or small nodules on the trunk and proximal extremities, but in some cases only a few lesions may be present (Figs 4.1–4.3). Oral

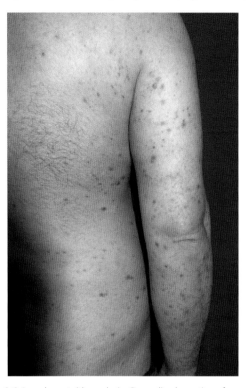

Figure 4.1 Lymphomatoid papulosis. Generalized eruption of papules and small nodules.

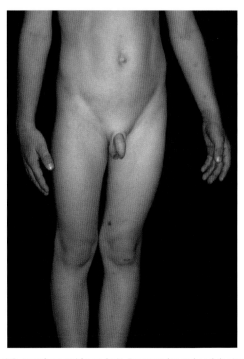

Figure 4.2 Lymphomatoid papulosis. Few papules and nodules in a 6-year-old child.

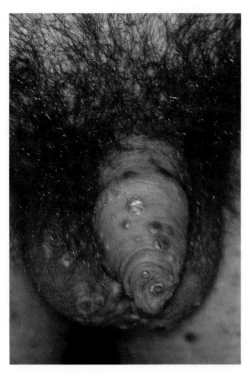

Figure 4.3 Lymphomatoid papulosis. Multiple papules and small nodules, some ulcerated, on the genital area.

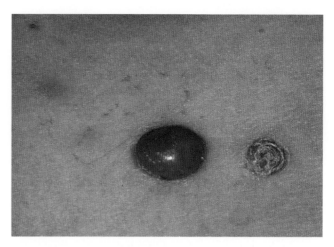

Figure 4.5 Lymphomatoid papulosis. Small erythematous nodule. Note a resolving lesion on the right side of the nodule.

or other mucosal involvement may be observed rarely [57–59]. The size of the lesions is variable but they are usually smaller than 1 cm. In a few patients large, rapidly growing nodules, sometimes with ulceration, may be the first manifestation of the disease (Fig. 4.4) [11]. The onset of large

tumors with complete spontaneous resolution has also been observed during the course of the disease but prognosis seems not to be affected and the disease runs the usual course, suggesting that large tumors may represent a morphologic variation of lymphomatoid papulosis rather than transformation into a more aggressive lymphoma [11].

The clinical picture is usually polymorphic, due to the presence of lesions in different stages of evolution (Fig. 4.5). Ulceration is common (Fig. 4.6). Spontaneous resolution is observed within a few weeks or, rarely, months. The time

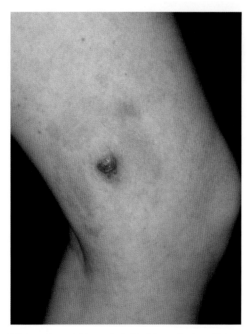

Figure 4.4 Lymphomatoid papulosis. Nodule on the leg with two small satellite papules at presentation of the disease. The patient then developed a "conventional" lymphomatoid papulosis.

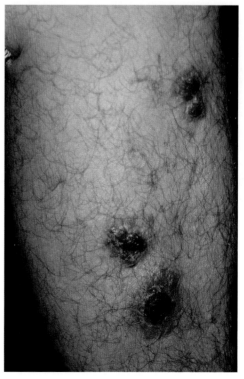

Figure 4.6 Lymphomatoid papulosis. Ulcerated erythematous nodules.

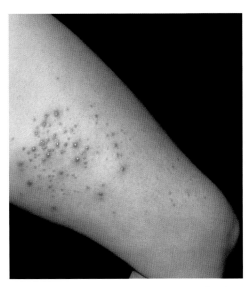

Figure 4.7 Regional lymphomatoid papulosis. Cluster of erythematous papules restricted to the median aspect of the left thigh.

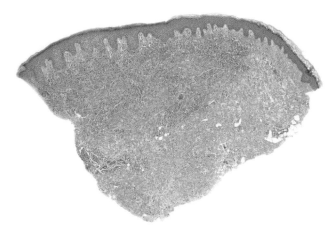

Figure 4.8 Lymphomatoid papulosis, type A. Wedge-shaped infiltrate in the dermis.

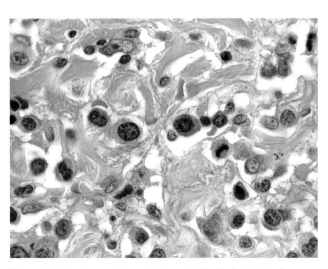

Figure 4.9 Lymphomatoid papulosis, type A. Detail of atypical cells.

interval between two episodes is variable: some patients may experience several eruptions within short periods of time, whereas others may have only a few lesions over several years.

Occasionally lesions of lymphomatoid papulosis are localized to just one area (regional lymphomatoid papulosis) (Fig. 4.7) [60–62]. Similar cases have been reported also as "persistent agmination" of lymphomatoid papulosis [63]. In these cases, differentiation from anaplastic large cell lymphoma can be extremely difficult, as this last can present with nodules surrounded by satellite lesions of smaller dimensions clinically simulating lymphomatoid papulosis. Association with pregnancy and with severe hypereosinophilic syndrome has also been reported [64,65]. Other unusual clinical variants of lymphomatoid papulosis include a type characterized by lesions clinically resembling hydroa vacciniforme, and one by presence of predominant pustular lesions [66,67].

Histopathology, immunophenotype and molecular genetics

Histopathology

The histopathologic features of lymphomatoid papulosis are variable. Three main histologic subtypes have been described. It is important to recognize that these variants can all be observed in one patient at the same time or during the course of the disease, and that the histopathologic picture is not associated with any prognostic implications. Sometimes, single lesions with features of different histological types have been referred to as lymphomatoid papulosis type A/B. We prefer to classify lesions into one of the following three groups according to the predominant histopathologic features.

Type A ("histiocytic" type)

This is the "conventional" and most frequent type of lymphomatoid papulosis, characterized by wedge-shaped lesions with the presence of scattered or clustered large atypical cells admixed with small lymphocytes, histiocytes, neutrophils and eosinophils (Figs 4.8, 4.9). Epidermotropism is variable.

Type B (mycosis fungoides-like)

This is a rare type of lymphomatoid papulosis that reveals a wedge-shaped or, more rarely, band-like infiltrate of small- to medium-sized pleomorphic (cerebriform) cells with epidermotropism (Figs 4.10, 4.11). It is crucial to understand that differentiation of lymphomatoid papulosis type B from mycosis fungoides can only be achieved by clinicopathologic correlation, and that a diagnosis of lymphomatoid papulosis type B should never be established without a complete clinical history.

Although large atypical cells are the hallmark of lymphomatoid papulosis, and the existence of a "small cell" variant

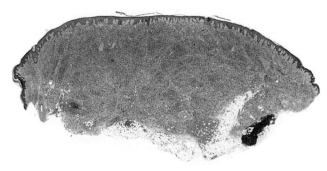

Figure 4.10 Lymphomatoid papulosis, type B. Wedge-shaped infiltrate of lymphocytes within the entire dermis. Note epidermotropism of solitary lymphocytes aligned along the basal layer.

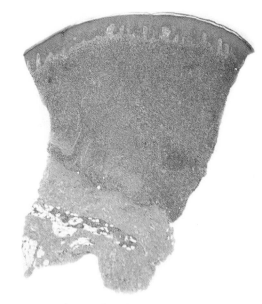

Figure 4.12 Lymphomatoid papulosis, type C. Dense infiltrate of atypical lymphocytes arranged in sheets.

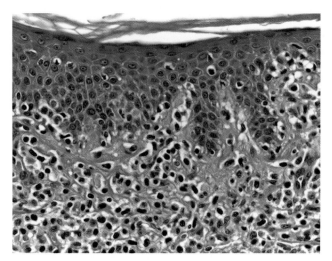

Figure 4.11 Lymphomatoid papulosis, type B. Note epidermotropism of solitary lymphocytes with small nuclei resembling the histopathologic features of mycosis fungoides.

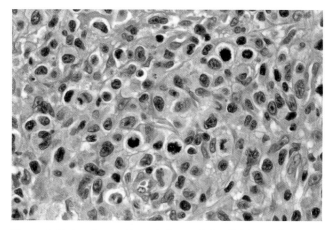

Figure 4.13 Lymphomatoid papulosis, type C. Detail of the atypical lymphocytes arranged in sheets, simulating the histopathologic features of anaplastic large cell lymphoma.

has been called into question, lymphomatoid papulosis type B composed of small- to medium-sized cells may be compared to the small/medium-cell variant of anaplastic large cell lymphoma (see later in this chapter), which is now a well-established morphologic subtype of that lymphoma.

We have recently observed several patients with a particular variant of type B lymphomatoid papulosis, characterized histopathologically by marked epidermotropism of CD8+ cytotoxic T lymphocytes within a hyperplastic epidermis, similar to what can be observed in pagetoid reticulosis. The clinical features in all patients were typical of lymphomatoid papulosis, but in most of these cases a first diagnosis of cutaneous aggressive epidermotropic CD8+ cytotoxic T-cell lymphoma was made due to the peculiar histopathologic presentation. An accurate clinicopathologic correlation in these cases is crucial.

Type C (anaplastic large cell lymphoma-like)
There is a nodular infiltrate characterized by sheets of cohesive, large atypical cells admixed with a few small lymphocytes, neutrophils, and eosinophils (Figs 4.12, 4.13). The histopatho-

logic features are indistinguishable from those of anaplastic large cell lymphoma, and a definitive diagnosis can be achieved only upon clinicopathologic correlation.

Other histologic variants
A variant of lymphomatoid papulosis characterized by lesions centered around a hair follicle has been termed "follicular lymphomatoid papulosis" (Fig. 4.14) [68–70]. Other unusual histopathologic findings in lymphomatoid papulosis include the presence of myxoid changes, eccrinotropic and neurotropic infiltrates, follicular mucinosis, and subepidermal blisters (Fig. 4.15) [32,71,72]. Rarely, angiocentricity and angiodestruction may be observed.

In some cases of lymphomatoid papulosis, a prominent acanthosis of the epidermis can be observed [73,74]. Rarely,

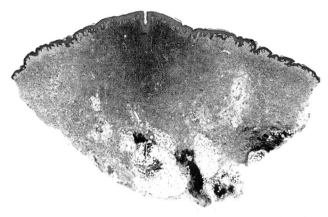

Figure 4.14 Follicular lymphomatoid papulosis. Note a wedge-shaped infiltrate disposed symmetrically around a hair follicle.

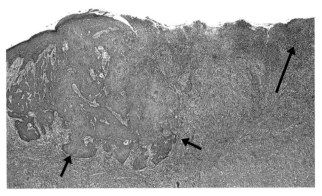

Figure 4.16 Lymphomatoid papulosis associated with multiple keratoacanthomas. The remnant of a keratoacanthoma is visible on the left side of this lesion (*short arrows*), whereas most atypical cells of the lymphomatoid papulosis are located on the right part of it (*long arrow*). The patient, a 79-year-old male, had concomitant typical lesions of keratoacanthoma without infiltrating CD30 atypical cells, as well as conventional lesions of lymphomatoid papulosis without epidermal hyperplasia.

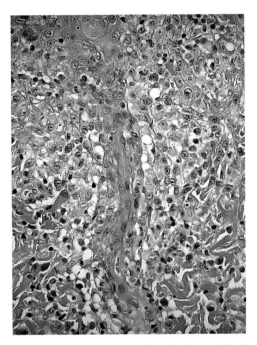

Figure 4.15 Syringotropic lymphomatoid papulosis. Atypical cells are disposed around an eccrine duct, in part infiltrating it.

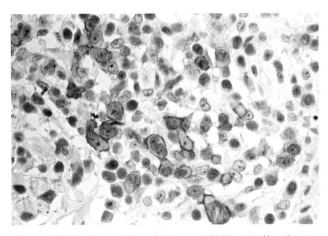

Figure 4.17 Lymphomatoid papulosis, type A. CD30 atypical lymphocytes disposed as solitary units and in small clusters.

the association with multiple keratoacanthomas has been documented (Fig. 4.16) [75]. In this context, it is interesting to note that in a recent study CD30⁺ cells could be observed in the inflammatory infiltrate of the vast majority of 21 randomly selected keratoacanthomas, suggesting that some of the cases reported as association of lymphomatoid papulosis and keratoacanthoma or as lymphomatoid papulosis with keratoacanthomatous changes may represent in truth keratoacanthomas with CD30⁺ cells [76].

Immunophenotype

The hallmark of lymphomatoid papulosis is the expression of CD30 by neoplastic cells (Fig. 4.17) [10,77–79]. Although the infiltrate of type B lymphomatoid papulosis has often been reported as being CD30⁻, most cases do in fact express the

antigen (Fig. 4.18) [32]. In this context, care should be taken to avoid misinterpreting the papular variant of mycosis fungoides as type B lymphomatoid papulosis (see also Chapter 2). CD30⁺ lymphocytes are often arranged in small clusters (type A) or in sheets (type C), a feature useful in the differential diagnosis of lymphomatoid papulosis from benign inflammatory skin diseases where CD30⁺ cells are usually (but not always!) scattered and isolated (however, this pattern can also be observed occasionally in cases of lymphomatoid papulosis).

Neoplastic cells express the phenotypic markers of T-helper lymphocytes (CD3⁺, CD4⁺, CD8⁻) in some cases, and of T cytotoxic cells (CD8⁺) in others [32,78–82]. Expression of CD56 is usually absent, but may be observed in some cases (Fig. 4.19) [32,83–86]. Pan-T-cell antigens may be lost, at least partially, in some cases.

The anaplastic lymphoma kinase (ALK) is not expressed [29,87]. Positivity for JunB was observed in a recent study in

71

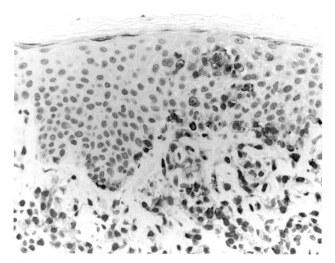

Figure 4.18 Lymphomatoid papulosis, type B. Intraepidermal lymphocytes positive for CD30.

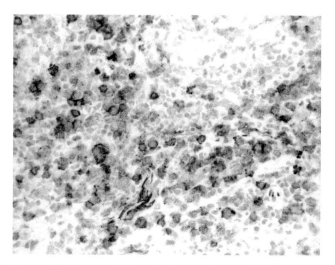

Figure 4.19 Lymphomatoid papulosis, type A. Large atypical lymphocytes positive for CD56.

all 18 cases of lymphomatoid papulosis tested [88], and c-Jun expression was observed in about 50% of tested cases [89]. Expression of fascin was found in a minority of cases [90], as well as of survivin and Bcl-2 [91]. It has been suggested that CD56 or fascin expression by neoplastic cells may be helpful in the distinction between lymphomatoid papulosis and anaplastic large cell lymphoma [90,92], but data on large series are lacking.

A recent report suggested that neoplastic cells in lymphomatoid papulosis are positive for the multiple myeloma oncogene 1 (MUM-1), whereas cells in anaplastic large cell lymphoma are negative [93]. Variability in MUM-1 staining of lymphomatoid papulosis and anaplastic large cell lymphoma, however, exists, and all cases of anaplastic large cell lymphoma were positive for MUM-1 in another study [94]. In our experience the value of this marker in the differential diagnosis between the two entities should not be overemphasized, and MUM-1 (or any other marker) expression cannot replace clinicopathologic correlation (the only valuable "tool" to distinguish lymphomatoid papulosis from cutaneous anaplastic large cell lymphoma).

Molecular genetics

There are no specific genetic abnormalities reported for lymphomatoid papulosis. Rearrangement of the T-cell receptor (TCR) is found in the majority of lesions [95]. Studies on single cells after microdissection of the specimens showed that the atypical CD30+ large cells have a common clonal origin [96].

Clinicopathologic differential diagnosis

Besides anaplastic large cell lymphoma, the differential diagnosis of lymphomatoid papulosis includes mainly papulonecrotic eruptions such as pityriasis lichenoides et varioliformis acuta (PLEVA). This distinction can be particularly difficult as overlapping clinicopathologic features can be seen. However, in the proper clinical background the presence of large atypical CD30+ cells is diagnostic of lymphomatoid papulosis. Cases reported as "pityriasis lichenoides et varioliformis with atypical CD30+ cells" [97,98] most likely represent examples of lymphomatoid papulosis [99].

Clusterin expression, originally thought to be specific for systemic anaplastic large cell lymphoma as opposed to cutaneous cases, was found in half of tested cases of lymphomatoid papulosis in a recent study, as well as in tumor cells of cutaneous anaplastic large cell lymphoma and CD30+ large cell transformation of mycosis fungoides, but only in a small minority of cases of reactive infiltrates with CD30+ cells, thus representing a potential tool in differential diagnosis of lymphomatoid papulosis from CD30+ pseudolymphomas [100]. As with all other small studies, however, these results, too, should not be overemphasized unless confirmed on larger numbers of cases.

For a detailed discussion of the differential diagnosis of lymphomatoid papulosis from cutaneous inflammatory infiltrates with large atypical CD30+ cells, see Chapter 22.

Treatment

As the disease is self-limiting, most patients with lymphomatoid papulosis will not require specific treatment [11]. Therapy should be directed mainly at controling symptoms in widespread eruptions or slowing down the frequency of recurrences [1,11]. Systemic steroids, psoralen + UV-A (PUVA), UV-A1, interferon-α2a, interferon-γ, and retinoids (alone or in combination) have been used with partial success [11,16,101–106]. The administration of low-dose methotrexate over a longer period of time may be beneficial in patients with frequent crops and large numbers of lesions [11,107]. Methotrexate has also been administered topically [108]. Some patients have been treated with imiquimod cream [109] or 308 nm excimer laser [110]. Recurrences after discontinuation of any type of treatment are the rule.

Analysis of data on different treatment modalities in lymphomatoid papulosis is hindered by the fact that lesions resolve spontaneously by definition; thus usually a "shorter" time to resolution and/or a decrease of the frequency of the eruptions are considered significant in judging the value of a given treatment. However, resolution time is variable in the absence of any treatment and it may be very subjective to calculate whether a given lesion has resolved earlier because of treatment, or not. In addition, the number of eruptions that a single patient experiences is variable.

At present, there are no data to support the efficacy of any given treatment scheme in diminishing the number and frequency of recurrences, or to demonstrate a preventive effect on the development of a second lymphoma.

Prognosis

Lymphomatoid papulosis is characterized by an excellent prognosis, and the expected 5-year survival is 100% [1,32, 33,111]. Some patients may experience very few recurrences of the disease over the years, whereas others may have lesions appearing almost continuously. At present there are no prognostic features that can help in predicting the course of the disease in a given patient. It is also still unclear whether complete remissions may occur; in a recent study, 9/21 patients who received a diagnosis of lymphomatoid papulosis were in complete remission after a follow-up time variable between 1 and 18 years (median 6 years) [112]. However, the authors did not specify whether the patients experienced long-standing remissions or were just symptom free at time of last follow-up control. In our experience, genuine lymphomatoid papulosis may show long periods of clinical remission, but recurrences are the rule rather than the exception.

Higher numbers of forkhead box protein P3 (FOX-P3)⁺ T regulatory (Treg) lymphocytes were observed in lymphomatoid papulosis as compared to cutaneous anaplastic large cell lymphoma, suggesting that these components of the reactive infiltrate may play a role in the better prognosis of patients with lymphomatoid papulosis [113].

The knowledge that 10–20% of the patients develop an associated malignant lymphoma means that regular follow-up is required for these patients. Unfortunately, clinicopathologic, phenotypic or molecular features provide no clues for the early identification of patients who will progress to a more aggressive lymphoma. In addition, as already mentioned there are no data to support a preventive effect of any given treatment scheme on the progression or transformation into high-grade lymphoma.

As already discussed, it seems that the occurrence of large CD30⁺ tumors limited to the skin at onset of lymphomatoid papulosis or during the course of the disease does not worsen the prognosis of these patients [11,31].

Résumé

Lymphomatoid papulosis

Clinical	Young adults. Chronic, recurrent eruption of papules and nodules that heal within 3–6 weeks without treatment. Excellent prognosis.
Morphology	Three histopathologic types: Type A: large, atypical, CD30⁺ cells admixed with small lymphocytes, eosinophils and neutrophils. Type B: wedge-shaped or band-like infiltrate of small/medium-sized atypical cells with epidermotropism. CD30⁺/⁻; a subset shows a pagetoid reticulosis-like picture. Type C: sheets of large, atypical, CD30⁺ cells.
Immunology	CD2, 3, 4, 5, 45 (+) CD30 + CD15 – CD8 – (+) TIA-1 (+) CD56 – (+) MUM-1 +
Genetics	No specific abnormalities. Monoclonal rearrangement of the TCR detected in the majority of the cases.
Treatment guidelines	Systemic steroids; PUVA, interferon-α2a (alone or in combination); methotrexate. Watchful waiting (waxing and waning of the lesions).

CUTANEOUS ANAPLASTIC LARGE CELL LYMPHOMA

Cutaneous anaplastic large cell lymphoma is defined as a CD30⁺ large T-cell lymphoma presenting primary in the skin and characterized by a good prognosis and response to treatment [1,2].

The differences in biologic behavior and prognosis between primary cutaneous and nodal anaplastic large cell lymphoma have been known for some time. Although earlier reports suggested that the interchromosomal (2;5) translocation, typical of nodal anaplastic large cell lymphoma, could also be found in cutaneous cases [114,115], it has been subsequently shown that it is absent in most primary cutaneous anaplastic large cell lymphomas confirming the distinction between the cutaneous and extracutaneous forms of this disease [1,28,29]. In fact, the new WHO classification of tumors of hematopoietic and lymphoid tissues lists the primary cutaneous form as a distinct entity, separate from the nodal counterpart [2]. Complete staging investigations are mandatory before definitive diagnosis, in order to exclude secondary involvement from nodal disease. The value of sentinel lymph node biopsy as a routine staging procedure has yet to be evaluated in large numbers of patients [116]. In our opinion, though, it should not be performed.

It should be emphasized that CD30⁺ tumors with anaplastic large cell morphology may be seen in patients with mycosis fungoides as a consequence of large cell transformation (see also Chapter 2). Thus, a diagnosis of primary cutaneous anaplastic large cell lymphoma should be made only when an accurate clinical history and clinical examination exclude the presence of mycosis fungoides. In addition, as mentioned before, large ulcerated tumors may be the presenting sign of lymphomatoid papulosis and these lesions should not be misinterpreted as tumors of anaplastic large cell lymphoma. CD30 expression can be observed also in tumors of aggressive cytotoxic NK/T-cell lymphomas. In this context, it should also be noted that expression of CD30 and anaplastic large cell morphology can be observed rarely in diffuse large B-cell lymphomas (see Chapter 12), and that complete phenotypic and genotypic analyses are necessary before classifying any given case.

The association of cutaneous anaplastic large cell lymphoma and lymphomatoid papulosis has been observed in several instances (see also previous paragraph on lymphomatoid papulosis) [64,117,118]. Distinction between the two entities may be very difficult as the histologic and immunophenotypic features may overlap. In this context, in 1995 LeBoit wrote: "... if one could line up 100 patients with lymphomatoid papulosis, primary cutaneous anaplastic large cell lymphoma, and cutaneous dissemination of Hodgkin's disease, a skilled clinician could more accurately sort the patients into diagnostic groups than a pathologist could by looking only at the immunophenotype of the large atypical cells" [119]. In addition it seems that progression to an anaplastic large cell lymphoma confined to the skin does not affect the favorable prognosis of lymphomatoid papulosis [31].

Cutaneous anaplastic large cell lymphoma has been observed in patients with severe immunodeficiency, due to both human immunodeficiency virus (HIV) infection and therapeutic-induced immunosuppression [120–124]. In cases arising in HIV patients, an association with human herpesvirus 8 (HHV-8) infection has been described in some cases [125]. A more detailed discussion of these cases is presented in the Chapter on cutaneous lymphomas in immunosuppressed individuals (Chapter 15).

Clinical features

Cutaneous anaplastic large cell lymphoma occurs mostly in adults of both sexes, but cases in children have been reported [33,126–128]. Clinically, patients present with solitary or localized, often ulcerated reddish-brown tumors (Fig. 4.20). Mucosal regions can be affected. Complete spontaneous regres-

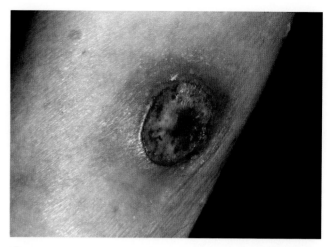

Figure 4.20 Cutaneous anaplastic large cell lymphoma. Solitary ulcerated tumor on the arm.

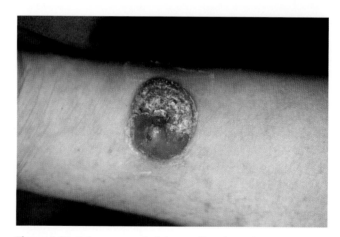

Figure 4.21 Cutaneous anaplastic large cell lymphoma. Large tumor on the arm showing partial regression. (Courtesy of I. Höpfel-Kreiner, Linz, Austria.)

sion has been observed in a few cases [129], but regression is more commonly partial (Fig. 4.21).

Clinical variants of the disease include the presence of satellite lesions around the primary tumor, simulating the clinical picture of regional lymphomatoid papulosis. Rarely, a few neoplastic cells can be detected in the peripheral blood in primary cutaneous cases [130]. This finding is similar to what has been observed in some cases of lymphomatoid papulosis (see previous section), and the clinical value is unclear.

Histopathology, immunophenotype and molecular genetics

Histopathology

Several different patterns and cell morphologies have been observed in lesions of cutaneous anaplastic large cell lymphoma [131]. At scanning power there is a nodular or diffuse infiltrate within the entire dermis and superficial part of the subcutis, composed of sheets of cohesive, large CD30⁺ atypical cells (Fig. 4.22). Most cases are composed of large anaplastic cells (large rounded or irregularly shaped nuclei with prominent nucleoli and abundant cytoplasm; giant cells with features of Reed–Sternberg cells), but large pleomorphic cells or immunoblasts can also be observed (Fig. 4.23a–c). In addition, cases with a predominant small/medium-sized pleomorphic cell morphology can be seen occasionally (Fig. 4.23d). Although a "small-to-medium" variant of a large cell lymphoma may seem an oxymoron, similar cases are well known in the lymph nodes, and can be observed in the skin as well. Sometimes anaplastic cells show epithelioid-like cytomorphologic features resembling undifferentiated carcinoma (Fig. 4.23e). Epidermotropism may be present.

Ulcerated lesions usually show epidermal hyperplasia and a prominent reactive infiltrate with small lymphocytes, neutrophils, and eosinophils (Fig. 4.23f). These cases may be indistinguishable histologically from lesions of lymphomatoid papulosis, and have sometimes been referred to as the "inflammatory" type of anaplastic large cell lymphoma. Staining for CD30 may help by highlighting the clusters of CD30⁺ cells. Cases with prominent neutrophils have been termed "neutrophil-rich" anaplastic large cell lymphoma [132, 133]. The number of eosinophils, too, may be extremely large (Fig. 4.24).

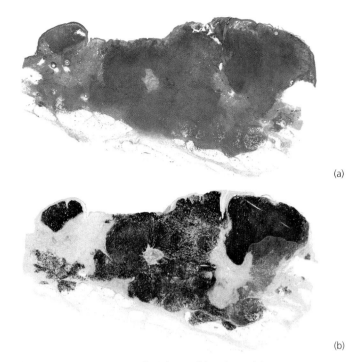

Figure 4.22 Cutaneous anaplastic large cell lymphoma. (a) Large tumor with sheets of cells infiltrating the entire dermis until the superficial part of the subcutaneous fat. (b) Most cells strongly express CD30. (Courtesy of Esmeralda Vale, Lisboa, Portugal.)

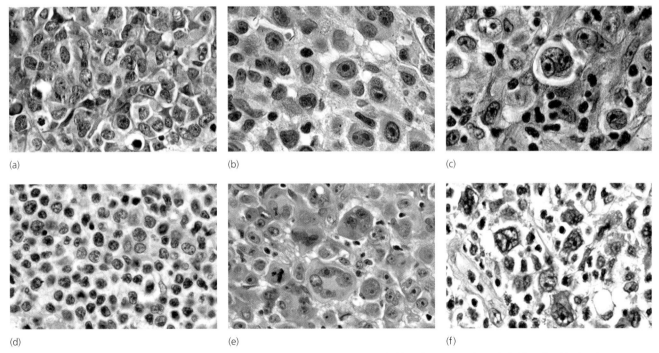

Figure 4.23 Cutaneous anaplastic large cell lymphoma. (a) Large pleomorphic and anaplastic cells. (b) Immunoblasts predominate in this case. (c) Presence of multinucleated cells resembling Reed–Sternberg cells of Hodgkin lymphoma. (d) Predominance of small- to medium-sized pleomorphic lymphocytes (so-called "small cell variant" of anaplastic large cell lymphoma). (e) Predominance of "epithelioid" cells with abundant eosinophilic cytoplasm. Some multinucleated cells are present. (f) Large anaplastic cells, some multinucleated, admixed with several neutrophils and eosinophils (so-called "neutrophilic-rich" variant of anaplastic large cell lymphoma).

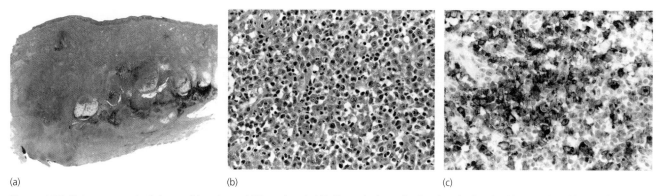

(a)   (b)   (c)

Figure 4.24 Cutaneous anaplastic large cell lymphoma. (a) Dense lymphoid infiltrates in the entire dermis and subcutis with necrosis and haemorrhage; (b) anaplastic cells admixed with numerous eosinophils; (c) positivity for CD30.

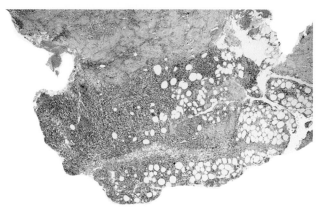

Figure 4.25 Cutaneous anaplastic large cell lymphoma confined to the subcutaneous fat.

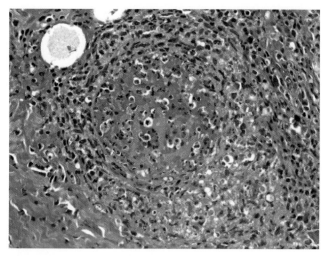

Figure 4.26 Cutaneous anaplastic large cell lymphoma. Note angiocentricity and angiodestruction.

Other rare histopathologic variants include prominent involvement of the subcutaneous fat (Fig. 4.25), and of a myxoid stroma resembling a sarcomatous lesion [134,135]. Angiocentricity and angiodestruction and, rarely, a signet-ring morphology of the neoplastic cells may be observed (Figs 4.26, 4.27). Necrosis may be prominent (Fig. 4.28a, b). In some cases, prominent tumor necrosis and peripheral palisading of neoplastic cells around necrotic areas may mimic the picture of a palisading granuloma. However, usually many eosinophils are present in the inflammatory infiltrate, a feature unusual for skin diseases in the spectrum of the palisading granulomas. Strong positivity for CD30 and for T-cell markers in palisading cells allows to make a correct diagnosis in these cases. More generally, presence of prominent necrosis in the context of an infiltrate rich in eosinophils should always arise the suspicion of a cutaneous anaplastic large cell lymphoma. Pseudoepitheliomatous epidermal hyperplasia can be observed in some cases, and may simulate the picture of a squamous cell carcinoma (Fig. 4.29).

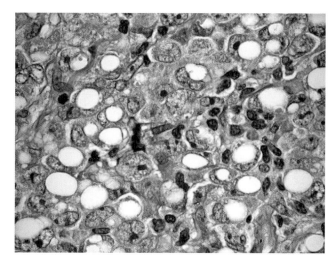

Figure 4.27 Cutaneous anaplastic large cell lymphoma with signet-ring cell morphology of neoplastic cells.

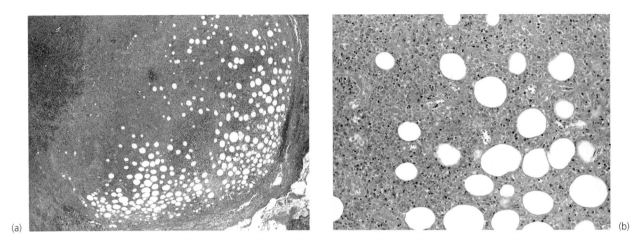

Figure 4.28 Cutaneous anaplastic large cell lymphoma. (a) Infiltration of the subcutaneous tissues with prominent necrosis. (b) Detail of necrotic part with "ghosts" of atypical lymphocytes admixed with adipocytes and debris.

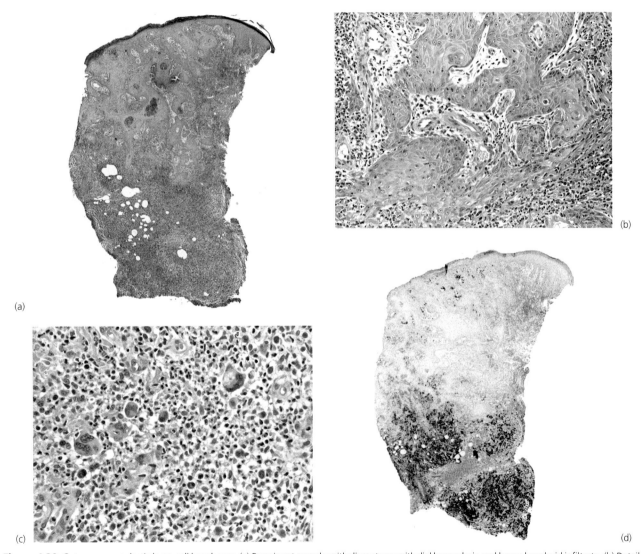

Figure 4.29 Cutaneous anaplastic large cell lymphoma. (a) Prominent pseudoepitheliomatous epithelial hyperplasia and heavy lymphoid infiltrate. (b) Detail of the pseudoepitheliomatous hyperplasia. (c) Detail of the lymphoid infiltrate with atypical, anaplastic cells admixed with neutrophils and a few eosinophils. (d) Positivity for CD30 highlights large numbers of neoplastic cells at the base of the the pseudoepitheliomatous hyperplasia.

Immunophenotype

The majority of neoplastic cells are CD30$^+$ and generally have a T-helper phenotype (CD3$^+$, CD4$^+$, CD8$^-$) (see Fig. 4.23) [71], though CD8$^+$ cases with a cytotoxic phenotype are not uncommon [82,136–138]. Expression of pan-T-cell antigens may be partially lost. CD15 and epithelial membrane antigen (EMA) are usually negative.

Expression of ALK protein is not found in purely cutaneous cases (see also molecular genetics, below) but is present in systemic disease with secondary cutaneous manifestations [87,139,140]. Unusual phenotypic variations have been described [141].

Expression of CD56 and fascin seems to be more frequent in anaplastic large cell lymphoma than in lymphomatoid papulosis; other markers studied give comparable results between the two entities (see section on lymphomatoid papulosis) [92]. Similarly, there are no clear-cut data supporting the suggestion that MUM-1 expression may be of differential diagnostic value. In fact, a recent study demonstrated a similar pattern of expression of this antigen in lymphomatoid papulosis and anaplastic large cell lymphoma [142]. In this context, it should be remembered that only small numbers of cases have been studied with any given marker, and that results are often largely overlapping between lymphomatoid papulosis and cutaneous anaplastic large cell lymphoma. In addition, as differentiation of lymphomatoid papulosis from anaplastic large cell lymphoma can be very difficult, stratification of cases may be arbitrary, and results should be interpreted with caution.

Molecular genetics

Monoclonal rearrangement of the TCR genes is observed in most cases. Single cell PCR analysis has demonstrated that most of the large CD30$^+$ cells are monoclonal [143]. There is good evidence that the interchromosomal (2;5) translocation seen in many nodal anaplastic large cell lymphomas is not present in primary cutaneous lesions [1,29].

No specific genetic alterations have been detected repeatably in cutaneous anaplastic large cell lymphoma. Some cases revealed chromosome imbalances by comparative genomic hybridization and cDNA microarray studies [144]. An allelic deletion at the chromosome region 9p21, containing the tumor suppressor gene p16, has been shown in some cases [145]. Translocations involving *MUM1* were detected by fluorescence *in situ* hybridization (FISH) studies using a breakapart *MUM1* probe [146].

Treatment

Solitary or localized lesions may be treated by surgical excision, radiotherapy or a combination of the two [1,11,147]. Patients presenting with extracutaneous involvement require systemic chemotherapy. The role of systemic chemotherapy in primary cutaneous lesions has been debated [128,148], but there is a widely accepted view that this treatment can be avoided in most patients with primary skin involvement [1,11].

Complete regression after effective specific antiviral treatment has been observed in patients with HIV-associated primary cutaneous anaplastic large cell lymphoma (see Chapter 15) [149].

Prognosis

Although the morphologic features are those of a high-grade non-Hodgkin lymphoma, the prognosis of patients with primary cutaneous anaplastic large cell lymphoma is generally favorable. The estimated 5-year survival is over 90% [1,33,111,150]. Spontaneous regression and absence of extracutaneous spread have been associated with a better prognosis [151]. A better prognosis has been found also in patients with lesions that showed a prominent pseudoepitheliomatous hyperplasia [152].

It seems that patients presenting with skin tumors and evidence of specific lesions within regional lymph nodes at staging (concomitant cutaneous and nodal anaplastic large cell lymphoma) have a prognosis similar to that of patients with disease confined to the skin [11].

Résumé		
Cutaneous anaplastic large cell lymphoma		
Clinical	Adults and younger patients. Solitary or regionally localized tumors, often ulcerated. Generally favorable prognosis.	
Morphology	Nodular infiltrates characterized by cohesive sheets of large, CD30$^+$ cells. Cytomorphology: large anaplastic cells; large pleomorphic cells or immunoblasts; small/medium and signet-ring cell morphology may be observed.	
Immunology	CD2, 3, 4, 5,	(+)
	CD30	+
	CD8	– (+)
	CD15, EMA	–
	TIA-1	(+)
	CD56	– (+)
	MUM-1	+
Genetics	Usually absence of t(2;5). Monoclonal rearrangement of the TCR detected in the majority of cases.	
Treatment guidelines	Solitary or localized lesions: surgical excision and/or radiotherapy. Systemic chemotherapy should probably be administered only in patients with extracutaneous involvement.	

"BORDERLINE" CASES

As mentioned before, the new WHO-EORTC classification of cutaneous lymphomas as well as the WHO 2008 classification of tumors of hematopoietic and lymphoid tissues consider lymphomatoid papulosis and cutaneous anaplastic large cell lymphoma as two ends of a spectrum of cutaneous CD30$^+$ lymphoproliferative disorders. In this spectrum there are cases that do not fit clearly into one or the other entity, and that are classified as "borderline." Most of the cases diagnosed in the past as "regressing atypical histiocytosis" probably belong to this category. In the WHO-EORTC classification, borderline cases are defined as follows: "The term 'borderline case' refers to cases in which, despite careful clinicopathologic correlation, a definite distinction between cutaneous anaplastic large cell lymphoma and lymphomatoid papulosis cannot be made. Clinical examination during further follow-up will generally disclose whether the patient has cutaneous anaplastic large cell lymphoma or lymphomatoid papulosis" [1].

We have seen patients presenting with solitary tumors diagnosed as cutaneous anaplastic large cell lymphoma, developing afterwards typical lesions of lymphomatoid papulosis, as well as patients with cutaneous anaplastic large cell lymphoma and small satellites in the surrounding skin, where a distinction between regional lymphomatoid papulosis and cutaneous anaplastic large cell lymphoma was not possible on clinicopathologic grounds. It should be underlined that a precise distinction between the two entities is not always necessary for proper classification and management of the patients. In addition, it is important to mention that pathologists and dermatopathologists should avoid generating confusion by classifying cases without proper clinicopathologic correlation.

When a precise classification is not possible on histopathologic grounds, we use the following phrasing: "cutaneous CD30$^+$ lymphoproliferative disorder with histopathologic features more likely suggesting –" and then adding the most likely histologic diagnosis – that is, lymphomatoid papulosis or cutaneous anaplastic large cell lymphoma. In this way, clinicians know exactly how to manage the patients, and any misunderstanding is avoided.

Résumé	
"Borderline" lesions of cutaneous CD30$^+$ lymphoproliferative disorders	
Clinical	Cases that do not fit clearly into one of the two categories of lymphomatoid papulosis or cutaneous anaplastic large cell lymphoma. Precise classification possible only on follow-up.
Morphology	Most cases show cohesive sheets of large, CD30$^+$ cells, thus resembling cutaneous anaplastic large cell lymphoma histopathologically.
Immunology	As in lymphomatoid papulosis and cutaneous anaplastic large cell lymphoma. There are no studies demonstrating the value of specific stainings for precise histopathologic classification of these cases.
Genetics	As in lymphomatoid papulosis and anaplastic large cell lymphoma.
Treatment guidelines	Management should follow the guidelines for cutaneous anaplastic large cell lymphoma.

TEACHING CASE

A biopsy specimen taken from this 26-year-old man was referred for histopathologic examination. Histology revealed a superficial, markedly epidermotropic infiltrate of atypical pleomorphic lymphocytes (Fig. 4.30a, b). Immunohistologic investigations showed a cytotoxic phenotype of the epidermotropic cells (Fig. 4.30c: staining for CD8). A tentative diagnosis of mycosis fungoides, cytotoxic phenotype versus other epidermotropic cytotoxic lymphoma was made.

The patient was subsequently referred to our outpatient unit for cutaneous lymphoma for clinicopathologic correlation and further management. He presented with several partly necrotic papules that, according to clinical history, were waxing and waning (Fig. 4.30d).

The clinical presentation was diagnostic of lymphomatoid papulosis. A staining for CD30 showed weak expression of the antigen in many intraepidermal cells (Fig. 4.30e).

Comment: This case exemplifies the need for clinicopathologic correlation for precise diagnosis and classification of cutaneous lymphoproliferative disorders. In spite of a histopathologic picture that was strongly suggestive of pagetoid reticulosis or cutaneous aggressive epidermotropic CD8+ cytotoxic T-cell lymphoma, this patient had an unusual variant of lymphomatoid papulosis. This case also shows that with proper staining technique, type B lymphomatoid papulosis is not negative for CD30, although the antigen's level within neoplastic cells may be low (thus the staining may be weak).

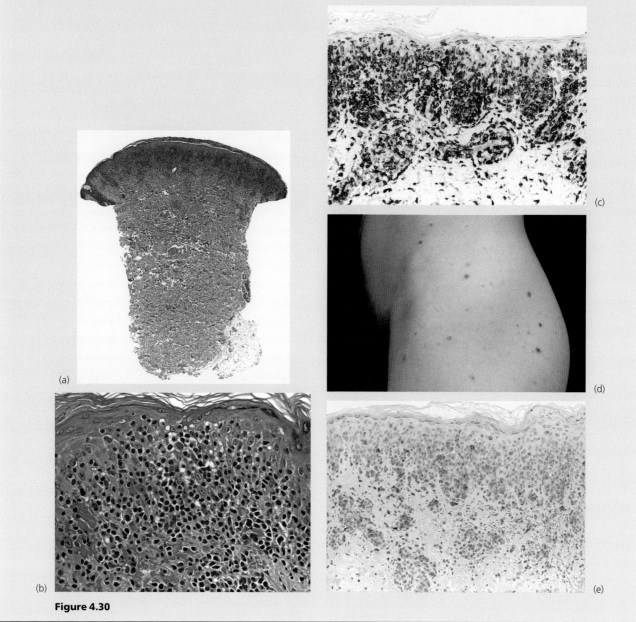

Figure 4.30

TEACHING CASE

This 80-year-old man presented with multiple papules and small nodules restricted to the lower part of the right leg (Fig. 4.31a). A biopsy revealed a well-circumscribed, nodular infiltrate in the dermis consisting of sheets of atypical, pleomorphic and anaplastic cells (Fig. 4.31b, c). Staining for CD30 revealed strong positivity of all cells (Fig. 4.31d). A diagnosis of "borderline" cutaneous CD30⁺ lymphoproliferative disorder was made. All lesions disappeared without treatment within 3 months.

Comment: This case shows the difficulty of classifying cutaneous CD30⁺ lymphoproliferative disorders on the basis of the

histopathologic features only. The lesions in this patient were restricted to one area of the body (like in regional lymphomatoid papulosis), but had histopathologic features of anaplastic large cell lymphoma. Borderline cases are often difficult to classify precisely as either lymphomatoid papulosis or cutaneous anaplastic large cell lymphoma; in these cases, short-term follow-up controls often help in establishing a precise diagnosis (in this patient, due to the complete spontaneous resolution, a final diagnosis of regional lymphomatoid papulosis was made).

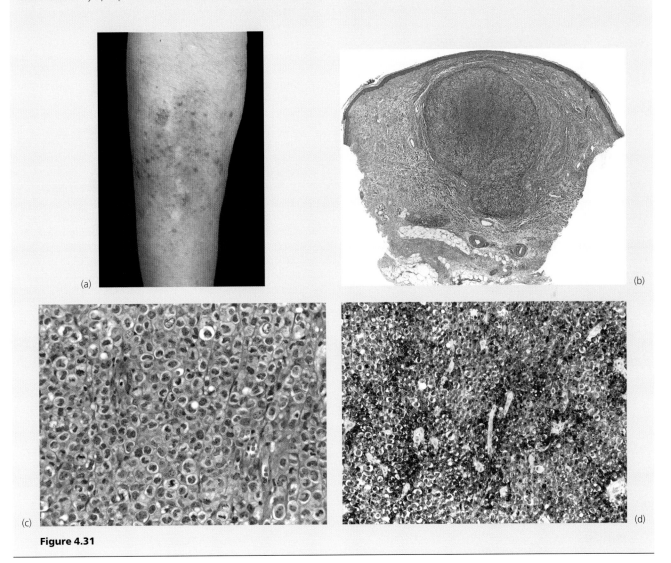

(a) (b) (c) (d)

Figure 4.31

References

1. Willemze R, Jaffe ES, Burg G et al. WHO-EORTC classification for cutaneous lymphomas. *Blood* 2005;**105**:3768–3785.

2. Ralfkiaer E, Willemze R, Paulli M, Kadin ME. Primary cutaneous CD30-positive T-cell lymphoproliferative disorders. In: Swerdlow SH, Campo E, Harris NL et al., eds. *WHO Classification of Tumours of Haematopoietic and Lymphoid Tissues*. Lyon: IARC Press, 2008: 300–301.

3. Stein H, Gerdes J, Schwab U et al. Identification of Hodgkin and Sternberg–Reed cells as a unique cell type derived from a newly detected small-cell population. *Int J Cancer* 1982;**30**:445–459.

4. Stein H, Mason DY, Gerdes J et al. The expression of the Hodgkin's disease associated antigen Ki1 in reactive and neoplastic lymphoid tissue: evidence that Reed–Sternberg cells and histiocytic malignancies are derived from activated lymphoid cells. *Blood* 1985;**66**:848–858.

5. Beljaards RC, Meijer CJLM, Scheffer E et al. Prognostic significance of CD30 (Ki-1/Ber-H2) expression in primary cutaneous large-cell lymphomas of T-cell origin. *Am J Pathol* 1989;**135**:1169–1178.

6. Beljaards RC, Kaudewitz P, Berti E et al. Primary cutaneous CD30-positive large cell lymphoma: definition of a new type of cutaneous lymphoma with a favorable prognosis. *Cancer* 1993;**71**:2097–2104.

7. Feller AC, Sterry W. Large cell anaplastic lymphoma of the skin. *Br J Dermatol* 1989;**121**:593–602.

8. Kaudewitz P, Stein H, Dallenbach F et al. Primary and secondary cutaneous Ki1 (CD30) anaplastic large cell lymphomas. *Am J Pathol* 1989;**135**:359–367.

9. Krishnan J, Tomaszewski MM, Kao GF. Primary cutaneous CD30-positive anaplastic large cell lymphoma: report of 27 cases. *J Cutan Pathol* 1993;**20**:193–202.

10. Ralfkiaer E, Bosq J, Gatter KC et al. Expression of Hodgkin and Reed–Sternberg cell associated antigen (Ki1) in cutaneous lymphoid infiltrates. *Arch Dermatol Res* 1987;**279**:285–292.

11. Bekkenk MW, Geelen FAMJ, van Voorst-Vader PC et al. Primary and secondary cutaneous CD30 lymphoproliferative disorders: a report from the Dutch Cutaneous Lymphoma Group on the long-term follow-up data of 219 patients and guidelines for diagnosis and treatment. *Blood* 2000;**95**:3653–3661.

12. Kadin ME. The spectrum of Ki1 cutaneous lymphomas. In: Van Vloten WA, Willemze R, Lange Vejlsgaard G, Thomsen K, eds. *Cutaneous Lymphomas and Pseudolymphomas*. Basel: Karger, 1990: 132–143.

13. Kaudewitz P, Burg G. Lymphomatoid papulosis and Ki1 (CD30) positive cutaneous large cell lymphomas. *Semin Diagn Pathol* 1991;**8**:117–124.

14. LeBoit PE. Lymphomatoid papulosis and cutaneous CD30 lymphoma. *Am J Dermatopathol* 1996;**18**:221–235.

15. Paulli M, Berti E, Rosso R et al. CD30/Ki-1-positive lymphoproliferative disorders of the skin: clinicopathologic correlation and statistical analysis of 86 cases. A multicentric study from the European Organization for Research and Treatment of Cancer Cutaneous Lymphoma project group. *J Clin Oncol* 1995;**13**:1343–1354.

16. Willemze R, Beljaards RC. The spectrum of primary cutaneous CD30 (Ki-1) positive lymphoproliferative disorders: a proposal for classification and guidelines for management and treatment. *J Am Acad Dermatol* 1993;**28**:973.

17. Flynn KJ, Dehner LP, Gajl-Peczalska KJ et al. Regressing atypical histiocytosis: a cutaneous proliferation of atypical neoplastic histiocytes with unexpectedly indolent biologic behaviour. *Cancer* 1982;**49**:959–970.

18. Cerio R, Black MM. Regressing atypical histiocytosis and lymphomatoid papulosis: variants of the same disorder? *Br J Dermatol* 1990;**123**:515–521.

19. Levi E, Wang Z, Petrogiannis-Haliotis T et al. Distinct effects of CD30 and Fas signaling in cutaneous anaplastic lymphomas: a possible mechanism for disease progression. *J Invest Dermatol* 2000;**115**:1034–1040.

20. Mori M, Manuelli C, Pimpinelli N et al. CD30-CD30 ligand interaction in primary cutaneous CD30 T-cell lymphomas: a clue to the pathophysiology of clinical regression. *Blood* 1999;**94**:3077–3083.

21. Nevala H, Karenko L, Vakeva L, Banki A. Proapoptotic and antiapoptotic markers in cutaneous T-cell lymphoma skin infiltrates and lymphomatoid papulosis. *Br J Dermatol* 2001;**145**:928–937.

22. Paulli M, Berti E, Boveri E et al. Cutaneous CD30 lymphoproliferative disorders: expression of bcl-2 and proteins of the tumor necrosis factor receptor superfamily. *Hum Pathol* 1998;**29**:1223–1230.

23. Vermeer MH, de Vries E, van Beek P, Meijer CJLM, Willemze R. Expression of Fas and Fas-ligand in primary cutaneous T-cell lymphoma (CTCL): association between lack of Fas expression and aggressive types of CTCL. *Br J Dermatol* 2000;**143**:313–319.

24. Greisser J, Doebbeling U, Roos M et al. Apoptosis in CD30-positive lymphoproliferative disorders of the skin. *Exp Dermatol* 2005;**14**:380–385.

25. Thakuria M, Agarwal S, Saffold OE, Jaworsky C. Fulminant cutaneous eruption in a 51-year-old man. *Arch Dermatol* 2007;**143**:255–260.

26. MacAulay WL. Lymphomatoid papulosis: a continuing self-healing eruption, clinically benign-histologically malignant. *Arch Dermatol* 1968;**97**:23–30.

27. Kim YC, Yang WI, Lee MG et al. Epstein–Barr virus in CD30+ anaplastic large cell lymphoma involving the skin and lymphomatoid papulosis in South Korea. *Int J Dermatol* 2006;**45**:1312–1316.

28. Wood GS, Hardman DL, Boni R et al. Lack of the t(2;5) or other mutations resulting in expression of anaplastic lymphoma kinase catalytic domain in CD30 primary cutaneous lymphoproliferative disorders and Hodgkin's disease. *Blood* 1996;**88**:1765–1770.

29. DeCoteau JF, Butmarc JR, Kinney MC, Kadin ME. The t(2;5) chromosomal translocation is not a common feature of primary cutaneous CD30 lymphoproliferative disorders: comparison with anaplastic large-cell lymphoma of nodal origin. *Blood* 1996;**87**:3437–3441.

30. Basarab T, Fraser-Andrews EA, Orchard G, Whittaker S, Russell-Jones R. Lymphomatoid papulosis in association with mycosis fungoides: a study of 15 cases. *Br J Dermatol* 1998;**139**:630–638.

31. Beljaards RC, Willemze R. The prognosis of patients with lymphomatoid papulosis associated with malignant lymphomas. *Br J Dermatol* 1992;**126**:596–602.

32. El Shabrawi-Caelen L, Kerl H, Cerroni L. Lymphomatoid papulosis: reappraisal of clinicopathologic presentation and classification into subtypes A, B and C. *Arch Dermatol* 2004; **140**:441–447.

33. Fink-Puches R, Zenahlik P, Bäck B et al. Primary cutaneous lymphomas: applicability of current classification schemes (European Organization for Research and Treatment of Cancer, World Health Organization) based on clinicopathologic features observed in a large group of patients. *Blood* 2002;**99**:800–805.

34. Harabuchi Y, Kataura A, Kobayashi K et al. Lethal midline granuloma (peripheral T-cell lymphoma) after lymphomatoid papulosis. *Cancer* 1992;**70**:835–839.

35. Karp DL, Horn TD. Lymphomatoid papulosis. *J Am Acad Dermatol* 1994;**30**:379–395.

36. Kaudewitz P, Stein H, Plewig G et al. Hodgkin's disease followed by lymphomatoid papulosis: immunophenotypic evidence for a close relationship between lymphomatoid papulosis and Hodgkin's disease. *J Am Acad Dermatol* 1990;**22**:999–1006.

37. Thomsen K, Lange Wantzin G. Lymphomatoid papulosis: a follow-up study of 30 patients. *J Am Acad Dermatol* 1987;**17**:632–636.

38. Weinman VF, Ackerman AB. Lymphomatoid papulosis: a critical review and new findings. *Am J Dermatopathol* 1981;**3**:129–162.

39. Aronsson A, Jonsson N, Tegner E. Transient lymphomatoid papulosis in mycosis fungoides. *Acta Derm Venereol (Stockh)* 1982;**62**:529.

40. Lish KM, Ramsay DL, Raphael BG, Jacobson M, Gottesman SRS. Lymphomatoid papulosis followed by acute myeloblastic leukemia. *J Am Acad Dermatol* 1993;**29**:112–115.

41. Chott A, Vonderheid EC, Olbricht S et al. The same dominant T cell clone is present in multiple regressing skin lesions and associated T cell lymphomas of patients with lymphomatoid papulosis. *J Invest Dermatol* 1996;**106**:696–700.

42. Davis TH, Morton CC, Miller-Cassman R, Balk SP, Kadin ME. Hodgkin's disease, lymphomatoid papulosis, and cutaneous T-cell lymphoma derived from a common T-cell clone. *N Engl J Med* 1992;**326**:1115–1122.

43. Wood GS, Crooks CF, Uluer AZ. Lymphomatoid papulosis and associated cutaneous lymphoproliferative disorders exhibit a common clonal origin. *J Invest Dermatol* 1995;**105**:51–55.

44. Zackheim HS, Jones C, LeBoit PE et al. Lymphomatoid papulosis associated with mycosis fungoides: a study of 21 patients including analyses for clonality. *J Am Acad Dermatol* 2003;**49**:620–623.

45. Zackheim HS, LeBoit PE, Gordon BI, Glassberg AB. Lymphomatoid papulosis followed by Hodgkin's lymphoma: differential response to therapy. *Arch Dermatol* 1993;**129**:86–91.

46. Wolf P, Cerroni L, Smolle J, Kerl H. PUVA-induced lymphomatoid papulosis in a patient with mycosis fungoides. *J Am Acad Dermatol* 1991;**25**:422–426.

47. Wang HH, Myers T, Lach LJ, Hsieh CC, Kadin ME. Increased risk of lymphoid and non-lymphoid malignancies in patients with lymphomatoid papulosis. *Cancer* 1999;**86**:1240–1245.

48. Schultz JC, Granados S, Vonderheid EC, Hwang ST. T-cell clonality of peripheral blood lymphocytes in patients with lymphomatoid papulosis. *J Am Acad Dermatol* 2005;**53**:152–155.

49. Ota M, Sawamura D, Shibaki A, Shimizu H. Bone marrow clonal T-cell population in lymphomatoid papulosis. *J Am Acad Dermatol* 2005;**52**:710–711.

50. Humme D, Lukowsky A, Steinhoff M, et al. Dominance of non-malignant T-cell clones and distortion of the TCR repertoire in the peripheral blood of patients with cutaneous CD30+ lymphoproliferative disorders. *J Invest Dermatol* 2009;**129**:89–98.

51. Aoki E, Aoki M, Kono M, Kawana S. Two cases of lymphomatoid papulosis in children. *Pediatr Dermatol* 2003;**20**:146–149.

52. el-Azhary RA, Gibson LE, Kurtin PJ, Pittelkow MR, Muller SA. Lymphomatoid papulosis: a clinical and histopathologic review of 53 cases with leukocyte immunophenotyping, DNA flow cytometry, and T-cell receptor gene rearrangement studies. *J Am Acad Dermatol* 1994;**30**:210–218.

53. Rogers M, de Launey J, Kemp A, Bishop A. Lymphomatoid papulosis in an 11-month-old infant. *Pediatr Dermatol* 1984;**2**:124–130.

54. Sanchez NP, Pittelkow MR, Muller SA, Banks PM, Winkelmann RK. The clinicopathologic spectrum of lymphomatoid papulosis: study of 31 cases. *J Am Acad Dermatol* 1983;**8**:81–94.

55. van Neer FJMA, Toonstra J, van Voorst Vader PC, Willemze R, van Vloten WA. Lymphomatoid papulosis in children: a study of 10 children registered by the Dutch cutaneous lymphoma working group. *Br J Dermatol* 2001;**144**:351–354.

56. Willemze R, Meijer CJLM, van Vloten WA, Scheffer E. The clinical and histological spectrum of lymphomatoid papulosis. *Br J Dermatol* 1982;**107**:131–144.

57. Serra-Guillen C, Requena C, Alfaro A et al. Oral involvement in lymphomatoid papulosis. *Actas Dermosifiliogr* 2007;**98**:265–267.

58. Allabert C, Esteve E, Joly P et al. Mucosal involvement in lymphomatoid papulosis: four cases. *Ann Dermatol Venereol* 2008;**135**:273–278.

59. Kagaya M, Kondo S, Kamada A et al. Localized lymphomatoid papulosis. *Dermatology* 2002;**204**:72–74.

60. Scarisbrick JJ, Evans AV, Woolford AJ, Black MM, Russell-Jones R. Regional lymphomatoid papulosis: a report of four cases. *Br J Dermatol* 1999;**141**:1125–1128.

61. Thomas GJ, Conejo-Mir JS, Ruiz AP, Barrios ML, Navarrete M. Lymphomatoid papulosis in childhood with exclusive acral involvement. *Pediatr Dermatol* 1998;**15**:146–147.

62. Heald P, Subtil A, Breneman D, Wilson LD. Persistent agmination of lymphomatoid papulosis: an equivalent of limited plaque mycosis fungoides type of cutaneous T-cell lymphoma. *J Am Acad Dermatol* 2007;**57**:1005–1011.

63. Kato N, Tomita Y, Yoshida K, Hisai H. Involvement of the tongue by lymphomatoid papulosis. *Am J Dermatopathol* 1998;**20**:522–526.

64. Yamamoto O, Tajiri M, Asahi M. Lymphomatoid papulosis associated with pregnancy. *Clin Exp Dermatol* 1997;**22**:141–143.

65. Granel B, Serratrice J, Swiader L et al. Lymphomatoid papulosis associated with both severe hypereosinophilic syndrome and CD30 positive large T-cell lymphoma: a case report. *Cancer* 2000;**89**:2138–2143.

66. Tabata N, Aiba S, Ichinohazama R et al. Hydroa vacciniforme-like lymphomatoid papulosis in a Japanese child: a new subset. *J Am Acad Dermatol* 1995;**32**:378–381.

67. Barnadas MA, Lopez D, Pujol RM et al. Pustular lymphomatoid papulosis in childhood. *J Am Acad Dermatol* 1992;**27**:627.

68. Kato N, Matsue K. Follicular lymphomatoid papulosis. *Am J Dermatopathol* 1997;**19**:189–196.

69. Pierard GE, Ackerman AB, Lapiere CM. Follicular lymphomatoid papulosis. *Am J Dermatopathol* 1980;**2**:173–180.

70. Requena L, Sanchez M, Coca S, Sanchez Yus E. Follicular lymphomatoid papulosis. *Am J Dermatopathol* 1990;**12**:67–75.

71. Atkins KA, Dahlem MM, Kohler S. A case of lymphomatoid papulosis with prominent myxoid change resembling a mesenchymal neoplasm. *Am J Dermatopathol* 2003;**25**:62–65.

72. Baschinsky D, Magro CM, Kovatich A, Crowson AN. Eccrinotropic and neurotropic lymphomatoid papulosis (LyP): a novel variant. *Mod Pathol* 2001;**14**:65.

73. Cespedes YP, Rockley PF, Flores F *et al.* Is there a special relationship between CD30-positive lymphoproliferative disorders and epidermal proliferation? *J Cutan Pathol* 2000;**27**:271–275.

74. Scarisbrick JJ, Calonje E, Orchard G, Child FJ, Russell-Jones R. Pseudocarcinomatous change in lymphomatoid papulosis and primary cutaneous CD30 lymphoma: a clinicopathologic and immunohistochemical study of 6 patients. *J Am Acad Dermatol* 2001;**44**:239–247.

75. Guitart J, Gordon K. Keratoacanthomas and lymphomatoid papulosis. *Am J Dermatopathol* 1998;**20**:430–432.

76. Fernandez-Flores A. CD30+ cell population in common keratoacanthomas: a study of 21 cases. *Romanian J Morphol Embryol Physiol* 2008;**49**:159–162.

77. Kaudewitz P, Stein H, Burg G, Mason DY, Braun-Falco O. Atypical cells in lymphomatoid papulosis express the Hodgkin cell-associated antigen Ki-1. *J Invest Dermatol* 1986;**86**:350–354.

78. Kadin ME. Characteristic immunologic profile of large atypical cells in lymphomatoid papulosis. *Arch Dermatol* 1986;**122**:1388–1390.

79. Kadin ME, Nasu K, Sako D, Said J, Vonderheid EC. Lymphomatoid papulosis: a cutaneous proliferation of activated helper T cells expressing Hodgkin's disease-associated antigens. *Am J Pathol* 1985;**119**:315–325.

80. Kummer JA, Vermeer MH, Dukers D, Meijer CJLM, Willemze R. Most primary cutaneous CD30-positive lymphoproliferative disorders have a CD4-positive cytotoxic T-cell phenotype. *J Invest Dermatol* 1997;**109**:636–640.

81. Jang KA, Choi JC, Choi JH. Expression of cutaneous lymphocyte-associated antigen and TIA-1 by lymphocytes in pityriasis lichenoides et varioliformis acuta and lymphomatoid papulosis: immunohistochemical study. *J Cutan Pathol* 2001;**28**:453–459.

82. Boulland ML, Wechsler J, Bagot M *et al.* Primary CD30-positive cutaneous T-cell lymphomas and lymphomatoid papulosis frequently express cytotoxic proteins. *Histopathology* 2000;**36**:136–144.

83. Harvell JD, Vaseghi M, Natkunam Y, Kohler S, Kim Y. Large atypical cells of lymphomatoid papulosis are CD56-negative: a study of 18 cases. *J Cutan Pathol* 2002;**29**:88–92.

84. Bekkenk MW, Kluin PM, Jansen PM, Meijer CJLM, Willemze R. Lymphomatoid papulosis with a natural killer-cell phenotype. *Br J Dermatol* 2001;**145**:318–322.

85. Natkunam Y, Warnke RA, Haghighi B *et al.* Co-expression of CD56 and CD30 in lymphomas with primary presentation in the skin: clinicopathologic, immunohistochemical and molecular analyses of seven cases. *J Cutan Pathol* 2000;**27**:392–399.

86. Flann S, Orchard GE, Wain EM, Russell-Jones R. Three cases of lymphomatoid papulosis with a CD56+ immunophenotype. *J Am Acad Dermatol* 2006;**55**:903–906.

87. Herbst H, Sander C, Tronnier M *et al.* Absence of anaplastic lymphoma kinase (ALK) and Epstein–Barr virus gene products in primary cutaneous anaplastic large cell lymphoma and lymphomatoid papulosis. *Br J Dermatol* 1997;**137**:680–686.

88. Rassidakis GZ, Thomaides A, Atwell C *et al.* JunB expression is a common feature of CD30+ lymphomas and lymphomatoid papulosis. *Mod Pathol* 2005;**18**:1365–1370.

89. Drakos E, Leventaki V, Schlette EJ *et al.* c-Jun expression and activation are restricted to CD30+ lymphoproliferative disorders. *Am J Surg Pathol* 2007;**31**:447–453.

90. Kempf W, Levi E, Kamarashev J *et al.* Fascin expression in CD30-positive cutaneous lymphoproliferative disorders. *J Cut Pathol* 2002;**29**:295–300.

91. Goteri G, Simonetti O, Rupoli S *et al.* Differences in survivin location and Bcl-2 expression in CD30+ lymphoproliferative disorders of the skin compared with systemic anaplastic large cell lymphomas: an immunohistochemical study. *Br J Dermatol* 2007;**157**:41–48.

92. Droc C, Cualing HD, Kadin ME. Need for an improved molecular/genetic classification for CD30+ lymphomas involving the skin. *Cancer Control* 2007;**14**:124–132.

93. Kempf W, Kutzner H, Cozzio A *et al.* MUM1 expression in cutaneous CD30+ lymphoproliferative disorders: a valuable tool for the distinction between lymphomatoid papulosis and primary cutaneous anaplastic large-cell lymphoma. *Br J Dermatol* 2008; **158**:1280–1287.

94. Wasco MJ, Fullen D, Su L, Ma L. The expression of MUM1 in cutaneous T-cell lymphoproliferative disorders. *Hum Pathol* 2008;**39**:557–563.

95. Weiss LM, Wood GS, Trela M, Warnke RA, Sklar JL. Clonal T-cell populations in lymphomatoid papulosis: evidence for a lymphoproliferative origin for a clinically benign disease. *N Engl J Med* 1986;**315**:475–479.

96. Steinhoff M, Hummel M, Anagnostopoulos I *et al.* Single-cell analysis of CD30 cells in lymphomatoid papulosis demonstrates a common clonal T-cell origin. *Blood* 2002;**100**:578–584.

97. Panhans A, Bodemer C, Macinthyre E *et al.* Pityriasis lichenoides of childhood with atypical CD30-positive cells and clonal T-cell receptor gene rearrangements. *J Am Acad Dermatol* 1996;**35**: 489–490.

99. Herron MD, Bohnsack JF, Vanderhooft SL. Septic, CD-30 positive febrile ulceronecrotic pityriasis lichenoides et varioliformis acuta. *Ped Dermatol* 2005;**22**:360–365.

99. Cerroni L. Lymphomatoid papulosis, pityriasis lichenoides et varioliformis acuta, and anaplastic large cell (Ki-1) lymphoma. *J Am Acad Dermatol* 1997;**37**:287.

100. Olsen SH, Ma L, Schnitzer B, Fullen DR. Clusterin expression in cutaneous CD30-positive lymphoproliferative disorders and their histologic simulants. *J Cut Pathol* 2009;**36**:302–307.

101. Proctor SJ, Jackson GH, Lennard AL, Marks J. Lymphomatoid papulosis: response to treatment with recombinant interferon α-2b. *J Clin Oncol* 1992;**10**:270.

102. Schmuth M, Topar G, Illersperger B *et al.* Therapeutic use of interferon-γ for lymphomatoid papulosis. *Cancer* 2000;**89**:1603–1610.

103. Volkenandt M, Kerscher M, Sander CA, Meurer M, Rocken M. PUVA-bath photochemotherapy resulting in rapid clearance of lymphomatoid papulosis in a child. *Arch Dermatol* 1995;**131**:1094.

104. Wyss M, Dummer R, Dommann SN *et al.* Lymphomatoid papulosis: treatment with recombinant interferon α-2a and etretinate. *Dermatology* 1995;**190**:288–291.

105. Yagi H, Tokura Y, Furukawa F, Takigawa M. Th2 cytokine mRNA expression in primary cutaneous CD30-positive lymphoproliferative disorders: successful treatment with recombinant interferon-γ. *J Invest Dermatol* 1996;**107**:827–832.

106. Calzavara Pinton P, Venturini M, Sala R. Medium-dose UVA1 therapy of lymphomatoid papulosis. *J Am Acad Dermatol* 2005; **52**:530–532.

107. Vonderheid EC, Sajjadian A, Kadin ME. Methotrexate is effective therapy for lymphomatoid papulosis and other primary cutaneous CD30-positive lymphoproliferative disorders. *J Am Acad Dermatol* 1996;**34**:470–481.

108. Bergstrom JS, Jaworsky C. Topical methotrexate for lymphomatoid papulosis. *J Am Acad Dermatol* 2003;**49**:937–939.

109. Hughes PS. Treatment of lymphomatoid papulosis with imiquimod 5% cream. *J Am Acad Dermatol* 2006;**54**:546–547.

110. Kontos AP, Kerr HA, Malick F, Fivenson DP, Lim HW, Wong HK. 308-nm Excimer laser for the treatment of lymphomatoid stage IA mycosis fungoides. *Photodermatol Photoimmunol Photomed* 2006;**22**:168–171.

111. Yu JB, Blitzblau RC, Decker RH, Housman DM, Wilson LD. Analysis of primary CD30 cutaneous lymphoproliferative disease and survival from the surveillance, epidemiology, and end results database. *J Clin Oncol* 2008;**26**:1483–1488.

112. Gruber R, Sepp NT, Fritsch PO, Schmuth M. Prognosis of lymphomatoid papulosis. *Oncologist* 2006;**11**:955–957.

113. Gjerdrum LM, Woetmann A, Odum N et al. FOXP3 positive regulatory T-cells in cutaneous and systemic CD30 positive T-cell lymphoproliferations. *Eur J Haematol* 2008;**80**:483–489.

114. Beylot-Barry M, Lamant L, Vergier B et al. Detection of t(2;5) (p23;q35) translocation by reverse transcriptase polymerase chain reaction and in situ hybridization in CD30-positive primary cutaneous lymphoma and lymphomatoid papulosis. *Am J Pathol* 1996;**149**:483–492.

115. Beylot-Barry M, Groppi A, Vergier B, Pulford K, Merlio JP. Characterization of t(2;5) reciprocal transcripts and genomic breakpoints in CD30+ cutaneous lymphoproliferations. *Blood* 1998;**91**:4668–4676.

116. Krämer KU, Starz H, Balda BR. Primary cutaneous CD30-positive large T-cell lymphoma with secondary lymph node involvement detected by sentinel lymphonodectomy. *Acta Derm Venereol (Stockh)* 2002;**82**:73–74.

117. McCarty MJ, Vukelja SJ, Sausville EA et al. Lymphomatoid papulosis associated with Ki-1-positive anaplastic large cell lymphoma. A report of two cases and a review of the literature. *Cancer* 1994;**74**:3051–3058.

118. Aoki M, Nhmi Y, Takezaki S, Azuma A, Seike M, Kawana S. CD30+ lymphoproliferative disorder: primary cutaneous anaplastic large cell lymphoma followed by lymphomatoid papulosis. *Br J Dermatol* 2001;**145**:123–126.

119. LeBoit PE. Hodgkin's disease, anaplastic large cell lymphoma, and lymphomatoid papulosis. Another scalpel blunted. *Am J Clin Pathol* 1995;**104**:3–4.

120. Corazza M, Zampino MR, Montanari A, Altieri E, Virgili A. Primary cutaneous CD30+ large T-cell lymphoma in a patient with psoriasis treated with cyclosporine. *Dermatology* 2003;**206**:330–333.

121. Kirby B, Owen CM, Blewitt RW, Yates VM. Cutaneous T-cell lymphoma developing in a patient on cyclosporin therapy. *J Am Acad Dermatol* 2002;**47**:s165–s167.

122. Beylot-Barry M, Vergier B, Masquelier B et al. The spectrum of cutaneous lymphomas in HIV infection. A study of 21 cases. *Am J Surg Pathol* 1999;**23**:1208–1216.

123. Chadburn A, Cesarman E, Jagirdar J, Subar M, Mir RN, Knowles DM. CD30 (Ki-1) positive anaplastic large cell lymphomas in individuals infected with the human immunodeficiency virus. *Cancer* 1993;**72**:3078–3090.

124. Jhala DN, Medeiros LJ, Lopez-Terrada D, Jhala NC, Krishnan B, Shahab I. Neutrophil-rich anaplastic large cell lymphoma of T-cell lineage. A report of two cases arising in HIV-positive patients. *Am J Clin Pathol* 2000;**114**:478–482.

125. Katano H, Suda T, Morishita Y et al. Human herpesvirus 8-associated solid lymphomas that occur in AIDS patients take anaplastic large cell morphology. *Mod Pathol* 2000;**13**:77–85.

126. Gould JW, Eppes RB, Gilliam AC et al. Solitary primary cutaneous CD30+ large cell lymphoma of natural killer cell phenotype bearing the t(2;5)(p23;q35) translocation and presenting in a child. *Am J Dermatopathol* 2000;**22**:422–428.

127. Meier F, Schaumburg-Lever G, Kaiserling E, Scheel-Walter H, Scherwitz C. Primary cutaneous large-cell anaplastic (Ki-1) lymphoma in a child. *J Am Acad Dermatol* 1992;**26**:813–817.

128. Tomaszewski MM, Moad JC, Lupton GP. Primary cutaneous Ki-1 (CD30) positive anaplastic large cell lymphoma in childhood. *J Am Acad Dermatol* 1999;**40**:857–861.

129. Bernier M, Bagot M, Broyer M, Farcet JP, Gaulard P, Wechsler J. Distinctive clinicopathologic features associated with regressive primary CD30 positive cutaneous lymphomas: analysis of 6 cases. *J Cutan Pathol* 1997;**24**:157–163.

130. Dereure O, Portales P, Balavoine M et al. Rare occurrence of CD30+ circulating cells in patients with cutaneous CD30+ anaplastic large cell lymphoma: a study of nine patients. *Br J Dermatol* 2003;**148**:246–251.

131. Massone C, El Shabrawi-Caelen L, Kerl H, Cerroni L. The morphologic spectrum of primary cutaneous anaplastic large T-cell lymphoma: a histopathologic study on 66 biopsy specimens from 47 patients with report of rare variants. *J Cutan Pathol* 2008;**35**:46–53.

132. Burg G, Kempf W, Kazakov DV et al. Pyogenic lymphoma of the skin: a peculiar variant of primary cutaneous neutrophil-rich CD30+ anaplastic large-cell lymphoma. Clinicopathological study of four cases and review of the literature. *Br J Dermatol* 2003;**148**:580–586.

133. Kato N, Mizuno O, Ito K, Kimura K, Shibata M. Neutrophil-rich anaplastic large cell lymphoma presenting in the skin. *Am J Dermatopathol* 2003;**25**:142–147.

134. Monterroso V, Bujan W, Jaramillo O, Medeiros LJ. Subcutaneous tissue involvement by T-cell lymphoma. A report of 2 cases. *Arch Dermatol* 1996;**132**:1345–1350.

135. Chan JKC, Buchanan R, Fletcher CDM. Sarcomatoid variant of anaplastic large cell Ki1 lymphoma. *Am J Surg Pathol* 1990; **14**:983–988.

136. Kikuchi A, Sakuraoka K, Kurihara S, Akiyama M, Shimizu H, Nishikawa T. CD8+ cutaneous anaplastic large cell-lymphoma: report of two cases with immunophenotyping, T-cell receptor gene rearrangement and electron microscopic studies. *Br J Dermatol* 1992;**126**:404–408.

137. Stein H, Foss HD, Dürkop H et al. CD30+ anaplastic large cell lymphoma: a review of its histopathologic, genetic, and clinical features. *Blood* 2000;**96**:3681–3695.

138. Felgar RE, Salhany KE, MacOn WR, Pietra GG, Kinney MC. The expression of TIA-1+ cytolytic type granules and other cytolytic lymphocyte-associated markers in CD30+ anaplastic large cell lymphomas (ALCL): correlation with morphology, immunophenotype, ultrastructure, and clinical features. *Hum Pathol* 1999;**30**:228–236.

139. Su LD, Schnitzer B, Ross CW *et al.* The t(2;5)-associated p80 NPM/ALK fusion protein in nodal and cutaneous CD30+ lymphoproliferative disorders. *J Cutan Pathol* 1997;**24**:597–603.

140. ten Berge RL, Oudejans JJ, Ossenkoppele GJ *et al.* ALK expression in extranodal anaplastic large cell lymphoma favours systemic disease with (primary) nodal involvement and a good prognosis and occurs before dissemination. *J Clin Pathol* 2000;**53**:445–450.

141. Kadin ME, Pinkus JL, Pinkus GS *et al.* Primary cutaneous ALCL with phosphorylated/activated cytoplasmic ALK and novel phenotype: EMA/MUC1+, cutaneous lymphocyte antigen negative. *Am J Surg Pathol* 2008;**32**:1421–1426.

142. Hernandez-Machin B, de Misa RF, Montenegro T, *et al.* MUM1 expression does not differentiate primary cutaneous anaplastic large-cell lymphoma and lymphomatoid papulosis. *Br J Dermatol* 2009;**160**:713–714.

143. Gellrich S, Wilks A, Lukowsky A *et al.* T cell receptor-g gene analysis of CD30+ large atypical individual cells in CD30+ large primary cutaneous T cell lymphomas. *J Invest Dermatol* 2003;**120**:670–675.

144. Mao X, Orchard G, Lillington DM, Russell-Jones R, Young BD, Whittaker S. Genetic alterations in primary cutaneous CD30+ anaplastic large cell lymphoma. *Gene Chromos Cancer* 2003;**37**:176–185.

145. Böni R, Xin H, Kamarashev J *et al.* Allelic deletion at 9p21-22 in primary cutaneous CD30+ large cell lymphoma. *J Invest Dermatol* 2000;**115**:1104–1107.

146. Feldman AL, Law M, Remstein ED *et al.* Recurrent translocations involving the *MUM1* oncogene locus in peripheral T-cell lymphomas. *J Haematopathol* 2008;**1**:191.

147. Piccinno R, Caccialanza M, Berti E, Beretta M, Gnecchi L. Radiotherapy of primary cutaneous CD30-positive large cell lymphoma. A preliminary study of eight patients. *J Dermatol Treatm* 1996;**7**:183–185.

148. Vermeer MH, Bekkenk MW, Willemze R. Should primary cutaneous Ki-1(CD30)-positive anaplastic large cell lymphoma in childhood be treated with multiple-agent chemotherapy? *J Am Acad Dermatol* 2001;**45**:638–639.

149. Fatkenheuer G, Hell K, Roers A, Diehl V, Salzberger B. Spontaneous regression of HIV associated T-cell non-Hodgkin's lymphoma with highly active antiretroviral therapy. *Eur J Med Res* 2000;**5**:236–240.

150. Liu HL, Hoppe RT, Kohler S, Harvell JD, Reddy S, Kim YH. CD30+ cutaneous lymphoproliferative disorders: the Stanford experience in lymphomatoid papulosis and primary cutaneous anaplastic large cell lymphoma. *J Am Acad Dermatol* 2003;**49**:1049–1058.

151. Vergier B, Beylot-Barry M, Pulford K *et al.* Statistical evaluation of diagnostic and prognostic features of CD30+ cutaneous lymphoproliferative disorders. A clinicopathologic study of 56 cases. *Am J Surg Pathol* 1998;**22**:1192–1202.

152. Zayour M, Gilmore E, Heald P, Rose M, Poligone B, Lazova R. A distinct entity in the spectrum of the CD30+ cutaneous lymphoproliferative diseases: oligolesional nodules with pseudo-epitheliomatous hyperplasia followed by spontaneous resolution. *Am J Dermatopathol* 2009;**31**:37–43.

5   Subcutaneous "panniculitis-like" T-cell lymphoma

Subcutaneous "panniculitis-like" T-cell lymphoma has been included as a distinct entity in both the World Health Organization (WHO)-European Organization for Research and Treatment of Cancer (EORTC) classification of cutaneous lymphomas and the new WHO classification of tumors of hematopoietic and lymphoid tissues [1,2]. As a degree of involvement of subcutaneous fat by neoplastic lymphocytes is common in many primary or secondary cutaneous T- and B-cell lymphomas, however, it is necessary to strictly separate true subcutaneous T-cell lymphomas from other lymphomas with involvement of the subcutaneous fat.

The definition of subcutaneous "panniculitis-like" T-cell lymphoma includes exclusive involvement of the subcutaneous fat and α/β cytotoxic T-cell phenotype [1,3,4]. When properly used, the term subcutaneous T-cell lymphoma encompasses a group of patients with relatively homogeneous clinicopathologic, phenotypic, and prognostic features. As in former time different entities were included in this group, readers should understand that criteria used in the past (even the recent past) differ from those that are required today for a diagnosis of subcutaneous "panniculitis-like" T-cell lymphoma [1,3,4].

Some cases of subcutaneous "panniculitis-like" T-cell lymphoma were classified in the past as malignant histiocytosis or histiocytic cytophagic panniculitis [5–15]. Soon after the first description, it became clear that many cases of histiocytic cytophagic panniculitis showed a monoclonal population of T lymphocytes, proving the lymphoid origin of the disease [12]. It subsequently became clear that histiocytic cytophagic panniculitis was not always fatal as previously thought, and that cases with a good prognosis could be observed [9,13,16, 17]. Not all cases of histiocytic cytophagic panniculitis are examples of subcutaneous "panniculitis-like" T-cell lymphoma and some probably represent examples of cutaneous γ/δ T-cell lymphoma or of Epstein–Barr virus (EBV)-associated extranodal NK/T-cell lymphoma, nasal type. In fact, involvement of the subcutis is common in these types of lymphoma (see Chapter 6) [3,18–22]. It has also been demonstrated that

some cases classified in the past as Weber–Christian panniculitis represent in truth examples of subcutaneous "panniculitis-like" T-cell lymphoma [23,24].

It seems likely that at least some of the cases diagnosed in the past as lupus panniculitis (lupus erythematosus profundus) or "benign panniculitis evolving into overt lymphoma" represent examples of subcutaneous "panniculitis-like" T-cell lymphoma with a slow progression [24]. In this context, it has been proposed recently that lupus panniculitis and subcutaneous T-cell lymphoma represent two ends of a spectrum of the same entity [25]. We have seen some patients who presented with typical lesions of subcutaneous "panniculitis-like" T-cell lymphoma histopathologically but with clinical features of lupus erythematosus (positivity of antinuclear antibodies or other clinical and/or serologic markers of the disease), and believe that "overlapping" cases may exist. It may be that some patients with lupus erythematosus develop during the course of the disease lesions of subcutaneous "panniculitis-like" T-cell lymphoma. In this context, we don't believe that lupus panniculitis and subcutaneous T-cell lymphoma represent two ends of a spectrum, although cases with overlapping clinicopathologic features (that is, features of both diseases) exist.

The literature on subcutaneous "panniculitis-like" T-cell lymphoma is confusing. In the past, based only on the involvement of the subcutis, many different types of lymphoma with different clinicopathologic features and prognostic behavior have been lumped together in this group, and the exact definition and diagnostic criteria were unclear [20–22,24,26–40]. Moreover, any review of the literature is hindered by the fact that complete phenotypic investigations were not carried out in many of the cases described in the past (and even in recent years), thus relying often on the involvement of the subcutis only for diagnosis and classification. Association with EBV infection, too, has been observed irregularly. It must be clearly underlined that a purely subcutaneous pattern ("lobular panniculitis-like") can be observed rarely in various cutaneous lymphomas of T- and B-cell phenotype, and that a prominent involvement of the subcutis *per se* is not a sufficient criterion for the diagnosis of subcutaneous "panniculitis-like" T-cell lymphoma [3,41,42]. In this context, one should remember also that many overlapping features can be observed in the

Skin Lymphoma: The Illustrated Guide. By L. Cerroni, K. Gatter and H. Kerl. Published 2009 Blackwell Publishing. ISBN: 978-1-4051-8554-7.

group of so-called "cytotoxic lymphomas" (see Chapter 6), including subcutaneous involvement by neoplastic lympho-cytes, and that multiple parameters are required to classify a given case into a precise category [3,43]. Finally, lesions with exclusive subcutaneous involvement have also been observed in patients with mycosis fungoides [44]. An accurate clinical history should always be obtained in patients with a putative subcutaneous T-cell lymphoma, and any skin lesions clinically suspicious of mycosis fungoides (e.g. superficial patches) should be biopsied.

Transmission of subcutaneous "panniculitis-like" T-cell lymphoma by allogenic bone marrow transplantation has been documented in a single case [45], as well as onset in an immunosuppressed individual after cardiac transplantation [46].

Clinical features

Patients are adults of both sexes [1,2,47]. Reports in children exist but phenotypic data in some cases are incomplete [48,49]. However, we have rarely seen children with a con-vincing diagnosis of subcutaneous "panniculitis-like" T-cell lymphoma. A long history of "benign panniculitis" (particu-larly lupus panniculitis) is often present [24]. Clinically patients present with solitary or multiple erythematous tumors or plaques, which are usually not ulcerated and are located most commonly on the extremities, especially the lower ones (Figs 5.1, 5.2) [1,2,47]. Other sites of the body, including the head, may be affected (Fig. 5.3) [24,50]. Skin lesions reveal non-specific features of panniculitis, and may simulate ery-thema nodosum, lupus panniculitis or other pannicultic diseases. One patient with alopecic lesions on the scalp has also been described, and one with a lesion on the leg resembling venous stasis ulceration [51,52]. Spontaneous resolution of some of the lesions may be observed [22,35]. We must under-line that some of the clinical variants described in the past may represent in truth examples of other cytotoxic lymphomas with subcutaneous involvement, as in many cases phenotypic details presented were not sufficient to confirm beyond doubt the classification of these cases as genuine subcutaneous "panniculitis-like" T-cell lymphomas.

In one patient, neoplastic T lymphocytes have been detected in the peripheral blood [53], but the clinical relevance of this finding, if any, has not been elucidated.

In a subset of patients (probably a small minority) there are accompanying symptoms such as fever, malaise, fatigue, and weight loss. A hemophagocytic syndrome may be seen in advanced stages, and can be the cause of death in these patients. The hemophagocytic syndrome is probably more common in the aggressive lymphomas with a γ/δ T-cell or NK cell phenotype (see Chapter 6).

As mentioned before, clinical features of lupus erythe-matosus may be co-existent with those of subcutaneous

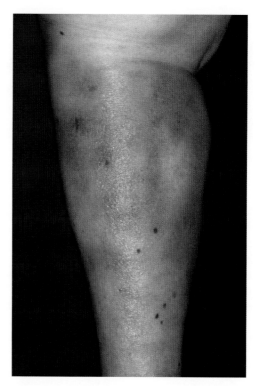

Figure 5.1 Subcutaneous T-cell lymphoma. Erythematous plaques ("panniculitis-like") on the leg.

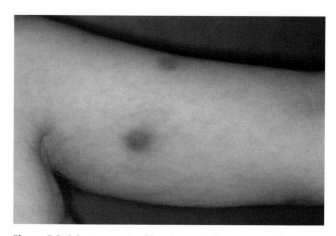

Figure 5.2 Subcutaneous T-cell lymphoma. Erythematous nodule ("erythema nodosum-like") on the arm.

"panniculitis-like" T-cell lymphoma in a small minority of patients. These features include positivity for antinuclear antibodies and subsets, hematologic changes (e.g. anemia, neutropenia), renal changes, and positive immunofluorescence test on lesional skin. In these cases we believe that a true association of both diseases exists, rather than a "trans-formation" of lupus erythematosus into subcutaneous T-cell lymphoma. Although patients with lupus erythematosus are at higher risk of developing hematologic malignancies, these are mostly of B-cell phenotype and the true risk (if any) of developing subcutaneous T-cell lymphoma is currently unclear.

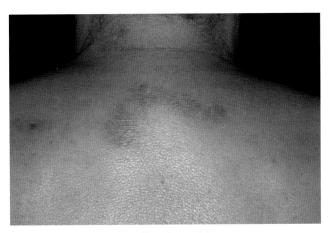

Figure 5.3 Subcutaneous T-cell lymphoma. Subcutaneous tumor on the back.

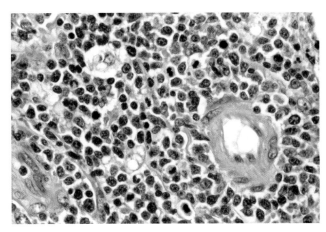

Figure 5.5 Subcutaneous T-cell lymphoma. Infiltration of subcutaneous fat by small- to medium-sized pleomorphic lymphocytes.

Histopathology, immunophenotype and molecular genetics

Histopathology

Histopathology reveals dense, nodular or diffuse infiltrates of small, medium and (rarely) large pleomorphic cells confined to the subcutaneous fat with the pattern of a lobular panniculitis (Figs 5.4, 5.5). Perivascular aggregates of non-neoplastic

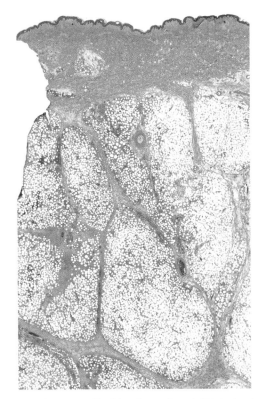

Figure 5.4 Subcutaneous T-cell lymphoma. Dense infiltrate showing prominent involvement of the subcutaneous fat, mimicking the histopathologic picture of a lobular panniculitis.

cells may be located within the reticular dermis, but clusters of neoplastic T lymphocytes are almost never situated outside the subcutaneous tissues. The epidermis is spared as a rule. Neoplastic cells within the subcutaneous fat are arranged in small clusters or as solitary units around the single adipocytes (so-called "rimming" of the adipocytes) (Fig. 5.6). Necrosis is often a prominent feature and may completely mask the specific histopathologic features (Fig. 5.7). A histiocytic infiltrate, often with the formation of granulomas, is also common [54,55]. In addition, reactive small lymphocytes can be admixed with the neoplastic cells but plasma cells and eosinophils are rare. Membranocystic (lipomembranous) lesions have been described in some cases [56,57].

Although "rimming" of adipocytes by neoplastic lymphocytes has been often described as a histopathologic feature diagnostic of subcutaneous "panniculitis-like" T-cell lymphoma, a similar phenomenon can be observed in virtually all lymphomas with prominent involvement of the subcutaneous fat, as well as in reactive subcutaneous infiltrates [58]. In fact,

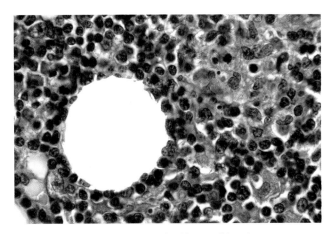

Figure 5.6 Subcutaneous "panniculitis-like" T-cell lymphoma. "Rimming" of an adipocyte by neoplastic lymphocytes. Note pleomorphism of the nuclei.

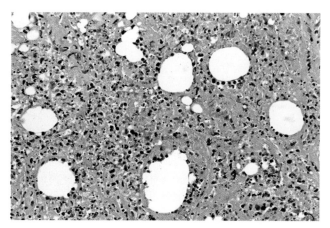

Figure 5.7 Subcutaneous T-cell lymphoma. Prominent necrosis with several atypical lymphocytes left within the infiltrate.

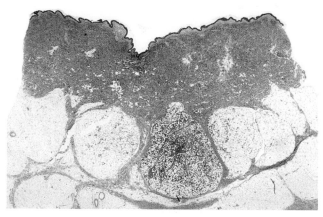

Figure 5.8 Subcutaneous T-cell lymphoma. Focal involvement of the fat restricted to one lobule of adipocytes. According to the patient, this lesion was only a few days old; clinically, the overlying epidermis was normal but one could detect a subcutaneous induration.

we have observed B-cell lymphomas showing both clinical and histopathologic features indistinguishable from those of subcutaneous T-cell lymphoma [41], and only accurate phenotypic investigations could allow a precise diagnosis. Necrosis and degenerative changes within the subcutaneous fat, though a feature often remarkable in subcutaneous T-cell lymphoma, are only rarely found in subcutaneous infiltration of B-cell lymphomas.

In some lesions the specific findings are confined to a small portion of the subcutaneous fat, thus rendering the examination of small biopsies (i.e. punch biopsies) problematic or even impossible (Fig. 5.8). In this context, it must be underlined that a diagnosis of subcutaneous "panniculitis-like" T-cell lymphoma can only be made when large, deep biopsies are available.

In rare cases we have observed conventional lesions of subcutaneous T-cell lymphoma showing changes of interface dermatitis at the dermoepidermal junction. Particularly in these cases, the differential diagnosis from lupus panniculitis is possible only upon precise phenotypic characterization of the subcutaneous infiltrate.

Immunohistology

Immunohistologic analysis shows an α/β T-suppressor phenotype (βF1+, CD3+, CD4−, CD8+) of neoplastic cells (Fig. 5.9a) [39,59,60]. Cytotoxic markers are always expressed (T-cell intracellular antigen (TIA)-1, granzyme B, perforin) [61], but CD56 is negative [4]. Staining for CD30 is consistently negative in true subcutaneous T-cell lymphoma. Proliferation markers (i.e. MIB-1) highlight a characteristic pattern of proliferating cells arranged in small clusters and around the adipocytes (Fig. 5.9b) [60]. *In situ* hybridization for EBV is negative.

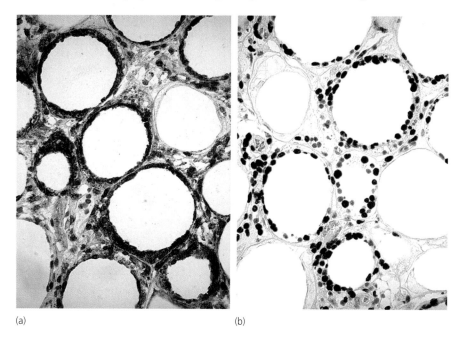

(a)　　　　　　　　(b)

Figure 5.9 Subcutaneous T-cell lymphoma. (a) Staining for CD8 demonstrates positivity of neoplastic lymphocytes around the adipocytes. (b) Staining for proliferating cells (MIB-1) is a helpful diagnostic tool, highlighting proliferating neoplastic lymphocytes around the adipocytes.

It should be emphasized that complete phenotypic analyses should always be performed in cases of malignant lymphoma with prominent involvement of the subcutis, and that only examination of a broad panel of antibodies allows a proper classification of the lesions. In fact, it is not uncommon to observe cases of B-cell lymphoma confined to the subcutaneous fat or cases of other T-cell lymphomas with similar architectural features (i.e. mycosis fungoides, cutaneous anaplastic large cell lymphoma, cutaneous γ/δ T-cell lymphoma, extranodal NK/T-cell lymphoma, nasal type). Cases of T-cell lymphoma with involvement of the subcutaneous tissue and positive for γ/δ T-cell markers or for CD30, or with a positive signal for EBV by *in situ* hybridization, should be more appropriately classified as cutaneous γ/δ T-cell lymphoma, cutaneous anaplastic large cell lymphoma, and extranodal NK/T-cell lymphoma, nasal type, respectively.

Molecular genetics

Molecular analysis of the T-cell receptor (TCR) genes shows a monoclonal rearrangement in the majority of cases [1,2, 62]. Single cell comparative genomic hybridization of laser-microdissected specimens revealed gains of chromosomes 2q and 4q and losses of chromosomes 1pter, 2pter, 10qter, 11qter, 12qter, 16, 19, 20, and 22 [63]. In the same study allelic *NAV3* aberrations were found by loss of heterozygosity and fluorescence *in situ* hybridization analyses in almost half of the cases [63]. It should be underlined that these results have been obtained in nine patients only, so confirmation by larger studies is necessary.

Differential diagnosis with other cutaneous NK and T-cell lymphomas with prominent involvement of the subcutaneous tissue

Rare cases of mycosis fungoides presenting with subcutaneous lesions can only be excluded by an accurate clinical history and by clinicopathologic correlation. In addition, mycosis fungoides usually shows a CD4+ phenotype, in contrast to the CD8+ one of subcutaneous "panniculitis-like" T-cell lymphoma (but a CD4−/CD8− or CD4−/CD8+ phenotype may be encountered in cases of mycosis fungoides). Examination of more than one skin biopsy usually is sufficient for a precise classification, as purely subcutaneous infiltration is only an occasional finding in mycosis fungoides. The following features favor a diagnosis of cutaneous γ/δ T-cell lymphoma: involvement of the dermis and/or epidermis (often with marked epidermotropism) in the same biopsy or in sequential biopsies taken at the same time or over time; negativity for α/β T-cell markers (markers for γ/δ T-cells are available at present only for investigation of frozen sections of tissue); positivity for CD56. Features that favor the diagnosis of extranodal NK/T-cell lymphoma, nasal type, are: marked involvement of the dermis, more rarely also of the epidermis in the same biopsy or in sequential biopsies

taken at the same time or over time; positivity for CD56; positive signal for EBV upon *in situ* hybridization; lack of monoclonal rearrangement of the TCR genes. Finally, features that favor a subcutaneous CD30+ anaplastic large cell lymphoma include presence of large pleomorphic or anaplastic cells strongly positive for CD30 and for CD4; it should be underlined, however, that purely subcutaneous anaplastic large cell lymphomas are exceedingly rare, and that CD30 expression may be observed in neoplastic cells of other T- and B-cell lymphomas, thus implying that such a diagnosis should be made only upon compelling evidence and after careful exclusion of other lymphoproliferative disorders.

Differential diagnosis with lupus panniculitis

As mentioned before, we have come across cases of genuine lupus erythematosus associated with subcutaneous "panniculitis-like" T-cell lymphoma, so evidence of one disease cannot be used to rule out presence of the second. Clinically, both lupus panniculitis and subcutaneous T-cell lymphoma present with panniculitic lesions located mostly on the limbs, thus not allowing a differential diagnosis. Histology also shows more overlapping than distinguishing features (particularly in later lesions!), and necrosis and degenerative changes may be prominent in both diseases. Plasma cells are often present within the inflammatory infiltrate in lupus panniculitis but not in subcutaneous T-cell lymphoma. Another distinguishing feature is the presence in lupus panniculitis of nodular aggregates of B cells, sometimes forming small germinal centers, characteristically located at the periphery of the lobules. We have never encountered similar aggregates in cases of clear-cut subcutaneous T-cell lymphoma. CD3+/CD8+ cells are the hallmark of subcutaneous "panniculitis-like" T-cell lymphoma and may be observed in lupus panniculitis as well, but proliferation rate is lower in the latter. We believe that a useful criterion for differential diagnosis is represented also by the finding in subcutaneous T-cell lymphoma of rimming of lymphocytes that are positive for MIB-1/Ki67. Finally, evidence of a clonal TCR gene rearrangement strongly supports a diagnosis of subcutaneous "panniculitis-like" T-cell lymphoma.

Treatment

Evaluation of different treatment schemes reported in the literature reflects the confusion concerning classification of these cases. In fact, extremely aggressive treatment modalities reported in some cases [64] are probably not necessary for patients with subcutaneous "panniculitis-like" T-cell lymphoma as defined in this chapter and in modern classification schemes. Systemic chemotherapy (CHOP or other schemes) and radiotherapy have been used in many instances [22,35,39,50,65]. Many patients can be controlled for long periods of time with systemic steroids [24]. A combination of steroids and cyclosporin has also been used [66]. Denileukin diftitox (Ontak, DAB_{389}-IL-2 fusion protein) has been used in one case, but phenotypic data were unavailable [67]. Complete remission has been achieved in one of two children treated by cyclosporin followed by chemotherapy [49]. The role of other treatment options (i.e. interferon, retinoids, low-dose methotrexate) has not been evaluated properly.

Recent reports have highlighted the efficacy of autologous or allogenic bone marrow/stem cell transplantation [68–70]. It is currently unclear when such an aggressive therapeutic option should be considered for the management of these patients.

Prognosis

In the past, due to the different classification of cases, it was believed that in most patients the course of subcutaneous "panniculitis-like" T-cell lymphoma is rapidly fatal (we also stated this in the first edition of this book). Recent experience contradicts this and shows that many patients follow a protracted course with recurrent subcutaneous lesions but without extracutaneous spread or hemophagocytic syndrome, indicating that at least two groups of patients with different prognostic features can be identified [24,71]. Once more, exact appreciation of the prognosis of subcutaneous T-cell lymphoma is hindered by the confusion existent in the literature, and by the lack of proper phenotypic investigations performed in many of the reported cases. Applying strictly the diagnostic criteria referred to in this chapter and in current classification schemes, the estimated 5-year survival is over 80% [4]. Angio-invasion has been recognized as a bad prognostic marker in one Chinese study [72].

The onset of a hemophagocytic syndrome is a bad prognostic sign. In the literature, a worse prognosis has been observed in cases characterized by a γ/δ T-cell phenotype or associated with EBV infection [16,24,27,30,37,73]. As already discussed, these cases should be classified as cutaneous γ/δ T-cell lymphoma and extranodal NK/T-cell lymphoma, nasal type, respectively.

Résumé	
Clinical	Adults, rarely children. Localized subcutaneous erythematous plaques and tumors arising preferentially on the extremities. Usually protracted course. In some patients a hemophagocytic syndrome occurs.
Morphology	Dense, nodular or diffuse infiltrates within the subcutaneous fat. "Rimming" of adipocytes by neoplastic lymphocytes. Cytomorphology characterized by small to medium-sized and (rarely) large pleomorphic cells admixed with variable numbers of macrophages. Necrosis prominent.
Immunology	CD2, 3, 5, + CD8 + βF1 + CD4, 30, 56 − TIA-1 +
Genetics	Monoclonal rearrangement of the TCR genes detected in the majority of the cases. No specific genetic alterations repeatably identified.
Treatment guidelines	Systemic steroids may be efficacious; systemic chemotherapy; radiotherapy.

TEACHING CASE

This 22-year-old woman had a long history of recurrent episodes of panniculitis on the limbs that resolved with lipoatrophy, and that was diagnosed as lupus panniculitis (lupus profundus) (Fig. 5.10a). A biopsy showed focal areas of lobular panniculitis (Fig. 5.10b) with prominent atypia of the lymphocytes (Fig. 5.10c). Immunohistologic stainings (performed retrospectively after death of the patient due to hemophagocytic syndrome) revealed the presence of an α/β cytotoxic population of T lymphocytes (Fig. 5.10d: CD8 staining).

Comment: This case shows the overlapping clinicopathologic features between lupus panniculitis and subcutaneous panniculitis-like T-cell lymphoma that can be observed in rare cases. It may be that a small subset of patients suffers from both diseases.

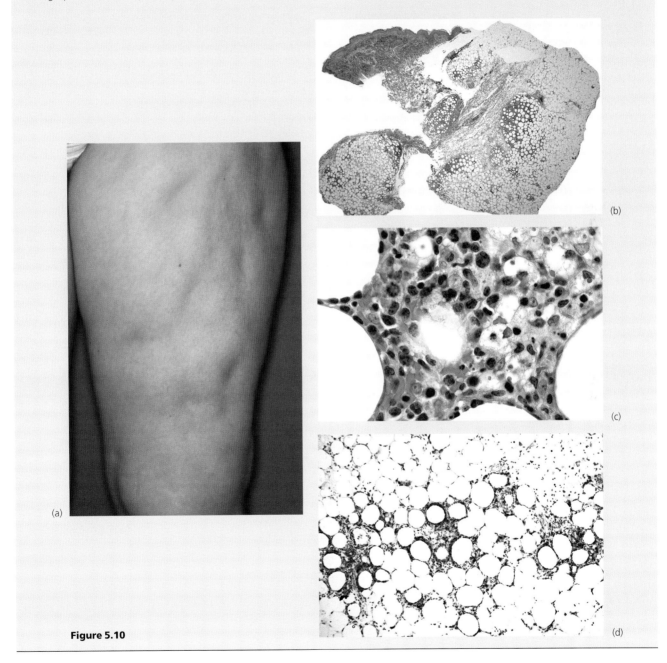

Figure 5.10

References

1. Willemze R, Jaffe ES, Burg G *et al.* WHO-EORTC classification for cutaneous lymphomas. *Blood* 2005;**105**:3768–3785.

2. Jaffe ES, Gaulard P, Ralfkiaer E, Cerroni L, Meijer CJLM. Subcutaneous panniculitis-like T-cell lymphoma. In: Swerdlow SH, Campo E, Harris NL *et al.*, eds. *WHO Classification of Tumours of Haematopoietic and Lymphoid Tissues*. Lyon: IARC Press, 2008: 294–295.

3. Massone C, Lozzi GP, Egberts F *et al.* The protean spectrum of non-Hodgkin lymphomas with prominent involvement of subcutaneous fat. *J Cutan Pathol* 2006;**33**:418–425.

4. Willemze R, Jansen PM, Cerroni L *et al.* Subcutaneous panniculitis-like T-cell lymphoma: definition, classification, and prognostic factors: an EORTC Cutaneous Lymphoma Group Study of 83 cases. *Blood* 2008;**111**:838–845.

5. Winkelmann RK, Bowie EJW. Hemorrhagic diathesis associated with benign histiocytic, cytophagic panniculitis and systemic histiocytosis. *Arch Intern Med* 1980;**140**:1460–1463.

6. Alegre VA, Winkelmann RK. Histiocytic cytophagic panniculitis. *J Am Acad Dermatol* 1989;**20**:177–185.

7. Aronson IK, West DP, Variakojis D *et al.* Panniculitis associated with cutaneous T-cell lymphoma and cytophagocytic histiocytosis. *Br J Dermatol* 1985;**112**:87–96.

8. Barron DR, Davis BR, Pomeranz JR, Hines JD, Park CH. Cytophagic histiocytic panniculitis: a variant of malignant histiocytosis. *Cancer* 1985;**55**:2538–2542.

9. Craig AJ, Cualing H, Thomas G, Lamerson C, Smith R. Cytophagic histiocytic panniculitis: a syndrome associated with benign and malignant panniculitis – case comparison and review of the literature. *J Am Acad Dermatol* 1998;**39**:721–736.

10. Crotty CP, Winkelmann RK. Cytophagic histiocytic panniculitis with fever, cytopenia, liver failure, and terminal hemorrhagic diathesis. *J Am Acad Dermatol* 1981;**4**:181–194.

11. Huilgol SC, Fenton D, Pambakian H *et al.* Fatal cytophagic panniculitis and haemophagocytic syndrome. *Clin Exp Dermatol* 1998;**23**:51–55.

12. Hytiroglou P, Phelps RG, Wattenberg DJ, Strauchen JA. Histiocytic cytophagic panniculitis: molecular evidence for a clonal T-cell disorder. *J Am Acad Dermatol* 1992;**27**:333–336.

13. Willis SM, Opal SM, Fitzpatrick JE. Cytophagic histiocytic panniculitis: systemic histiocytosis presenting as chronic, non-healing, ulcerative skin lesions. *Arch Dermatol* 1985;**121**:910–913.

14. Wick MR, Patterson JW. Cytophagic histiocytic panniculitis: a critical reappraisal. *Arch Dermatol* 2000;**136**:922–924.

15. Wick MR, Sanchez NP, Crotty CP, Winkelmann RK. Cutaneous malignant histiocytosis: a clinical and histopathologic study of eight cases, with immunohistochemical analysis. *J Am Acad Dermatol* 1999;**8**:50–62.

16. Iwatsuki K, Harada H, Ohtsuka M, Han G, Kaneko F. Latent Epstein–Barr virus infection is frequently detected in subcutaneous lymphoma associated with hemophagocytosis but not in non-fatal cytophagic histiocytic panniculitis. *Arch Dermatol* 1997;**133**:787–788.

17. White JW Jr, Winkelmann RK. Cytophagic histiocytic panniculitis is not always fatal. *J Cutan Pathol* 1989;**16**:137–144.

18. Arnulf B, Copie-Bergman C, Delfau-Larue MH *et al.* Nonhepatosplenic γ/δ T-cell lymphoma: a subset of cytotoxic lymphomas with mucosal or skin localization. *Blood* 1998;**91**:1723–1731.

19. Chan JKC. Peripheral T-cell and NK-cell neoplasms: an integrated approach to diagnosis. *Mod Pathol* 1999;**12**:177–199.

20. Kim YC, Kim SC, Yang WI, Go JH, Vandersteen DP. Extranodal NK/T-cell lymphoma with extensive subcutaneous involvement, mimicking subcutaneous panniculitis-like T cell lymphoma. *Int J Dermatol* 2002;**41**:919–921.

21. Munn SE, McGregor JM, Jones A *et al.* Clinical and pathological heterogeneity in cutaneous γ/δ T-cell lymphoma: a report of three cases and a review of the literature. *Br J Dermatol* 1996;**135**:976–981.

22. Santucci M, Pimpinelli N, Massi D *et al.* Cytotoxic natural killer cell cutaneous lymphomas: report of the EORTC cutaneous lymphoma task force workshop. *Cancer* 2003;**97**:610–627.

23. White JW Jr, Winkelmann RK. Weber–Christian panniculitis: a review of 30 cases with this diagnosis. *J Am Acad Dermatol* 1998;**39**:56–62.

24. Hoque SR, Child FJ, Whittaker SJ *et al.* Subcutaneous panniculitis-like T-cell lymphoma: a clinicopathological, immunophenotypic and molecular analysis of six patients. *Br J Dermatol* 2003;**148**:516–525.

25. Magro CM, Crowson AN, Kovatich AJ, Burns F. Lupus profundus, indeterminate lymphocytic lobular panniculitis and subcutaneous T-cell lymphoma: a spectrum of subcuticular T-cell lymphoid dyscrasia. *J Cutan Pathol* 2001;**28**:235–247.

26. Burg G, Dummer R, Wilhelm M *et al.* A subcutaneous δ-positive T cell lymphoma that produces interferon γ. *N Engl J Med* 1991;**325**:1078–1081.

27. Chang SE, Huh J, Choi JH *et al.* Clinicopathological features of CD56 nasal-type T natural killer cell lymphomas with lobular panniculitis. *Br J Dermatol* 2000;**142**:924–930.

28. Dargent JL, Roufosse C, Delville JP *et al.* Subcutaneous panniculitis-like T-cell lymphoma: further evidence for a distinct neoplasm originating from large granular lymphocytes of T/NK phenotype. *J Cutan Pathol* 1998;**25**:394–400.

29. Gonzalez CL, Medeiros LJ, Braziel RM, Jaffe ES. T-cell lymphoma involving subcutaneous tissue: a clinicopathologic entity commonly associated with hemophagocytic syndrome. *Am J Surg Pathol* 1991;**15**:17–27.

30. Avinoach I, Halevy S, Argov S, Sacks M. γ/δ T-cell lymphoma involving the subcutaneous tissue and associated with a hemophagocytic syndrome. *Am J Dermatopathol* 1994;**16**:426–433.

31. Jang KA, Choi JH, Sung KJ *et al.* Primary CD56 nasal-type T natural killer-cell subcutaneous panniculitic lymphoma: presentation as haemophagocytic syndrome. *Br J Dermatol* 1999;**141**:706–709.

32. Kumar S, Krenacs L, Medeiros J *et al.* Subcutaneous panniculitic T-cell lymphoma is a tumor of cytotoxic T lymphocytes. *Hum Pathol* 1998;**29**:397–403.

33. Mehregan DA, Su WPD, Kurtin PJ. Subcutaneous T-cell lymphoma: a clinical, histopathologic, and immunohistochemical study of six cases. *J Cutan Pathol* 1994;**21**:110–117.

34. Monterroso V, Bujan W, Jaramillo O, Medeiros LJ. Subcutaneous tissue involvement by T-cell lymphoma: a report of 2 cases. *Arch Dermatol* 1996;**132**:1345–1350.

35. Perniciaro C, Zalla MJ, White JW Jr, Menke DM. Subcutaneous T cell lymphoma: report of two additional cases and further observations. *Arch Dermatol* 1993;**129**:1171–1176.

36. Romero LS, Goltz RW, Nagi C, Shin SS, Ho AD. Subcutaneous T-cell lymphoma with associated hemophagocytic syndrome and terminal leukemic transformation. *J Am Acad Dermatol* 1996; **34**:904–910.

37. Salhany KE, MacOn WR, Choi JK *et al.* Subcutaneous panniculitis-like T-cell lymphoma: clinicopathologic, immunophenotypic, and genotypic analysis of alpha/beta and gamma/delta subtypes. *Am J Surg Pathol* 1998;**22**:881–893.

38. von den Driesch P, Staib G, Simon M Jr, Sterry W. Subcutaneous T-cell lymphoma. *J Am Acad Dermatol* 1997;**36**:285–289.

39. Wang CY, Su WP, Kurtin PJ. Subcutaneous panniculitic T-cell lymphoma. *Int J Dermatol* 1996;**35**:1–8.

40. Marzano AV, Berti E, Paulli M, Caputo R. Cytophagic histiocytic panniculitis and subcutaneous panniculitis-like T-cell lymphoma. *Arch Dermatol* 2000;**136**:889–896.

41. Cerroni L. Subcutaneous immunocytoma. *Dermatopathol Pract Concept* 2000;**6**:87–88.

42. Marzano AV, Alessi E, Berti E. CD30-positive multilobated peripheral T-cell lymphoma primarily involving the subcutaneous tissue. *Am J Dermatopathol* 1997;**19**:284–288.

43. Kinney MC. The role of morphologic features, phenotype, genotype, and anatomic site in defining extranodal T-cell or NK-cell neoplasms. *Am J Clin Pathol* 1999;**111**:S104–118.

44. Proctor MS, Price NM, Cox AJ, Hoppe RT. Subcutaneous mycosis fungoides. *Arch Dermatol* 1978;**114**:1326–1328.

45. Berg KD, Brinster NK, Huhn KM *et al.* Transmission of a T-cell lymphoma by allogeneic bone marrow transplantation. *N Engl J Med* 2001;**345**:1458–1463.

46. Bragman SG, Yeaney GA, Greig BW, Vnencak-Jones CL, Hamilton KS. Subcutaneous panniculitic T-cell lymphoma in a cardiac allograft recipient. *J Cutan Pathol* 2005;**32**:366–370.

47. Fink-Puches R, Zenahlik P, Bäck B *et al.* Primary cutaneous lymphomas: applicability of current classification schemes (European Organization for Research and Treatment of Cancer, World Health Organization) based on clinicopathologic features observed in a large group of patients. *Blood* 2002;**99**:800–805.

48. Taniguchi S, Kono T. Subcutaneous T-cell lymphoma in a child with eosinophilia. *Br J Dermatol* 2000;**142**:183–184.

49. Shani-Adir A, Lucky AW, Prendiville J *et al.* Subcutaneous panniculitic T-cell lymphoma in children: response to combination therapy with cyclosporine and chemotherapy. *J Am Acad Dermatol* 2004;**50**:s18–22.

50. Au WY, Ng WM, Choy C, Kwong YL. Aggressive subcutaneous panniculitis-like T-cell lymphoma: complete remission with fludarabine, mitoxantrone and dexamethasone. *Br J Dermatol* 2000;**143**:408–410.

51. Török L, Gurbity TP, Kirschner A, Krenacs L. Panniculitis-like T-cell lymphoma clinically manifested as alopecia. *Br J Dermatol* 2002;**147**:785–788.

52. Weenig RH, Su WPD. Subcutaneous panniculitis-like T-cell lymphoma presenting as venous stasis ulceration. *Int J Dermatol* 2006;**45**:1083–1085.

53. Nishie W, Yokota K, Sawamura D *et al.* Detection of circulating lymphoma cells in subcutaneous panniculitis-like T-cell lymphoma. *Br J Dermatol* 2003;**149**:1081–1082.

54. Scarabello A, Leinweber B, Ardigó M *et al.* Cutaneous lymphomas with prominent granulomatous reaction. A potential pitfall in the histopathologic diagnosis of cutaneous T- and B-cell lymphomas. *Am J Surg Pathol* 2002;**26**:1259–1268.

55. Prescott RJ, Banerjee SS, Cross PA. Subcutaneous T-cell lymphoma with florid granulomatous panniculitis. *Histopathology* 1992;**20**:535–537.

56. Ohtake N, Shimada S, Mizoguchi S, Setoyama M, Kanzaki T. Membranocystic lesions in a patient with cytophagic histiocytic panniculitis associated with subcutaneous T-cell lymphoma. *Am J Dermatopathol* 1998;**20**:276–280.

57. Weenig RH, Ng CS, Perniciaro C. Subcutaneous panniculitis-like T-cell lymphoma. An elusive case presenting as lipomembranous panniculitis and a review of 72 cases in the literature. *Am J Dermatopathol* 2001;**23**:206–215.

58. Lozzi GP, Massone C, Citarella L, Kerl H, Cerroni L. Rimming of adipocytes by neoplastic lymphocytes. A histopathologic feature not restricted to subcutaneous T-cell lymphoma. *Am J Dermatopathol* 2006;**28**:9–12.

59. El-Shabrawi-Caelen L, Cerroni L, Kerl H. The clinicopathologic spectrum of cytotoxic lymphomas of the skin. *Sem Cutan Med Surg* 2000;**19**:118–123.

60. Cerroni L, Kerl H. Diagnostic immunohistology: cutaneous lymphomas and pseudolymphomas. *Sem Cutan Med Surg* 1999;**18**: 64–70.

61. Felgar RE, MacOn WR, Kinney MC, Roberts S, Pasha T, Salhany KE. TIA-1 expression in lymphoid neoplasms. Identification of subsets with cytotoxic T lymphocyte or natural killer cell differentiation. *Am J Pathol* 1997;**150**:1893–1900.

62. Kadin ME. Genetic and molecular genetic studies in the diagnosis of T-cell malignancies. *Hum Pathol* 2003;**34**:322–329.

63. Hahtola S, Burghart E, Jeskanen L *et al.* Clinicopathological characterization and genomic aberrations in subcutaneous panniculitis-like T-cell lymphoma. *J Invest Dermatol* 2008;**128**: 2304–2309.

64. Haycox CL, Back AL, Raugi GJ, Piepkorn M. Subcutaneous T-cell lymphoma treated with systemic chemotherapy, autologous stem cell support, and limb amputation. *J Am Acad Dermatol* 1997;**37**:832–835.

65. McGinnis KS, Shapiro M, Junkins-Hopkins JM *et al.* Denileukin diftitox for the treatment of panniculitic lymphoma. *Arch Dermatol* 2002;**138**:740–742.

66. Tsukamoto Y, Katsumobu Y, Omura Y *et al.* Subcutaneous panniculitis-like T-cell lymphoma: Successful initial treatment with prednisolone and cyclosporin A. *Intern Med* 2006;**45**:21–24.

67. Cho KH, Oh JK, Kim CW, Heo DS, Kim ST. Peripheral T-cell lymphoma involving subcutaneous tissue. *Br J Dermatol* 1995; **132**:290–295.

68. Alaibac M, Berti E, Pigozzi B *et al.* High-dose chemotherapy with autologous blood stem cell transplantation for aggressive subcutaneous panniculitis-like T-cell lymphoma. *J Am Acad Dermatol* 2005;**52**:s121–s123.

69. Ichii M, Hatanaka K, Imakita M, Ueda Y, Kishino B, Tamaki T. Successful treatment of refractory subcutaneous panniculitis-like T-cell lymphoma with allogeneic peripheral blood stem cell transplantation from HLA-mismatched sibling donor. *Leukem Lymph* 2006;**47**:2250–2252.

70. Perez-Persona E, Mateos-Mazon JJ, Lopez-Villar O *et al.* Complete remission of subcutaneous panniculitic T-cell lymphoma after allogeneic transplantation. *Bone Marrow Transpl* 2006;**38**:821–822.

71. Burg G, Dummer R, Nestle F. Distinct subtypes of subcutaneous T-cell lymphoma. *Arch Dermatol* 1994;**130**:1073.

72. Kong YY, Dai B, Kong JC *et al.* Subcutaneous panniculitis-like T-cell lymphoma. A clinicopathologic, immunophenotypic, and molecular study of 22 Asian cases according to WHO-EORTC classification. *Am J Surg Pathol* 2008;**32**:1495–1502.

73. Abe Y, Muta K, Ohshima K *et al.* Subcutaneous panniculitis by Epstein–Barr virus-infected natural killer (NK) cell proliferation terminating in aggressive subcutaneous NK cell lymphoma. *Am J Hematol* 2000;**64**:221–225.

6 Aggressive cutaneous cytotoxic lymphomas

Cytotoxic lymphomas are tumors derived from T or natural killer (NK) lymphocytes with a cytotoxic phenotype. Neoplastic cells typically express at least one cytotoxic protein such as T-cell intracellular antigen (TIA)-1, granzyme B, or perforin [1–7]. The World Health Organization (WHO)-European Organization for Research and Treatment of Cancer (EORTC) classification of primary cutaneous lymphomas lists them as distinct (extranodal NK/T-cell lymphoma, nasal type) or provisional entities (cutaneous γ/δ T-cell lymphoma, primary cutaneous aggressive epidermotropic CD8$^+$ cytotoxic T-cell lymphoma) [8]. The new WHO classification of tumors of hematopoietic and lymphoid tissues recognizes the first two as distinct and the last as provisional entities, and includes hydroa vacciniforme-like lymphoma as a provisional entity as well [9–11].

Although cytotoxic NK/T-cell lymphomas are commonly described as aggressive neoplasms, the expression of cytotoxic proteins themselves is not restricted to a specific group of lymphomas as they can be observed in many different cases, including mycosis fungoides (rarely in early lesions, more commonly in late stages of the disease) (see Chapter 2) and cutaneous CD30$^+$ lymphoproliferative disorders (see Chapter 4), among others. Expression of cytotoxic proteins is also the rule in cases of subcutaneous "panniculitis-like" T-cell lymphoma (see Chapter 5). In short, cytotoxic proteins do not have any diagnostic or prognostic value *per se*, and their expression should be evaluated in the context of the clinicopathologic and molecular features of the lesions. It has been shown that the expression of cytotoxic proteins and inhibitory receptors varies in different types of cytotoxic lymphomas, suggesting that they may differ with regard to their functional profiles [12].

We would also like to stress that these lymphomas show many overlapping clinicopathologic features, and that classification may be subjective in some cases. In particular, distinction from mycosis fungoides and from subcutaneous

Skin Lymphoma: The Illustrated Guide. By L. Cerroni, K. Gatter and H. Kerl. Published 2009 Blackwell Publishing, ISBN: 978-1-4051-8554-7.

"panniculitis-like" T-cell lymphoma can be difficult (see Chapters 2 and 5), and often impossible without proper history and complete clinical information. Moreover, in spite of extensive phenotypic and genotypic studies, a few cases defy precise classification [13].

It is important to underline that for most of these lymphomas cytomorphologic features are variable and are not associated with prognostic features. In addition, cytomorphology is similar in all these entities, and may be characterized by predominance of small-, medium- or large-sized cells (usually with pleomorphic nuclei). Thus, cytomorphologic aspects are neither useful for a specific diagnosis and classification of the lymphoma, nor are a feature associated with the biologic behavior, and should always be analyzed together with all other clinical, histopathologic, phenotypic, and molecular genetic features.

Finally, it should be emphasized that distinguishing between primary and secondary cutaneous involvement is less important for this group of tumors than for most other skin lymphomas [7,14]. In fact, cases with a primary cutaneous presentation often develop extracutaneous dissemination within a short period of time, and prognosis is usually very poor regardless of the results of staging investigations at presentation.

PRIMARY CUTANEOUS AGGRESSIVE EPIDERMOTROPIC CD8$^+$ CYTOTOXIC T-CELL LYMPHOMA

Primary cutaneous aggressive epidermotropic CD8$^+$ cytotoxic T-cell lymphoma is a disease characterized by aggressive behavior clinically and proliferation of epidermotropic CD8$^+$ T lymphocytes histopathologically [15]. Distinction from the rare cases of CD8$^+$ mycosis fungoides (see Chapter 2) and from a rare variant of lymphomatoid papulosis (CD8$^+$ pagetoid reticulosis-like lymphomatoid papulosis – see Chapter 4) is made mainly on the basis of the clinical presentation and behavior. In contrast to mycosis fungoides, patients with primary cutaneous aggressive epidermotropic CD8$^+$ cytotoxic T-cell lymphoma present with plaques and tumors, often ulcerated, at the onset of their disease [15–17].

In the past, cases of primary cutaneous aggressive epidermotropic CD8+ cytotoxic T-cell lymphoma were classified as either aggressive mycosis fungoides or generalized pagetoid reticulosis (Ketron–Goodman type), or mycosis fungoides "a tumeur d'emblee." In both the WHO-EORTC and the WHO 2008 classifications, this lymphoma is listed as a provisional entity [8,9]. Pediatric patients with a clinical presentation resembling hydroa vacciniforme would be better classified as hydroa vacciniforme-like lymphoma (see Chapter 6).

Clinical features

Patients are usually adults of both sexes possibly with a slight male predominance [5,15]. They present with generalized patches, plaques and tumors, almost invariably with ulceration (Figs 6.1, 6.2). The clinical features are indistinguishable from those observed in patients with cutaneous γ/δ-positive

T-cell lymphoma, and are identical to those of generalized pagetoid reticulosis (and of advanced mycosis fungoides). Involvement of the mucosal regions is common [15,18]. The tumor often spreads to the central nervous system [15].

For a diagnosis of primary cutaneous aggressive epidermotropic CD8+ cytotoxic T-cell lymphoma it is crucial to exclude a history of mycosis fungoides. Lesions of lymphomatoid papulosis with a CD8+ phenotype should also be ruled out clinically (see Chapter 4).

Histopathology, immunophenotype and molecular genetics

Histopathology
Histology reveals a nodular or diffuse proliferation of lymphocytes, usually with marked epidermotropism (Fig. 6.3). In spite of the name of this lymphoma, the epidermotropism may be less pronounced in some lesions, especially in advanced stages (Fig. 6.4). As in all aggressive cutaneous lymphomas, invasion and destruction of adnexal skin structures are common (Fig. 6.5). Cytomorphology is variable and can be characterized by small-, medium- or large-sized pleomorphic cells (Fig. 6.6). Some cases may show a predominance of immunoblasts. Intraepidermal vesiculation and necrosis can be seen. Angiocentricity and angiodestruction are uncommon.

As discussed before, cases of CD8+ T-cell lymphoma with exclusive involvement of the subcutis should be classified as subcutaneous "panniculitis-like" T-cell lymphomas. Distinction of primary cutaneous aggressive epidermotropic CD8+ cytotoxic T-cell lymphoma from cutaneous γ/δ T-cell lymphoma is difficult and often determined on an arbitrary basis. Cases with a γ/δ phenotype usually show a more prominent involvement of the subcutaneous fat than those of primary

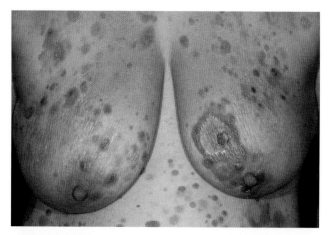

Figure 6.1 Cutaneous aggressive epidermotropic CD8+ cytotoxic T-cell lymphoma. Multiple papules, plaques, flat tumors and ulcerated lesions.

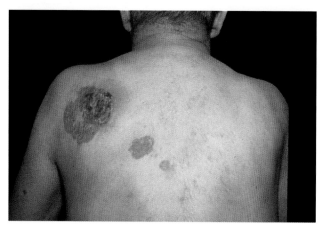

Figure 6.2 Cutaneous aggressive epidermotropic CD8 cytotoxic T-cell lymphoma. Multiple plaques and flat tumors with large erosions. The clinical presentation is identical to that described in the past as generalized pagetoid reticulosis (Ketron–Goodman type).

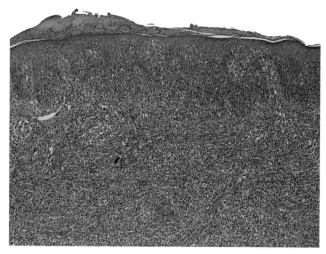

Figure 6.3 Cutaneous aggressive epidermotropic CD8+ cytotoxic T-cell lymphoma. Hyperplastic epidermis with many epidermotropic lymphocytes and diffuse lymphoid infiltrates in the dermis.

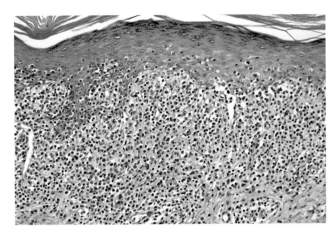

Figure 6.4 Cutaneous aggressive epidermotropic CD8 cytotoxic T-cell lymphoma. Epidermotropism is less marked in this case.

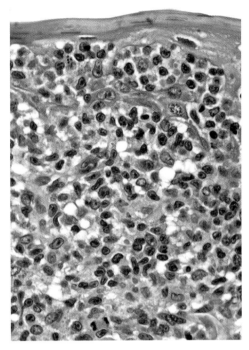

Figure 6.6 Cutaneous aggressive epidermotropic CD8 cytotoxic T-cell lymphoma. Medium–large pleomorphic lymphocytes with epidermotropism.

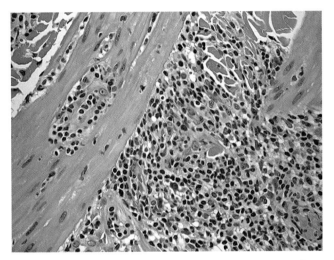

Figure 6.5 Cutaneous aggressive epidermotropic CD8 cytotoxic T-cell lymphoma. Pleomorphic lymphocytes predominate. Note invasion of a smooth muscle.

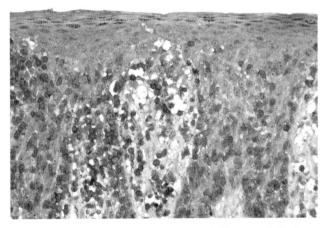

Figure 6.7 Cutaneous aggressive epidermotropic CD8 cytotoxic T-cell lymphoma. Staining for CD8 highlights the epidermotropic lymphocytes.

cutaneous aggressive epidermotropic CD8$^+$ cytotoxic T-cell lymphoma. Another differential feature is the presence of a marked interface dermatitis in many cases of cutaneous γ/δ T-cell lymphoma. However, it remains to be determined whether or not these two diseases represent phenotypic variations of the same entity of aggressive cutaneous cytotoxic T-cell lymphoma.

Immunophenotype

Immunohistology reveals a characteristic phenotypic profile of neoplastic lymphocytes (βF1$^+$, CD2$^{-/+}$, CD3$^+$, CD4$^-$, CD7$^+$, CD8$^+$, TIA-1$^+$, CD45Ra$^+$, CD45RO$^-$) (Fig. 6.7) [15]. Some pan-T-cell markers may be lost. In the original description by Berti *et al.*, CD56 was consistently negative [15], but CD56$^+$ cases classified as cutaneous aggressive epidermotropic CD8$^+$ cytotoxic T-cell lymphoma have been described by Santucci

et al. [2]. However, in this study cutaneous γ/δ T-cell lymphoma was not included as a specific category, and it may be that these cases represented examples of this type of lymphoma with CD8 positivity.

The Epstein–Barr virus (EBV) is not detectable in neoplastic cells.

Molecular genetics

Molecular biology shows a monoclonal rearrangement of the T-cell receptor (TCR) gene. No specific genetic alterations have been identified.

Treatment

As the disease is very rare, data on therapy are lacking, and double-blinded studies have not been carried out. At present the treatment of choice is systemic chemotherapy. The role of bone marrow or stem cell transplantation has not been evaluated.

Prognosis

The prognosis of patients with primary cutaneous aggressive epidermotropic CD8+ cytotoxic T-cell lymphoma is poor, and the estimated 5-year survival is 0% [5,8,15]. The disease often metastasizes to unusual sites such as the lung, testis and central nervous system.

Résumé

Primary cutaneous aggressive epidermotropic CD8+ cytotoxic T-cell lymphoma

Clinical	Adults. Generalized plaques and tumors, commonly ulcerated. Aggressive course. Involvement of mucosal sites common. No previous history of mycosis fungoides.
Morphology	Nodular or diffuse infiltrates characterized by small-, medium- or large-sized pleomorphic cells or immunoblasts. Prominent epidermotropism (may be lacking in some lesions).
Immunology	CD3, 7, 8, 45Ra + βF1 + CD4, 30 – CD56 – TIA-1 +
Genetics	Monoclonal rearrangement of the TCR genes detected in the majority of the cases. No specific genetic alteration identified yet.
Treatment guidelines	Systemic chemotherapy.

PRIMARY CUTANEOUS γ/δ T-CELL LYMPHOMA

Primary cutaneous γ/δ T-cell lymphoma is a tumor of γ/δ T lymphocytes with specific tropism for the skin [19–24]. The precise definition and characterization of this lymphoma are hindered by the overlapping features with many other cutaneous lymphoma entities, especially with subcutaneous "panniculitis-like" T-cell lymphoma and primary cutaneous aggressive epidermotropic CD8+ cytotoxic T-cell lymphoma (see Chapter 5 and previous section of this chapter). Even the existence of cutaneous γ/δ T-cell lymphoma as a specific entity is debated [25–27]. Cutaneous γ/δ T-cell lymphoma is included as a provisional entity in the WHO-EORTC classification, and as a distinct entity in the WHO 2008 classification [8,9].

A major problem for the precise characterization of this rare lymphoma is the lack of a reliable marker of γ/δ T-lymphocytes on routinely fixed, paraffin-embedded sections of tissue. The immunohistochemical marker δ1 works only on frozen material, thus hindering the evaluation of routine specimens. At present, cutaneous γ/δ T-cell lymphoma is often a diagnosis of exclusion, supported by negativity for βF1, a marker of α/β T-lymphocytes. However, βF1 expression may be lost by neoplastic α/β T lymphocytes.

In the past, cases of cutaneous γ/δ T-cell lymphoma were classified as either aggressive mycosis fungoides or generalized pagetoid reticulosis (Ketron–Goodman type), or mycosis fungoides "a tumeur d'emblee" [7,28]. Distinction from classic mycosis fungoides with a rare γ/δ T-cell phenotype (see Chapter 2) is made exclusively on the basis of the clinical presentation and behavior. In fact, in contrast to "classic" mycosis fungoides, patients with cutaneous γ/δ T-cell lymphoma present at the onset with rapidly growing, disseminated patches, plaques and tumors which are often ulcerated. For cutaneous T-cell lymphomas characterized by a proliferation of γ/δ T lymphocytes, as for cutaneous T-cell lymphomas with CD8 positivity, two main subtypes have been identified in the literature, the first characterized by rapidly progressive disease and poor prognosis (representing true cutaneous γ/δ T-cell lymphoma), the second showing a chronic course and better prognosis (this last representing mycosis fungoides with γ/δ phenotype) [27]. It must be stressed that the importance of an α/β versus a γ/δ T-cell subset antigen expression in the classification of peripheral T-cell lymphomas is still unclear.

Due to the frequent prominent involvement of subcutaneous tissues, many cases of cutaneous γ/δ T-cell lymphoma are incorrectly classified as subcutaneous "panniculitis-like" T-cell lymphoma (see Chapter 5). However, γ/δ T-cell lymphoma almost invariably shows prominent involvement of the epidermis either in the same biopsy specimen or in other biopsies taken at the same time or during the course of the disease. A typical example is represented by the patient pictured in Figure 6.8, who was included in the chapter on subcutaneous T-cell lymphomas in the first edition of this book (old figures 7.1, 7.2). The same patient was included as an example of "malignant histiocytosis" in the book on cutaneous lymphomas by Burg and Braun-Falco in 1983 [29]. This case clearly shows how these unusual lymphomas are reclassified over time, thanks to new phenotypic and molecular studies that allow us to define more specific categories and to classify the cases more precisely. As discussed previously, we believe that cutaneous γ/δ T-cell lymphoma should

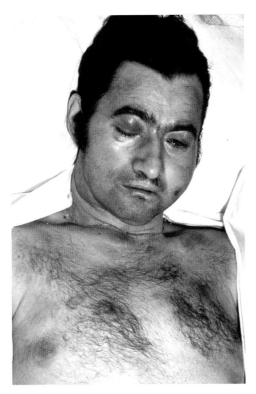

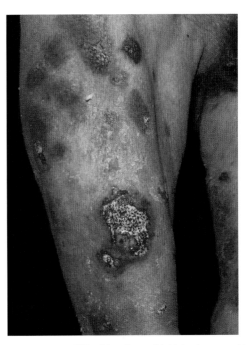

Figure 6.9 Cutaneous γ/δ T-cell lymphoma. Multiple plaques and tumors, some ulcerated, on the leg.

Figure 6.8 Cutaneous γ/δ T-cell lymphoma. Multiple erythematous plaques and tumors on the trunk and face. Histopathologic features of two lesions from this patient are depicted in Figs 6.12 and 6.13. This patient was included within the "subcutaneous T-cell lymphomas" in the first edition of our book (Figs 7.1, 7.2 of that edition), but reclassification of skin biopsies revealed the typical features of cutaneous γ/δ T-cell lymphoma.

be distinguished and separated from the less aggressive subcutaneous "panniculitis-like" T-cell lymphoma, and these disorders are classified separately in modern classification schemes [8,9].

Clinical features

Patients are adults, with an equal distribution of males and females. They present with generalized patches, plaques and tumors, which are often ulcerated (Figs 6.8, 6.9). Large, solitary tumors may also be seen. The clinical features are similar to those observed in patients with primary cutaneous aggressive epidermotropic CD8+ cytotoxic T-cell lymphoma. The patches of the disease, unlike the common patches of mycosis fungoides, reveal the clinical features of severe interface dermatitis with a red-brown aspect and small superficial erosions (Fig. 6.10). Involvement of the mucosal regions and other locations unusual for mycosis fungoides is common (Fig. 6.11). Hemophagocytic syndrome is a frequent complication.

For a diagnosis of cutaneous γ/δ T-cell lymphoma it is crucial to exclude a history of mycosis fungoides.

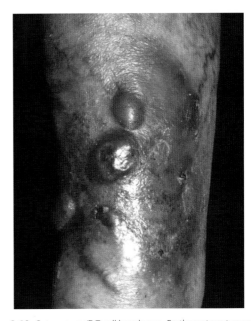

Figure 6.10 Cutaneous γ/δ T-cell lymphoma. Erythematous tumors surrounded by red–brownish flat lesions resembling clinically lesions of severe interface dermatitis.

Histopathology, immunophenotype and molecular genetics

Histopathology

Histology reveals a proliferation of lymphocytes, usually with both marked epidermotropism and involvement of the subcutaneous tissues (Figs 6.12, 6.13). Cytomorphology is variable

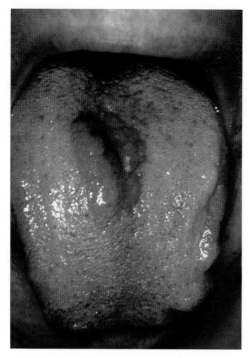

Figure 6.11 Cutaneous γ/δ T-cell lymphoma. Large tumor on the tongue.

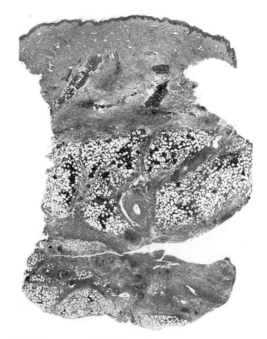

Figure 6.13 Cutaneous γ/δ T-cell lymphoma. Prominent involvement of the subcutaneous fat (same patient as Figs 6.8 and 6.12).

and can be characterized by small-, medium- or large-sized pleomorphic cells (Fig. 6.14). Intraepidermal vesiculation and necrosis can be seen. Angiocentricity and/or angiodestruction are commonly seen (Fig. 6.15). The presence of large macrophages engulfing neoplastic lymphocytes or other blood cells can be seen in cases with a hemophagocytic syndrome (Fig. 6.16).

Although epidermotropic lesions may resemble those observed in mycosis fungoides, unlike mycosis fungoides cutaneous γ/δ T-cell lymphoma is often characterized by the presence within the papillary dermis of prominent edema rather than of fibrosis and coarse bundles of collagen (see Fig. 6.12), probably reflecting the different biology of the

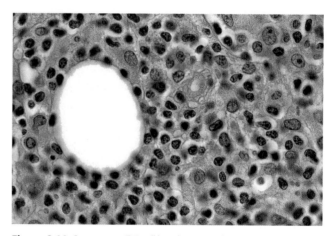

Figure 6.14 Cutaneous γ/δ T-cell lymphoma. Predominance of medium- and large-sized lymphocytes.

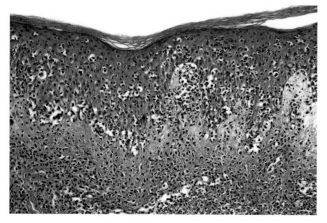

Figure 6.12 Cutaneous γ/δ T-cell lymphoma. Markedly epidermotropic infiltrate. Note edema of the papillary dermis (same patient as Figs 6.8 and 6.13).

lesions (acute, rapid onset in cutaneous γ/δ T-cell lymphoma, chronic lesions in mycosis fungoides).

As discussed previously in this chapter, the distinction of cutaneous γ/δ T-cell lymphoma from primary cutaneous aggressive epidermotropic CD8⁺ cytotoxic T-cell lymphoma is difficult, and can be subjective. We prefer to classify lesions with γ/δ T-cell phenotype as cutaneous γ/δ T-cell lymphoma; these cases usually show a more prominent involvement of the subcutaneous fat than those of primary cutaneous aggressive epidermotropic CD8⁺ cytotoxic T-cell lymphoma. Another differential feature is the presence of a marked interface dermatitis in many cases of cutaneous γ/δ T-cell lymphoma, but not in those of primary cutaneous aggressive epidermotropic CD8⁺ cytotoxic T-cell lymphoma.

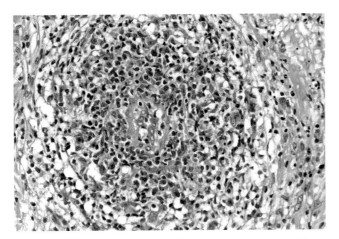

Figure 6.15 Cutaneous γ/δ T-cell lymphoma. Prominent angiocentricity with early angiodestruction. Note pleomorphic lymphocytes.

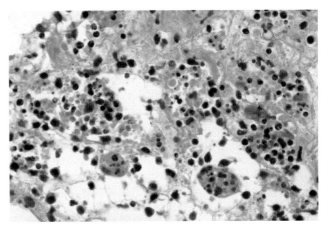

Figure 6.16 Cutaneous γ/δ T-cell lymphoma. Hemophagocytosis characterized by large histiocytes engulfing leukocytes. This histopathologic feature may be associated with overt hemophagocytic syndrome.

Immunophenotype

Immunohistology reveals a characteristic phenotypic profile of neoplastic lymphocytes (βF1$^-$, CD3$^+$, TIA-1$^+$, CD56$^+$, CD57$^-$) (Fig. 6.17). CD4 is absent though CD8 may be expressed in some cases. Immunohistology on frozen sections reveals positivity for δ1. Some pan-T-cell markers may be lost.

The Epstein–Barr virus (EBV) is not present in the neoplastic cells.

Molecular genetics

Molecular biology shows a monoclonal rearrangement of the TCR genes. A recent molecular study demonstrated that γ/δ T-cell lymphomas (including both cutaneous and extracutaneous forms) have a different molecular profile than

α/β T-cell lymphomas [30]. γ/δ T-cell lymphomas revealed overexpression of genes of NK-cell–associated molecules, such as killer cell immunoglobulin–like receptor (KIR) genes (KIR3DL1, KIR2DL4, and KIR2DL2), and killer cell lectin-like receptors (KLRC4, KLRD1, and KLRC2). In the same study it was shown that hepatosplenic γ/δ T-cell lymphoma represents a distinct subset of lymphoma distinct from other γ/δ T-cell lymphomas arising at other sites, including the skin [30].

Treatment

As already discussed for primary cutaneous aggressive epidermotropic CD8$^+$ cytotoxic T-cell lymphoma, data on therapy

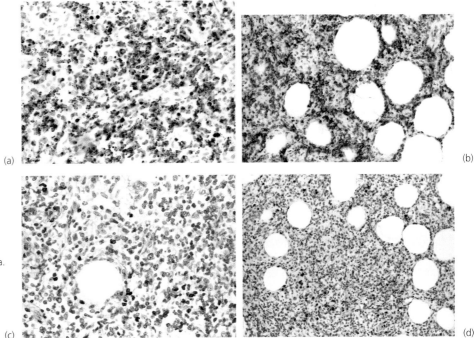

Figure 6.17 Cutaneous γ/δ T-cell lymphoma. Neoplastic cells are positive for TIA-1 (a) and CD56 (b), negative for βF1 (c) and CD8 (d). The few positive cells in plates (c) and (d) represent internal positive controls (reactive lymphocytes).

(a)
(b)
(c)
(d)

are lacking and double-blinded studies have not been carried out. At present the treatment of choice is systemic chemotherapy. The role of bone marrow or stem cell transplantation has not been evaluated.

Prognosis

The prognosis of patients with cutaneous γ/δ T-cell lymphoma is poor. Occasional patients may show a prolonged course [31]. It has been suggested that expression of the γ/δ phenotype is a bad prognostic indicator in cutaneous T-cell lymphomas, irrespective of the classification [32]. However, in our experience a cytotoxic phenotype does not have prognostic implications in mycosis fungoides (see Chapter 2) [33]. In patients with cutaneous γ/δ T-cell lymphoma, involvement of the subcutaneous fat tissues seems to be a bad prognostic factor [32]. However, as already discussed, in the heterogeneous and confusing group of cutaneous cytotoxic NK/T-cell lymphomas, prognostic features of cases reported in the literature may be related to mistakes in the classification rather than to genuine features of the neoplasms described.

It has recently been proposed that expression of human leukocyte antigen G (HLA-G) and of interleukin 10 (IL-10) may be one of the factors accounting for evasion of immunosurveillance by neoplastic cells in CD8+ and CD56+ cutaneous T-cell lymphomas, thus contributing to their aggressive behavior [34].

Résumé		
Cutaneous g/δ T-cell lymphoma		
Clinical	Adults, rarely children. Generalized plaques and tumors, commonly ulcerated. Aggressive course. No previous history of mycosis fungoides.	
Morphology	Nodular or diffuse infiltrates characterized by small/medium- to large-sized pleomorphic cells. Subcutaneous fat commonly involved. Prominent epidermotropism.	
Immunology	CD3, 5,	+
	δ1 (frozen)	+
	βF1	–
	CD4, 30	–
	CD8	–(+)
	TIA-1	+
Genetics	Monoclonal rearrangement of the TCR-γ gene detected in the majority of the cases. Overexpression of NK-cell-associated molecules; genetic differences from α/β T-cell lymphomas.	
Treatment guidelines	Systemic chemotherapy.	

EXTRANODAL NK/T-CELL LYMPHOMA, NASAL TYPE

Extranodal NK/T-cell lymphoma, nasal type, is a well-defined cytotoxic lymphoma [8,10,35]. This lymphoma is commonly located in the upper respiratory tract, especially the nasal cavity, but involvement of other organs can be observed, particularly the skin. The disease may be primary cutaneous, that is, staging investigations can be negative at presentation [2,7, 36,37]. It is more common in particular areas of the globe such as Asia, Mexico, and Central and South America.

In the past, similar cases were reported as "lethal midline granuloma" or "granuloma gangrenescens" [38–41]. Over many years, it has become recognized that lethal midline granuloma is a term encompassing various diseases with different etiologies and pathogenesis, and that the majority of cases are associated with EBV, have a lymphoid differentiation, and an aggressive course [42–46]. Lethal midline granuloma represents direct extension of the lymphoma from the nasal cavity to the overlying skin, with destruction of the bone and soft tissues. Some cases of extranodal NK/T-cell lymphoma, nasal type, were also included in the past in the groups of angiocentric lymphoma and polymorphic reticulosis [47,48].

As for all lymphomas listed in this chapter, overlapping clinicopathologic features are common and classification can be arbitrary. Most cases have an NK phenotype and are associated with EBV infection [6]. Negativity for T-cell markers and germline rearrangement of T lymphocytes, together with positivity for EBV in neoplastic cells, should be interpreted as a strong hint towards a diagnosis of extranodal NK/T cell lymphoma, nasal type.

Clinical features

Patients are adults with a predominance of males. Children are rarely affected [49]. The skin lesions are erythematous or violaceous plaques and tumors, which are sometimes ulcerated (Fig. 6.18). The oral cavity and upper respiratory tract should be checked carefully at presentation and during follow-up, as involvement of these regions is common. Symptoms of nasal obstruction and/or epistaxis should be thoroughly investigated for evidence of nasal lymphoma. The variant described in the past as lethal midline granuloma is associated with large ulcers of the nose and adjacent tissues (Figs 6.19, 6.20). Hemophagocytic syndrome is a possible complication.

Besides conventional presentation with plaques and tumors, we have observed rarely young patients who presented with marked swelling of the head and neck area that at biopsy represented a specific infiltrate of extranodal NK/T-cell lymphoma, nasal-type. The clinical impression was that of edematous swelling but the lesions did not resolve with conventional

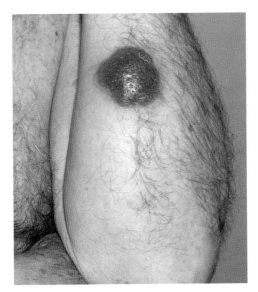

Figure 6.18 Extranodal NK/T-cell lymphoma, nasal type. Erythematous tumor on the arm. The patient had more tumors on the upper and lower extremities. (Courtesy of Esmeralda Vale, Lisboa, Portugal.)

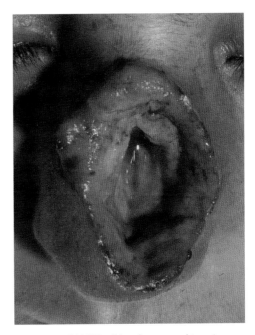

Figure 6.20 Extranodal NK/T-cell lymphoma, nasal type. Large ulcerated tumor on the nose in a 15-year-old girl (so-called "lethal midline granuloma," late lesion).

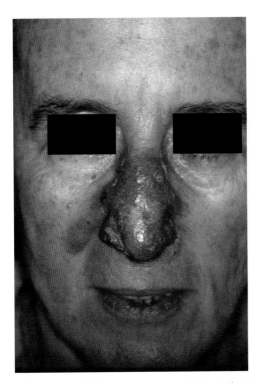

Figure 6.19 Extranodal NK/T-cell lymphoma, nasal type. Erythematous, partly crusted plaques on the nose and cheek (so-called "lethal midline granuloma," early lesion).

treatment, and histologic examination revealed an aggressive lymphoma.

In some cases of extranodal NK/T-cell lymphoma, nasal type, the clinical features of cutaneous manifestations can be similar to those seen in mycosis fungoides, and only phenotypic and molecular analyses allow these cases to be classified

correctly. An accurate clinical history to rule out mycosis fungoides is mandatory before establishing the diagnosis.

A case of "lethal midline granuloma" in a patient with lymphomatoid papulosis has been described in the past [50]. In this case, the nasal lesion had a CD30+ phenotype and showed the same monoclonal rearrangement of the TCR gene as the skin lesions of the lymphomatoid papulosis. This case probably represented progression of the lymphomatoid papulosis to an anaplastic large cell lymphoma rather than to a true extranodal NK/T-cell lymphoma, nasal type. In this context, one needs to remember that lymphomas of both B- and T-cell origin other than the extranodal NK/T-cell lymphoma, nasal type, can develop in the mucosa of the nasal and upper respiratory tract.

Histopathology, immunophenotype and molecular genetics

Histopathology

Histology reveals a diffuse proliferation of lymphocytes involving the dermis and, often, the subcutaneous tissues (Fig. 6.21). Epidermotropism may be present (Fig. 6.22), being a possible source of error in the differential diagnosis with mycosis fungoides. Usually there is prominent angiocentricity and/or angiodestruction; necrosis may also be found [51]. The cytomorphologic features are variable: some cases show a predominance of small, some of medium-sized and some of large pleomorphic lymphocytes (Fig. 6.23) [51]. Azurophilic granules are commonly observed in Giemsa-stained sections of tissue.

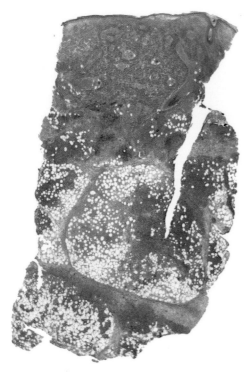

Figure 6.21 Extranodal NK/T-cell lymphoma, nasal type. Neoplastic infiltrate in the dermis and subcutis. Note similarities to the cutaneous γ/δ T-cell lymphoma depicted in Fig. 6.13.

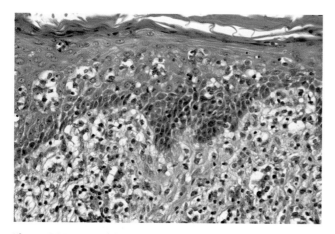

Figure 6.22 Extranodal NK/T-cell lymphoma, nasal type. Epidermotropism of small-sized lymphocytes, mimicking the histopathologic picture of mycosis fungoides.

In some cases a prominent involvement of the subcutaneous tissues can be observed, resembling the morphologic picture of subcutaneous "panniculitis-like" T-cell lymphoma or of lupus panniculitis [52–54]. However, the same biopsy or other biopsies invariably show involvement of the dermis, and sometimes of the epidermis, as well. Involvement of the vessels is not infrequent.

Reactive cells, including small lymphocytes, histiocytes, and eosinophils, are admixed with the neoplastic lymphocytes in

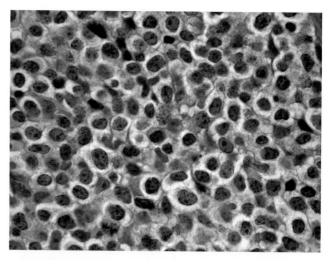

Figure 6.23 Extranodal NK/T-cell lymphoma, nasal type. Predominance of large pleomorphic lymphocytes.

many cases. A granulomatous reaction may also be present, as well as pseudo-epitheliomatous epidermal hyperplasia.

Immunophenotype

Neoplastic cells are characterized in the great majority of cases by negativity for T-cell markers such as TCRβ, TCRδ, CD3, CD4, CD5, CD7, and CD8 [10,55]. The ε chain of the CD3 molecule is usually expressed intracytoplasmically [56]. CD2, CD56 and cytotoxic proteins (TIA-1, granzyme B, perforin) are positive in practically all cases, but CD57 is negative (Fig. 6.24a). Aberrant expression of B-cell markers (CD79a) has been detected in one case, underlining the need for complete phenotypic investigations [57].

EBV can be demonstrated by *in situ* hybridization in practically all cases in the majority of the neoplastic cells (Fig. 6.24b), and a negative result casts serious doubts on the diagnosis. Immunohistochemical staining for EBV latent membrane protein (LMP) is inconsistent.

Molecular genetics

Molecular analyses reveal a germline configuration of the TCR genes in most of the cases. A restricted killer cell immunoglobulin-like receptor repertoire has been found by the reverse transcriptase polymerase chain reaction (RT-PCR) technique indicating the presence of a monoclonal or possibly oligoclonal NK cell proliferation [58]. Rare cases of extranodal NK/T-cell lymphoma, nasal type, show a true T-cell phenotype with a monoclonal TCR gene rearrangement.

Mutations of the *Fas* gene have been described in nasal-type extranodal NK/T-cell lymphoma [59]. Oncogene copy number gains and other chromosomal alterations have also been detected in a few cases [60]. Comparative genomic hybridization studies revealed recurrent abnormalities characteristic of the extranodal NK/T-cell lymphoma, nasal type, namely gain of 2q and loss of 6q16.1-q27, 11q22.3-q23.3,

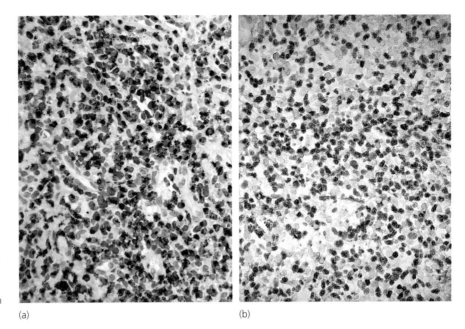

Figure 6.24 Extranodal NK/T-cell lymphoma, nasal type. (a) Positivity of neoplastic cells for the cytotoxic marker TIA-1. (b) Positive signal within neoplastic cells after *in situ* hybridization for the Epstein–Barr virus (EBER–1).

(a)

(b)

5p14.1-p14.3, 5q34-q35.3, 1p36.23-p36.33, 2p16.1-p16.3, 4q12, and 4q31.3-q32.1 [61]. Gene expression profiling revealed a distinct molecular signature, confirming the origin from activated NK cells and showing overexpression of genes involved in cell–cell interactions (integrins, E-cadherin, *VCAM1*), extracellular matrix (*TIMP1, TIMP2, TIMP3*), innate immune responses (Toll-like receptors), chemokine encoding (*CXCL9/Mig, CXCL10/IP-10, CXCL12/SDF-1*), oncogenes such as c-myc among others, and EBV-related gene (*EBI3*) [62].

Treatment

Cases with involvement limited to the skin should be treated like those with extracutaneous involvement. The therapy of choice is systemic chemotherapy. A case treated by denileukin diftitox and bexarotene showed a good response initially, but relapsed with rapid dissemination and death [63].

Prognosis

The prognosis of extranodal NK/T-cell lymphoma, nasal type, is poor and most patients die a few months after the diagnosis [5,51]. The estimated 5-year survival is 0% [5]. A better prognosis has been described in patients who have primary skin involvement, as opposed to those with nasal lymphoma and secondary skin manifestations [64]. Patients reported to have better prognosis and co-expression of CD30 and CD56 may have had examples of cutaneous CD30+ anaplastic large cell lymphoma [65].

Résumé

Extranodal NK/T-cell lymphoma, nasal type

Clinical	Adults. Solitary, regionally localized or generalized plaques and tumors, sometimes ulcerated. Aggressive course. No previous history of mycosis fungoides.
Morphology	Nodular or diffuse infiltrates characterized by small-, medium- or large-sized pleomorphic cells.
Immunology	CD2, 3ε, 56 +
	CD3, 4, 5, 8 – (some cases CD3+)
	CD30 –
	TIA-1 +
	EBER-1 +
Genetics	TCR genes in germline in the majority of the cases. Gain of 2q, and loss of 6q16.1–q27, 11q22.3–q23.3, 5p14.1–p14.3, 5q34–q35.3, 1p36.23–p36.33, 2p16.1–p16.3, 4q12, and 4q31.3–q32.1.
Treatment guidelines	Systemic chemotherapy.

HYDROA VACCINIFORME-LIKE LYMPHOMA

A rare, peculiar NK/T-cell lymphoma affecting mainly children and resembling hydroa vacciniforme clinically has been described in Latin American (particularly Mexico, Guatemala and Peru) and some Asiatic countries (Japan, Korea and Taiwan) [66–73]. A putative case occurring in a Caucasian patient has also been reported [74]. Other terms used for this unusual lymphoproliferative disorder are hydroa-like lymphoma, hydroa vacciniforme-like T-cell lymphoma, atypical hydroa vacciniforme, angiocentric T-cell lymphoma of childhood, and edematous, scarring vasculitic panniculitis. This lymphoma is not listed in the WHO-EORTC classification of cutaneous lymphomas; in the WHO 2008 classification of tumors of hematopoietic and lymphoid tissues it is listed as hydroa vacciniforme-like lymphoma, included as a provisional entity in the group of EBV+ lymphoproliferative disorders of childhood [11].

The relationship of this disorder to conventional hydroa vacciniforme is unclear, but cases with intermediate features have been described [75–78]. EBV is implicated in the genesis of both disorders, and it may be that hydroa vacciniforme-like T-cell lymphoma represents the malignant end of a spectrum of EBV-associated hydroa vacciniforme, perhaps arising only in genetically predisposed individuals.

Clinical features, histopathology, immunophenotype and molecular genetics

Most reported patients are children, but rarely adults with a similar clinical presentation have been observed. Lesions arise especially on sun-exposed areas, particularly the face and ears, the lower parts of the arms and back of the hands, but other lesions are found on sun-covered skin, too. Sun sensitivity is invariably found. Clinically there are infiltrated plaques, often crusted and/or ulcerated, associated with blisters, edema, and varioliform scars (Fig. 6.25). Large tumors

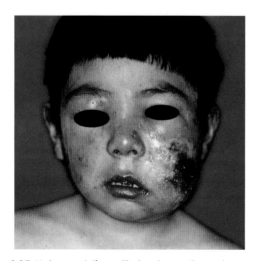

Figure 6.25 Hydroa vacciniforme-like lymphoma. Ulcerated, crusted lesions on the face with large mass on the cheek and prominent swelling. (Courtesy of Dr Mario Magana, Mexico City, Mexico.)

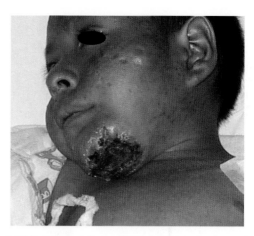

Figure 6.26 Hydroa vacciniforme-like lymphoma. Large ulcerated tumor on the chin; note several varioliform scars. (Courtesy of Dr O. Sangueza, Winston Salem, USA.)

may be present (Fig. 6.26). Systemic symptoms are present in the vast majority of the patients and include malaise, fever, weight loss, and often lymphadenopathy and hepatosplenomegaly. Laboratory investigations may reveal decreased levels of hemoglobin and a low hematocrit level, in addition to other alterations.

Histology is characterized by relatively dense lymphoid infiltrates with variably atypical lymphocytes (atypia may be minimal in some cases, however) involving the entire dermis and in some cases the subcutaneous tissues (Fig. 6.27). Angiocentricity is frequently found, as well as infiltration of adnexal structures. The epidermis shows variable degrees of necrosis, spongiosis, and ulceration.

Neoplastic cells are positive for CD2 and CD3. Most cases reported expressed CD8 or were CD4−/CD8−, and were positive for cytotoxic proteins (TIA-1, granzyme B, perforin). CD30 and CD56 expression have been observed in a proportion of cases [79,80]. A putative NK phenotype has been described rarely. *In situ* hybridization for EBV shows a positive signal in practically all tested cases. Two of two tested cases were negative for T-cell receptor-γ chain rearrangement by PCR.

Treatment and prognosis

The majority of patients with a diagnosis of hydroa vacciniforme-like lymphoma have been treated by systemic polychemotherapy, but it is not clear what the treatment of choice for "borderline" cases should be. Most cases published in the literature are either alive with specific manifestations of the disease or dead of systemic lymphoma. However, long-term follow-up data are missing, and the published series are very small. It seems that hydroa vacciniforme-like lymphoma has a relatively bad prognosis, probably intermediate between cutaneous aggressive cytotoxic T-cell lymphomas and more indolent types of cutaneous T-cell lymphoma.

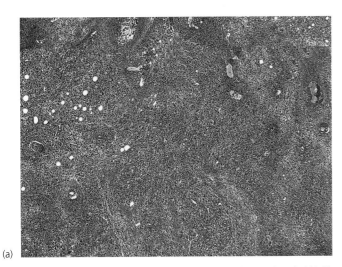
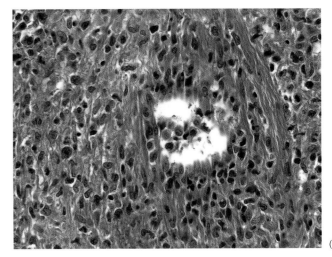

(a)
(b)

Figure 6.27 Hydroa vacciniforme-like lymphoma. (a) Dense lymphoid infiltrates in the dermis. (b) Small to medium-sized pleomorphic lymphocytes predominate. (Courtesy of Dr. O. Sangueza, Winston Salem, USA.)

Résumé

Hydroa vacciniforme-like T-cell lymphoma

Clinical	Mostly children. Lesions resemble hydroa vacciniforme clinically. Sun sensitivity.
Morphology	Atypical lymphocytes with angiocentricity.
Immunology	CD2, 3 +
	CD4 –
	CD8 +(–)
	EBER-1 +
	CD30, 56 +/–
Genetics	Data not sufficient for conclusive interpretation.
Treatment guidelines	Probably systemic chemotherapy should be administered.

TEACHING CASE

A 58-year-old man presented with a solitary tumor on the trunk. A biopsy was obtained, and histology showed dense, diffuse infiltrates of atypical lymphocytes with clear-cut epidermotropism and formation of Darier's nests (Pautrier's microabscesses) (Fig. 6.28a). The cells were positive for CD2, CD3ε and cytotoxic proteins TIA-1 (Fig. 6.28b), granzyme B and perforin, but negative for CD4, CD5, CD7, CD8, βF1 (Fig. 6.28c), CD30, and CD56 (Fig. 6.28b, c). *In situ* hybridization for EBV (EBER-1) showed a strong signal in all cells (Fig. 6.28d). Molecular analyses of the TCR-γ gene by PCR revealed a polyclonal smear. A diagnosis of extranodal NK/T-cell lymphoma, nasal type, was established.

Comment: This case shows the overlapping histopathologic features of extranodal NK/T-cell lymphoma, nasal type, with mycosis fungoides and with other epidermotropic cytotoxic lymphomas. A precise classification can be obtained only by integration of clinical data with histopathologic features and complete phenotypic and gene rearrangement studies. In the past, a similar case would have been categorized as "mycosis fungoides a tumeur d'emblee". Demonstration of EBV positivity by *in situ* hybridization is crucial for the diagnosis of extranodal NK/T-cell lymphoma, nasal type.

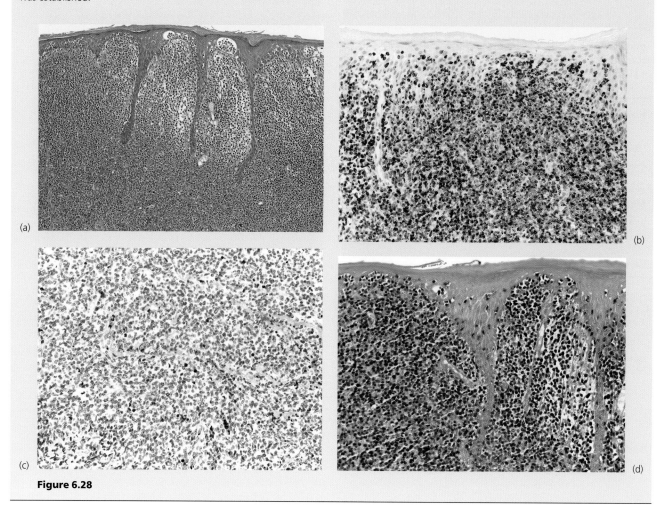

(a)　(b)　(c)　(d)

Figure 6.28

References

1. Chan JKC. Peripheral T-cell and NK-cell neoplasms: an integrated approach to diagnosis. *Mod Pathol* 1999;**12**:177–199.

2. Santucci M, Pimpinelli N, Massi D *et al.* Cytotoxic natural killer cell cutaneous lymphomas: report of the EORTC cutaneous lymphoma task force workshop. *Cancer* 2003;**97**:610–627.

3. Cerroni L, Kerl H. Diagnostic immunohistology: cutaneous lymphomas and pseudolymphomas. *Semin Cutan Med Surg* 1999;**18**: 64–70.

4. El-Shabrawi-Caelen L, Cerroni L, Kerl H. The clinicopathologic spectrum of cytotoxic lymphomas of the skin. *Semin Cutan Med Surg* 2000;**19**:118–123.

5. Fink-Puches R, Zenahlik P, Bäck B *et al.* Primary cutaneous lymphomas: applicability of current classification schemes (European Organization for Research and Treatment of Cancer, World Health Organization) based on clinicopathologic features observed in a large group of patients. *Blood* 2002;**99**:800–805.

6. Kluin PM, Feller A, Gaulard P *et al.* Peripheral T/NK-cell lymphoma: a report of the IXth Workshop of the European Association for Haematopathology. *Histopathology* 2001;**38**:250–270.

7. Massone C, Chott A, Metze D *et al.* Subcutaneous, blastic natural killer (NK) NK/T-cell and other cytotoxic lymphomas of the skin: a morphologic, immunophenotypic and molecular study of 50 patients. *Am J Surg Pathol* 2004;**28**:719–735.

8. Willemze R, Jaffe ES, Burg G *et al.* WHO-EORTC classification for cutaneous lymphomas. *Blood* 2005;**105**:3768–3785.

9. Gaulard P, Berti E, Willemze R, Jaffe ES. Primary cutaneous peripheral T-cell lymphomas, rare subtypes. In: Swerdlow SH, Campo E, Harris NL *et al.*, eds. *WHO Classification of Tumours of Haematopoietic and Lymphoid Tissues.* Lyon: IARC Press, 2008: 302–305.

10. Chan JKC, Quintanilla-Martinez L, Ferry JA, Peh SC. Extranodal NK/T-cell lymphoma, nasal-type. In: Swerdlow SH, Campo E, Harris NL *et al.*, eds. *WHO Classification of Tumours of Haematopoietic and Lymphoid Tissues.* Lyon: IARC Press, 2008: 285–288.

11. Quintanilla-Martinez L, Kimura H, Jaffe ES. EBV-positive T-cell lymphoproliferative disorders of childhood. In: Swerdlow SH, Campo E, Harris NL *et al.*, eds. *WHO Classification of Tumours of Haematopoietic and Lymphoid Tissues.* Lyon: IARC Press, 2008: 278–280.

12. Kamarashev J, Burg G, Mingari MC *et al.* Differential expression of cytotoxic molecules and killer cell inhibitory receptors in CD8 and CD56 cutaneous lymphomas. *Am J Pathol* 2001;**158**:1593–1598.

13. Tao J, Shelat SG, Jaffe ES, Bagg A. Aggressive Epstein–Barr virus-associated, CD8, CD30, CD56, surface CD3 natural killer (NK)-like cytotoxic T-cell lymphoma. *Am J Surg Pathol* 2002;**26**:111–118.

14. Bekkenk MW, Vermeer MH, Jansen PM *et al.* Peripheral T-cell lymphomas unspecified presenting in the skin: analysis of prognostic factors in a group of 82 patients. *Blood* 2003;**102**:2213–2219.

15. Berti E, Tomasini D, Vermeer MH, Meijer CJLM, Alessi E, Willemze R. Primary cutaneous CD8-positive epidermotropic cytotoxic T cell lymphomas. A distinct clinicopathological entity with an aggressive clinical behaviour. *Am J Pathol* 1999;**155**: 483–492.

16. Agnarsson BA, Vonderheid EC, Kadin ME. Cutaneous T cell lymphoma with suppressor/cytotoxic (CD8) phenotype: identification of rapidly progressive and chronic subtypes. *J Am Acad Dermatol* 1990;**22**:569–577.

17. Lu D, Patel KA, Duvic M, Jones D. Clinical and pathological spectrum of CD8-positive cutaneous T-cell lymphomas. *J Cutan Pathol* 2002;**29**:465–472.

18. Quarterman MJ, Lesher JL Jr, Davis LS, Pantazis CG, Mullins S. Rapidly progressive CD8-positive cutaneous T-cell lymphoma with tongue involvement. *Am J Dermatopathol* 1995;**17**:287–291.

19. Arnulf B, Copie-Bergman C, Delfau-Larue MH *et al.* Nonhepatosplenic γ/δ T-cell lymphoma: a subset of cytotoxic lymphomas with mucosal or skin localization. *Blood* 1998;**91**:1723–1731.

20. Heald P, Buckley P, Gilliam A *et al.* Correlations of unique clinical, immunotypic, and histologic findings in a cutaneous gamma/delta T-cell lymphoma. *J Am Acad Dermatol* 1992;**26**:865–870.

21. Jones D, Vega F, Sarris AH, Medeiros LJ. CD4- CD8-'double-negative' cutaneous T-cell lymphomas share common histologic features and an aggressive clinical course. *Am J Surg Pathol* 2002; **26**:225–231.

22. Kadin ME. Cutaneous γδ T-cell lymphomas – how and why should they be recognized? *Arch Dermatol* 2000;**136**:1052–1054.

23. Ralfkiaer E, Wollf-Sneedorff A, Thomsen K, Geisler C, Lange Vejlsgaard G. T-cell receptor gamma-delta-positive peripheral T-cell lymphomas presenting in the skin: a clinical, histological and immunophenotypic study. *Exp Dermatol* 1992;**1**:31–36.

24. Toro JR, Beaty M, Sorbara L *et al.* γδ T-cell lymphoma of the skin. A clinical, microscopic, and molecular study. *Arch Dermatol* 2000; **136**:1024–1032.

25. de Wolf-Peeters C, Achten R. Gamma/delta T-cell lymphomas: a homogeneous entity? *Histopathology* 2000;**36**:294–305.

26. Kinney MC. The role of morphologic features, phenotype, genotype, and anatomic site in defining extranodal T-cell or NK-cell neoplasms. *Am J Clin Pathol* 1999;**111**:s104–s118.

27. Munn SE, McGregor JM, Jones A *et al.* Clinical and pathological heterogeneity in cutaneous gamma-delta T-cell lymphoma: a report of three cases and a review of the literature. *Br J Dermatol* 1996;**135**:976–981.

28. Berti E, Cerri A, Cavicchini S *et al.* Primary cutaneous gamma-delta T-cell lymphoma presenting as disseminated pagetoid reticulosis. *J Invest Dermatol* 1991;**96**:718–723.

29. Burg G, Braun-Falco O. *Cutaneous Lymphomas.* Berlin: Springer Verlag, 1983: 391–392.

30. Miyazaki K, Yamaguchi M, Imai H, *et al.* Gene expression profiling of peripheral T-cell lymphoma including gamma-delta T-cell lymphoma. *Blood* 2009;**113**:1071–1074.

31. Hosler GA, Liegeois N, Anhalt GJ, Moresi JM. Transformation of cutaneous gamma/delta T-cell lymphoma following 15 years of indolent behavior. *J Cutan Pathol* 2008;**35**:1063–1067.

32. Toro JR, Liewehr DJ, Pabby N *et al.* Gamma-delta T-cell phenotype is associated with significantly decreased survival in cutaneous T-cell lymphoma. *Blood* 2003;**101**:3407–3412.

33. Massone C, Crisman G, Kerl H, Cerroni L. The prognosis of early mycosis fungoides is not influenced by phenotype and T-cell clonality. *Br J Dermatol* 2008;**159**:881–886.

34. Urosevic M, Kamarashev J, Burg G, Dummer R. Primary cutaneous CD8+ and CD56+ T-cell lymphomas express HLA-G and killer-cell inhibitory ligand, ILT2. *Blood* 2004;**103**:1796–1798.

35. Chan JKC, Jaffe ES, Ralfkiaer E. Extranodal NK/T-cell lymphoma, nasal type. In: Jaffe ES, Harris NL, Stein H, Vardiman JW, eds. *World Health Organization Classification of Tumours of Haematopoietic and Lymphoid Tissues.* Lyon: IARC press, 2001: 204–207.

36. Miyamoto T, Yoshino T, Takehisa T, Hagari Y, Mihara M. Cutaneous presentation of nasal/nasal type T/NK cell lymphoma: clinicopathological findings of four cases. *Br J Dermatol* 1998; **139**:481–487.

37. Natkunam Y, Smoller BR, Zehnder JL, Dorfman RF, Warnke RA. Aggressive cutaneous NK and NK-like T-cell lymphomas. Clinicopathologic, immunohistochemical, and molecular analyses of 12 cases. *Am J Surg Pathol* 1999;**23**:571–581.

38. Schafer RJ, Schuster HH. Granuloma gangraenescens als maligne Retikulose. *Zentralbl Allg Pathol* 1975;**119**:111–115.

39. Chott A, Rappersberger K, Schlossarek W, Radaszkiewicz T. Peripheral T cell lymphoma presenting primarily as lethal midline granuloma. *Hum Pathol* 1988;**19**:1093–1101.

40. Kassel SH, Echevarria RA, Guzzo FP. Midline malignant reticulosis (so-called lethal midline granuloma). *Cancer* 1969;**23**:920–935.

41. Fechner RE, Lamppin DW. Midline malignant reticulosis. A clinicopathologic entity. *Arch Otolaryngol* 1972;**95**:467–476.

42. Gaulard P, Henni T, Marolleau JP *et al.* Lethal midline granuloma (polymorphic reticulosis) and lymphomatoid granulomatosis. Evidence for a monoclonal T-cell lymphoproliferative disorder. *Cancer* 1988;**62**:705–710.

43. Eichel BS, Harrison EG Jr, Devine KD, Scanlon PW, Brown HA. Primary lymphoma of the nose including a relationship to lethal midline granuloma. *Am J Surg* 1966;**112**:597–605.

44. Ishii Y, Yamanaka N, Ogawa K *et al.* Nasal T-cell lymphoma as a type of so-called "lethal midline granuloma". *Cancer* 1982;**50**: 2336–2344.

45. Harabuchi Y, Yamanaka N, Kataura A *et al.* Epstein–Barr virus in nasal T-cell lymphomas in patients with lethal midline granuloma. *Lancet* 1990;**335**:128–130.

46. Vilde JL, Perronne C, Huchon A *et al.* Association of Epstein–Barr virus with lethal midline granuloma. *N Engl J Med* 1985; **313**:1161.

47. Aozasa K, Ohsawa M, Tomita Y, Tagawa S, Yamamura T. Polymorphic reticulosis is a neoplasm of large granular lymphocytes with CD3+ phenotype. *Cancer* 1995;**75**:894–901.

48. Strickler JG, Meneses MF, Habermann TM *et al.* Polymorphic reticulosis: a reappraisal. *Hum Pathol* 1994;**25**:659–665.

49. Sandner A, Helmbold P, Winkler M, Gattenlöhner S, Müller-Hermelink HK, Holzhausen HJ. Cutaneous dissemination of nasal NK/T-cell lymphoma in a young girl. *Clin Exp Dermatol* 2008;**33**:615–618.

50. Harabuchi Y, Kataura A, Kobayashi K *et al.* Lethal midline granuloma (peripheral T-cell lymphoma) after lymphomatoid papulosis. *Cancer* 1992;**70**:835–839.

51. Chan JKC, Sin VC, Wong KF *et al.* Nonnasal lymphoma expressing the natural killer marker CD56: a clinicopathologic study of 49 cases of an uncommon aggressive neoplasm. *Blood* 1997;**89**: 4501–4513.

52. Jang KA, Choi JH, Sung KJ *et al.* Primary CD56+ nasal-type T/natural killer-cell subcutaneous panniculitic lymphoma: presentation as haemophagocytic syndrome. *Br J Dermatol* 1999; **141**:706–709.

53. Chang SE, Huh J, Choi JH, Sung KJ, Moon KC, Koh JK. Clinicopathological features of CD56+ nasal-type T/natural killer cell lymphomas with lobular panniculitis. *Br J Dermatol* 2000;**142**: 924–930.

54. Aguilera P, Mascaro JM Jr, Martinez A *et al.* Cutaneous γ/δ T-cell lymphoma: a histopathologic mimicker of lupus erythematosus profundus (lupus panniculitis). *J Am Acad Dermatol* 2007;**56**: 643–647.

55. Schwartz EJ, Molina-Kirsch H, Zhao S, Marinelli RJ, Warnke RA, Natkunam Y. Immunohistochemical characterization of nasal-type extranodal NK/T-cell lymphoma using a tissue microarray. An analysis of 84 cases. *Am J Clin Pathol* 2008;**130**:343–351.

56. Ohno T, Yamaguchi M, Oka K, Miwa H, Kita K, Shirakawa S. Frequent expression of CD3 epsilon in CD3 (Leu 4)-negative nasal T-cell lymphomas. *Leukemia* 1995;**9**:44–52.

57. Blakolmer K, Vesely M, Kummer JA, Jurecka W, Mannhalter C, Chott A. Immunoreactivity of B-cell markers (CD79a, L26) in rare cases of extranodal cytotoxic peripheral T (NK/T-) cell lymphomas. *Mod Pathol* 2000;**13**:766–772.

58. Lin CW, Lee WH, Chang CL, Yang SY, Hsu SM. Restricted killer cell immunoglobulin-like receptor repertoire without T-cell receptor g rearrangement supports a true natural killer-cell lineage in a subset of sinonasal lymphomas. *Am J Pathol* 2001;**159**:1671–1679.

59. Takakuwa T, Dong Z, Nakatsuka S *et al.* Frequent mutations of Fas gene in nasal NK/T cell lymphoma. *Oncogene* 2002;**21**: 4702–4705.

60. Mao X, Onadim Z, Price EA *et al.* Genomic alterations in blastic natural killer/extranodal natural killer-like T cell lymphoma with cutaneous involvement. *J Invest Dermatol* 2003;**121**:618–627.

61. Nakashima Y, Tagawa H, Suzuki R *et al.* Genome-wide array-based comparative genomic hybridization of natural killer cell lymphoma/leukemia: different genomic alteration patterns of aggressive NK-cell leukemia and extranodal NK/T-cell lymphoma, nasal type. *Genes Chromosomes Cancer* 2005;**44**: 247–255.

62. Huang Y, de Reynies A, de Leval L *et al.* Gene expression profiling reveals a distinct molecular signature for nasal NK/T-cell lymphomas. *J Haematopathol* 2008;**1**:248.

63. Kerl K, Prins C, Cerroni L, French LE. Regression of extranodal natural killer/T-cell lymphoma, nasal type with denileukin diftitox (Ontak®) and bexarotene (Targretin®): report of a case. *Br J Dermatol* 2006;**154**:988–991.

64. Choi YL, Park JH, Namkung JH, *et al.* Extranodal NK. T-cell lymphoma with cutaneous involvement: 'nasal' vs. 'nasal-type' subgroups – A retrospective study of 18 patients. *Br J Dermatol* 2009;**160**:333–337.

65. Mraz-Gernhard S, Natkunam Y, Hoppe RT, LeBoit P, Kohler S, Kim YH. Natural killer/natural killer-like T-cell lymphoma, CD56+, presenting in the skin: an increasingly recognized entity with an aggressive course. *J Clin Oncol* 2001;**19**:2179–2188.

66. Ruiz-Maldonado R, Parrilla F, Orozco-Covarrubias M, Ridaura C, Sanchez LT, McKinster CD. Edematous, scarring vasculitic panniculitis: a new multisystemic disease with malignant potential. *J Am Acad Dermatol* 1995;**32**:37–44.

67. Magana M, Sangueza OP, Cervantes M. Linfoma cutaneo de celulas-T angiocentrico de la ninez. *Actas Dermatol Dermatopatol* 2003;**3**:5–10.

68. Magana M, Sangueza P, Gil-Beristain J *et al.* Angiocentric cutaneous T-cell lymphoma of childhood (hydroa-like lymphoma): a distinctive type of cutaneous T-cell lymphoma. *J Am Acad Dermatol* 1998;**38**:574–579.

69. Chen HH, Hsiao CH, Chiu HC. Hydroa vacciniforme-like primary cutaneous CD8-positive T-cell lymphoma. *Br J Dermatol* 2002; **147**:587–591.

70. Barrionuevo C, Anderson VM, Zevallos-Giampietri E *et al.* Hydroa-like cutaneous T-cell lymphoma: a clinicopathologic and molecular genetic study of 16 pediatric cases from Peru. *Appl Immunohistochem Mol Morph* 2002;**10**:7–14.

71. Cho KH, Kim CW, Heo DS *et al.* Epstein–Barr virus-associated peripheral T-cell lymphoma in adults with hydroa vacciniforme-like lesions. *Clin Exp Dermatol* 2001;**26**:242–247.

72. Cho KH, Lee SH, Kim CW *et al.* Epstein-Barr virus-associated lymphoproliferative lesions presenting as a hydroa vacciniforme-like eruption: an analysis of six cases. *Br J Dermatol* 2004;**151**: 372–380.

73. Oono T, Arata J, Masuda T *et al.* Coexistence of hydroa vacciniforme and malignant lymphoma. *Arch Dermatol* 1986;**122**:1306–1309.

74. Steger GG, Dittrich C, Hönigsmann H, Moser K. Permanent cure of hydroa vacciniforme after chemotherapy for Hodgkin's disease. *Br J Dermatol* 1988;**119**:684–685.

75. Wu YH, Chen HC, Hsiao PF, Tu MI, Lin YC, Wang TY. Hydroa vacciniforme-like Epstein–Barr virus-associated monoclonal T-lymphoproliferative disorder in a child. *Int J Dermatol* 2007; **46**:1081–1086.

76. Iwatsuki K, Ohtsuka K, Harada JI *et al.* Clinicopathologic manifestations of Epstein–Barr virus-associated cutaneous lymphoproliferative disorders. *Arch Dermatol* 1997;**133**:1081–1086.

77. Iwatsuki K, Xu Z, Takata M *et al.* The association of latent Epstein–Barr virus infection with hydroa vacciniforme. *Br J Dermatol* 1999;**140**:715–721.

78. Iwatsuki K, Yamamoto T, Tsuji K *et al.* A spectrum of clinical manifestations caused by host immune responses against Epstein–Barr virus infections. *Acta Med Okayama* 2004;**58**:169–180.

79. Doeden K, Molina-Kirsch H, Perez E, Warnke R, Sundram U. Hydroa-like lymphoma with CD56 expression. *J Cutan Pathol* 2008;**35**:488–494.

80. Feng S, Jin P, Zeng X. Hydroa vacciniforme-like primary cutaneous CD8-positive T-cell lymphoma. *Eur J Dermatol* 2008;**18**: 364–365.

Cutaneous adult T-cell leukemia/lymphoma

Adult T-cell leukemia/lymphoma (ATLL) is a malignant lymphoproliferative disease associated with a retrovirus infection caused by the human T-cell lymphotropic virus I (HTLV-I). The disease is endemic in the south of Japan and in the Caribbean Islands and is rare in other regions, but reports on its occurrence have come from many different countries besides the endemic ones. Cutaneous manifestations and histopathologic features are identical to those of mycosis fungoides, so demonstration of retroviral infection is mandatory for the diagnosis. The cutaneous manifestations are included as a specific entity in the World Health Organization (WHO)-European Organization for Research and Treatment of Cancer (EORTC) classification of primary cutaneous lymphomas [1]. Four variants of ATLL are recognized in the new WHO classification of tumors of hematopoietic and lymphoid tissues [2]: acute and chronic leukemic, lymphomatous, and smoldering types. Although cutaneous manifestations are usually considered as a smoldering form of the disease, it has been suggested that patients with purely cutaneous lesions may have a better prognosis, and should be classified separately from those with smoldering ATLL [3].

Clinical features

Patients are usually adults of both genders, but rarely adolescents may be affected [4]. Specific skin manifestations can be observed in about half of the patients, especially those presenting with indolent forms of the disease [5–7]. Primary cutaneous involvement may also be seen [7]. Elderly men are affected more frequently. Anti-HTLV-I antibodies can be demonstrated in the serum of affected individuals.

The clinical presentation of the cutaneous form is indistinguishable from that of mycosis fungoides. Cutaneous lesions are localized or generalized macules and papules, patches, plaques, and tumors (Figs 7.1–7.3) [5,6,8,9]. Erythroderma may also develop. Rarely the disease may present with large solitary nodules [10]. A leukemic blood picture and

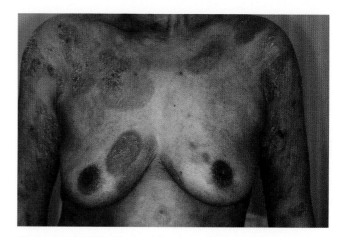

Figure 7.1 Adult T-cell leukemia/lymphoma. Disseminated patches, plaques and flat tumors. The clinical picture is indistinguishable from that of mycosis fungoides. (Courtesy of Dr T. Shiomi, Yonago, Japan.)

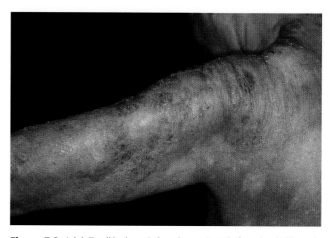

Figure 7.2 Adult T-cell leukaemia/lymphoma. Detail of erosive, infiltrated patches and plaques identical to those seen in mycosis fungoides. (Courtesy of Dr T. Shiomi, Yonago, Japan.)

Skin Lymphoma: The Illustrated Guide. By L. Cerroni, K. Gatter and H. Kerl. Published 2009 Blackwell Publishing, ISBN: 978-1-4051-8554-7.

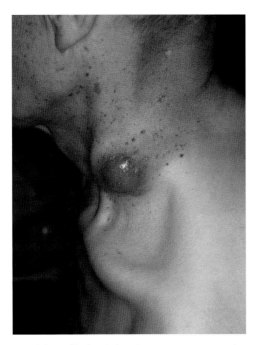

Figure 7.3 Adult T-cell leukemia/lymphoma. Large tumor on the neck. (Courtesy of Dr K. Kodama and Prof. H. Shimizu, Sapporo, Japan.)

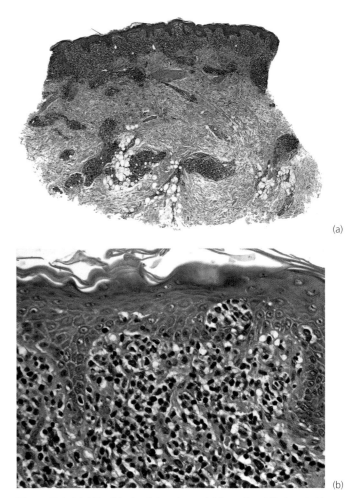

(a)

(b)

Figure 7.4 Adult T-cell leukemia/lymphoma. (a) Dense band-like lymphoid infiltrate in the superficial and mid-dermis with perivascular infiltrates in the deep dermis. (b) Epidermotropism with formation of Darier's nests (Pautrier's microabscesses). (Courtesy of Dr T. Shiomi, Yonago, Japan.)

involvement of the bone marrow are found in more than half of the patients. Spontaneous regression of skin lesions has been observed rarely [11].

Histopathology, immunophenotype and molecular genetics

Histology shows an infiltrate of small-to-medium- or medium-to-large pleomorphic lymphocytes with prominent epidermotropism (Fig. 7.4) [5,6]. The histopathologic picture is often indistinguishable from that of mycosis fungoides. Variants of ATLL with angiocentricity and/or angiodestruction or with bullous lesions have been observed [12,13].

Immunohistology usually reveals a T-helper (CD3⁺, CD4⁺, CD8⁻) phenotype, but some cases may be CD4⁻/CD8⁺ or CD4⁺/CD8⁺. The tumor cells are positive for CD25 and frequently positive for the T regulatory (T*reg*) molecule forkhead box protein P3 (FOX-P3), thus possibly deriving from T*reg* lymphocytes or showing aberrant expression of T*reg* markers [14–16]. FOX-P3-negativity of neoplastic cells in cases of mycosis fungoides may be a helpful differential diagnostic clue.

Molecular analyses show a monoclonal rearrangement of the TCR gene as well as the presence of the integrated genome of HTLV-I [17].

In this context, it should be underlined that, prompted by the clinicopathologic similarities to ATLL, several investig-

ators have looked for the presence of HTLV-I DNA in cases of "classic" mycosis fungoides and Sézary syndrome. So far, there is no convincing evidence of the involvement of HTLV-I in these diseases (see Chapter 2). Demonstration of monoclonal integration of HTLV-I DNA in neoplastic cells may therefore be used as a reliable means to distinguish ATLL from mycosis fungoides.

Treatment and prognosis

The prognosis is generally poor but indolent variants have been described. The smoldering type seems to have a better prognosis [18]. The treatment of choice is usually systemic chemotherapy but less aggressive therapeutic options such as psoralen + UV-A (PUVA) may be used for cases with an indolent behavior and restricted to the skin [5,6,19,20].

Résumé	
Clinical	Adults, rarely younger patients. Four variants recognized: acute and chronic leukemic, lymphomatous, and smoldering types. Primary cutaneous involvement may be seen.
Morphology	Histopathologic features similar to those observed in mycosis fungoides.
Immunology	CD3, 4 +
	CD8 −
	CD25 +
	FOX-P3 +/−
Genetics	Monoclonal integration of HTLV-I DNA.
Treatment guidelines	Systemic chemotherapy. PUVA may be used for cases restricted to the skin.

References

1. Willemze R, Jaffe ES, Burg G et al. WHO-EORTC classification for cutaneous lymphomas. *Blood* 2005;**105**:3768–3785.

2. Ohshima K, Jaffe ES, Kikuchi M et al. Adult T-cell leukaemia/ lymphoma. In: Swerdlow SH, Campo E, Harris NL et al., eds. *WHO Classification of Tumours of Haematopoietic and Lymphoid Tissues*. Lyon: IARC Press, 2008: 281–284.

3. Amano M, Kurokawa M, Ogata K, Itoh H, Kataoka H, Setoyama M. New entity, definition and diagnostic criteria of cutaneous adult T-cell leukemia/lymphoma: Human T-lymphotropic virus type 1 proviral DNA load can distinguish between cutaneous and smoldering types. *J Dermatol* 2008;**35**:270–275.

4. Lucas CT, Gillis KJ, Ness JM et al. Adult T-cell leukaemia/ lymphoma in an adolescent presenting with skin lesions. *Ped Dermatol* 2008;**25**:373–377.

5. DiCaudo DJ, Perniciaro C, Worrell JT, White JW Jr, Cockerell CJ. Clinical and histologic spectrum of human T-cell lympho- tropic virus type I-associated lymphoma involving the skin. *J Am Acad Dermatol* 1996;**34**:69–76.

6. Nagatani T, Miyazawa M, Matsuzaki T et al. Adult T-cell leukaemia–lymphoma (ATLL): clinical, histopathological, immu- nological and immunohistochemical characteristics. *Exp Dermatol* 1992;**1**:248–252.

7. Shimoyama M. Diagnostic criteria and classification of clinical subtypes of adult T-cell leukaemia–lymphoma: a report from the Lymphoma Study Group (1984–87). *Br J Haematol* 1991;**79**: 428–437.

8. Yamaguchi T, Ohshima K, Karube K et al. Clinicopathological features of cutaneous lesions of adult T-cell leukaemia/ lymphoma. *Br J Dermatol* 2005;**152**:76–81.

9. Pezeshkpoor F, Yazdanpanah MJ, Shirdel A. Specific cutaneous manifestations in adult T-cell leukemia/lymphoma. *Int J Dermatol* 2008;**47**:359–362.

10. Shimizu S, Yasui C, Koizumi K, Ikeda H, Tsuchiya K. Cutaneous- type adult T-cell leukemia/lymphoma presenting as a solitary large skin nodule: a review of the literature. *J Am Acad Dermatol* 2007;**57**:s115–s117.

11. Kawabata H, Setoyama M, Fukushige T, Kanzaki T. Spontane- ous regression of cutaneous lesions in adult T-cell leukaemia– lymphoma. *Br J Dermatol* 2001;**144**:434–435.

12. Manabe T, Hirokawa M, Sugihara K, Kohda M. Angiocentric and angiodestructive infiltration of adult T-cell leukaemia–lymphoma (ATLL) in the skin: report of two cases. *Am J Dermatopathol* 1988; **10**:487–496.

13. Michael EJ, Shaffer JJ, Collins HE, Grossman ME. Bullous adult T-cell lymphoma–leukemia and human T-cell lymphotropic virus-1 associated myelopathy in a 60-year-old man. *J Am Acad Dermatol* 2002;**46**:S137–141.

14. Kohno T, Yamada Y, Akamatsu N, et al. Possible origin of adult T- cell leukemia/lymphoma cells from human T lymphotropic virus type-1-infected regulatory T cells. *Cancer Sci* 2005;**96**:527–533.

15. Karube K, Aoki R, Sugita Y, et al. The relationship of FOXP3 expression and clinicopathological characteristics in adult T-cell leukemia/lymphoma. *Mod Pathol* 2008;**21**:617–625.

16. Abe M, Uchihashi K, Kazuto T, et al. Foxp3 expression on normal and leukemic CD4+CD25+ T cells implicated in human T-cell leukemia virus type-1 is inconsistent with Treg cells. *Eur J Haematol* 2008;**81**:209–217.

17. Kato N, Sugawara H, Aoyagi S, Mayuzumi M. Lymphoma-type adult T-cell leukaemia–lymphoma with a bulky cutaneous tumour showing multiple human T-lymphotropic virus-1 DNA integra- tion. *Br J Dermatol* 2001;**144**:1244–1248.

18. Ishitsuka K, Ikeda S, Utsonomiya A, et al. Smouldering adult T-cell leukaemia/lymphoma: a follow-up study in Kyushu. *Br J Haematol* 2008;**143**:442–444.

19. Chan EF, Dowdy YG, Lee B et al. A novel chemotherapeutic regimen (interferon-α, zidovudine, and etretinate) for adult T-cell lymphoma resulting in rapid tumor destruction. *J Am Acad Dermatol* 1999;**40**:116–121.

20. Takemori N, Hirai K, Onodera R et al. Satisfactory remission achieved by PUVA therapy in a case of crisis-type adult T-cell leukaemia–lymphoma with generalized cutaneous leukaemic cell infiltration. *Br J Dermatol* 1995;**133**:955–960.

8 Cutaneous small–medium pleomorphic T-cell lymphoma

This is probably one of the most controversial entities of cutaneous T-cell lymphoma, and the debate has not been settled yet. The existence of a primary cutaneous small–medium pleomorphic T-cell lymphoma distinct from mycosis fungoides and Sézary syndrome has been postulated in the past [1–3]. This lymphoma is listed as a provisional entity in both the original European Organization for Research and Treatment of Cancer (EORTC) and the World Health Organization (WHO)-EORTC classifications of primary cutaneous lymphomas, thus showing lack of progress in definition during the last years [4,5]. In the new WHO classification of tumors of hematopoietic and lymphoid tissues, cutaneous small–medium pleomorphic T-cell lymphoma has been included as a provisional entity as well [6]. In spite of the controversies, recent studies described groups of patients with putative cutaneous small–medium pleomorphic T-cell lymphoma [7,8], although in our opinion a heterogeneous group of patients may have been included in these studies.

Since mycosis fungoides and Sézary syndrome are cutaneous T-cell lymphomas characterized by the predominance of small–medium pleomorphic T lymphocytes, the diagnosis of cutaneous small–medium pleomorphic T-cell lymphoma can only be accepted if mycosis fungoides and Sézary syndrome are excluded by a complete clinical examination [9,10]. In fact, a careful re-examination of the clinical pictures of some of the cases reported previously as cutaneous small–medium pleomorphic T-cell lymphoma suggests that at least some of them were actually examples of mycosis fungoides.

As already mentioned, there is still no consensus on the existence, definition, and classification of cutaneous small–medium pleomorphic T-cell lymphomas as a distinct entity, nor is there agreement on the diagnosis of cases classified as such in the literature. Cases similar on clinical and histopathologic grounds have been reported in the past under different diagnoses, including "idiopathic pseudo T-cell lymphoma," "pseudolymphomatous folliculitis," "cutaneous lymphoid hyperplasia," "solitary lymphomatoid papule, nodule or tumor," and "monoclonal atypical T-cell hyperplasia" among others [11–16]. In addition, cases of aggressive cutaneous cytotoxic lymphomas may show a small–medium pleomorphic cytomorphology (see Chapter 6) [17], generating more disarray in an already confused field.

The diagnosis of cutaneous small–medium pleomorphic T-cell lymphoma should probably be restricted to those cases characterized by the following features:
- absence of other lesions and/or clinical history of mycosis fungoides
- nodular or diffuse infiltrates of small–medium pleomorphic (monoclonal) T lymphocytes admixed with many reactive cells
- absence of marked epidermotropism of neoplastic cells
- α/β phenotype
- absence of CD30 expression.

The presence of Epstein–Barr virus (EBV) DNA has been detected by polymerase chain reaction (PCR) techniques in cutaneous small–medium pleomorphic T-cell lymphomas, but the exact role (if any) of this virus in the pathogenesis of the disease is unclear [18].

Clinical features

Patients are adults or elderly without a clear-cut gender predilection. They present usually with solitary tumors, commonly located on the face and neck or upper trunk, but multiple tumors can be seen (Fig. 8.1). The surface of the tumors is erythematous or purplish; ulceration can be seen but is uncommon (Fig. 8.2).

Histopathology, immunophenotype and molecular genetics

Histopathology

Histology reveals dense, nodular or diffuse lymphoid infiltrates within the entire dermis, often involving the superficial part of the subcutaneous fat (Fig. 8.3). Cytomorphology shows a predominance of small/medium-sized lymphocytes with pleomorphic nuclei (Fig. 8.4). Large cells, when present, should not exceed 30% of the neoplastic infiltrate [5,19]. Epidermotropism is usually completely absent or present only focally.

Skin Lymphoma: The Illustrated Guide. By L. Cerroni, K. Gatter and H. Kerl. Published 2009 Blackwell Publishing, ISBN: 978-1-4051-8554-7.

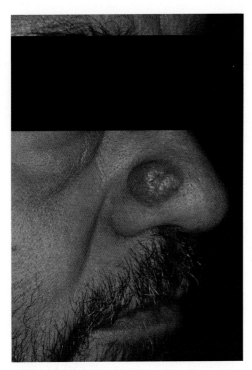

Figure 8.1 Cutaneous small–medium pleomorphic T-cell lymphoma. Solitary tumor on the nose.

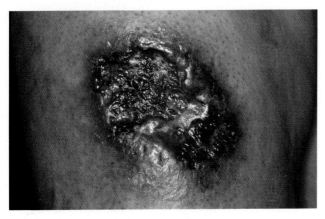

Figure 8.2 Cutaneous small–medium pleomorphic T-cell lymphoma. Large ulcerated lesion on the thigh.

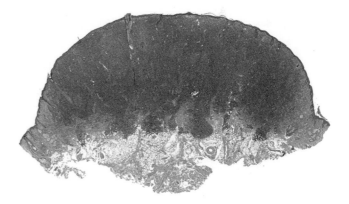

Figure 8.3 Cutaneous small–medium pleomorphic T-cell lymphoma. Dense infiltrate of lymphocytes extending throughout the dermis into the superficial part of the subcutaneous fat.

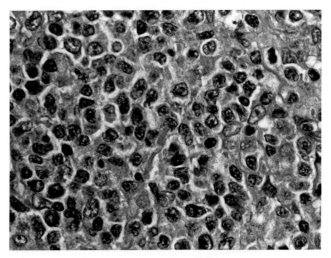

Figure 8.4 Cutaneous small–medium pleomorphic T-cell lymphoma. Small- and medium-sized pleomorphic lymphocytes predominate, admixed with a few larger cells.

Many reactive cells are commonly found admixed with the neoplastic ones. A granulomatous reaction can be observed in a proportion of the cases, and may sometimes cause diagnostic problems [20,21].

Immunophenotype

The neoplastic cells show usually a T-helper phenotype, sometimes with the loss of pan-T-cell antigens (e.g. CD5) (Fig. 8.5a, b). CD30 is not expressed by the neoplastic cells. A variably large, reactive infiltrate of B lymphocytes is commonly found (Fig. 8.5c). The proliferation rate is usually increased (Fig. 8.5d). A recent study showed that neoplastic cells express follicular T-cell markers such as PD-1 and CXCL13 [22].

Although cases with a CD8+ phenotype have been reported, care should be taken to distinguish cutaneous small–medium pleomorphic T-cell lymphoma from primary cutaneous aggressive epidermotropic CD8+ cytotoxic T-cell lymphoma, as they represent two completely distinct entities with different clinical presentation and behavior. An entity termed "indolent CD8+ lymphoid proliferation of the ear" described recently by Petrella *et al.* may represent a phenotypic variant of cutaneous small–medium pleomorphic T-cell lymphoma [23]. In fact, this lymphoid proliferation does not seem to be confined to the ears [24], and the distribution of lesions and clinical presentation is similar to the cutaneous solitary small–medium pleomorphic T-cell lymphoma. We have observed similar cases [25], but data are yet too scarce in order to establish whether these patients have a distinct entity of cutaneous T-cell lymphoma, or a phenotypic variation of the cutaneous small/medium pleomorphic T-cell lymphoma.

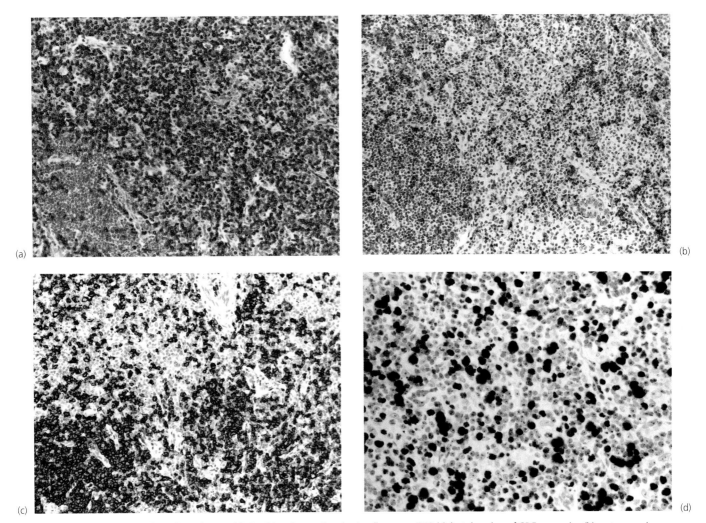

Figure 8.5 Cutaneous small–medium pleomorphic T-cell lymphoma. Neoplastic cells express CD3 (a), but show loss of CD5 expression (b); note several CD20⁺ B lymphocytes (c) and an increased proliferation rate (Ki67) (d).

Molecular genetics

Molecular analysis of the T-cell receptor (TCR) genes rearrangement shows monoclonality of T lymphocytes in the majority of the cases. Specific genetic aberrations have not been identified yet.

Treatment

Most patients present with solitary tumors that can be treated by surgical excision alone, local radiotherapy or a combination of the two [5]. In one study cyclophosphamide or interferon-α have been used for patients with generalized skin lesions [1].

Prognosis

The potential of cutaneous small–medium pleomorphic T-cell lymphomas to dissemination is unclear, and evaluation of

prognosis has been hindered by the difficulties in diagnosis and classification referred to at the beginning of this chapter. Provisionally, it seems that the prognosis is good, with an estimated 5-year survival of over 80% [4,5,26]. Patients with solitary tumors may be compared conceptually to those with solitary lesions in mycosis fungoides, and seem to have an excellent prognosis [27].

Final considerations

The main problem in the proper understanding of cutaneous small–medium pleomorphic T-cell lymphoma and related lesions is represented by the considerable confusion existing in the literature, with several names given to the same disease, and the same name given to what may well be different disorders. Most of the cases reported in the literature as cutaneous small–medium pleomorphic T-cell lymphoma are characterized by solitary lesions, but patients presenting with virtually identical solitary tumors have been classified as cutaneous pseudolymphoma (under many different names) in the past. On the other hand, rapidly progressive cutaneous small–medium pleomorphic T-cell lymphomas characterized by multiple tumors seem to be conceptually different from the indolent cases presenting with solitary lesions. In fact, in our experience no patient presenting with solitary nodules died of the disease, and in some patients the lesions had been present for several months or years before treatment [28–29].

In summary, at least four issues are still open at present.
• Whether a disease presenting with solitary tumors of small–medium pleomorphic lymphocytes, often with monoclonal rearrangement of the TCR genes, represents a low-grade variant of cutaneous T-cell lymphoma (that is, cutaneous small–medium pleomorphic T-cell lymphoma) or a cutaneous pseudolymphoma.
• Whether the very rare cases of "aggressive" cutaneous small–medium pleomorphic T-cell lymphoma presenting with rapidly evolving tumors should be classified in this same category or as peripheral T-cell lymphoma, not otherwise specified.
• Whether the phenotype plays a role in diagnosis and classification of these lesions (CD8+ cases?).
• How should we manage these patients?
We believe that, regardless of the controversies concerning diagnosis and classification, patients presenting with solitary, indolent tumors should be managed in a non-aggressive way. It seems likely that patients with multiple tumours at presentation, on the other hand, require a more aggressive treatment strategy.

Résumé

Clinical	Adults and elderly adults. Localized or, less commonly, multiple tumors. Preferential locations: head and neck, upper trunk. Usually non-aggressive course (rare cases with multiple lesions at presentation may have a worse prognosis).
Morphology	Small–medium pleomorphic cells.
Immunology	CD2, 3, 4 + CD5 +/– βF1 + CD8 –(+) CD7, 30 –
Genetics	No specific abnormalities detected. Monoclonal rearrangement of the TCR is present in most cases.
Treatment	*Solitary tumors:* surgical excision, local radiotherapy or a combination of the two. *Multiple lesions:* cyclophosphamide, interferon-α.

References

1. Friedmann D, Wechsler J, Delfan MH *et al.* Primary cutaneous pleomorphic small T-cell lymphoma: a review of 11 cases. *Arch Dermatol* 1995;**131**:1009–1015.
2. von den Driesch P, Coors EA. Localized cutaneous small to medium-sized pleomorphic T-cell lymphoma: a report of 3 cases stable for years. *J Am Acad Dermatol* 2002;**46**:531–535.
3. Sterry W, Siebel A, Mielke V. HTLV-I-negative pleomorphic T-cell lymphoma of the skin: the clinicopathological correlations and natural history of 15 patients. *Br J Dermatol* 1992;**126**:456–462.
4. Willemze R, Kerl H, Sterry W *et al.* EORTC classification for primary cutaneous lymphomas: a proposal from the Cutaneous Lymphoma Study Group of the European Organization for Research and Treatment of Cancer. *Blood* 1997;**90**:354–371.
5. Willemze R, Jaffe ES, Burg G *et al.* WHO-EORTC classification for cutaneous lymphomas. *Blood* 2005;**105**:3768–3785.
6. Gaulard P, Berti E, Willemze R, Jaffe ES. Primary cutaneous peripheral T-cell lymphoma, rare subtypes. In: Swerdlow SH, Campo E, Harris NL *et al.*, eds. *WHO Classification of Tumours of Haematopoietic and Lymphoid Tissues.* Lyon: IARC Press, 2008: 302–305.
7. Grogg KL, Jung S, Erickson LA, McClure RF, Dogan A. Primary cutaneous CD4-positive small/medium-sized pleomorphic T-cell lymphoma: a clonal T-cell lymphoproliferative disorder with indolent behavior. *Mod Pathol* 2008;**21**:708–715.
8. Garcia-Herrera A, Colomo L, Camos M *et al.* Primary cutaneous small/medium CD4 T-cell lymphomas: A heterogeneous group of tumors with different clinicopathologic features and outcome. *J Clin Oncol* 2008;**26**:1–11.
9. Kerl H, Cerroni L. Controversies in cutaneous lymphomas. *Semin Cutan Med Surg* 2000;**19**:157–160.
10. Kerl H, Cerroni L. Is small/medium-sized pleomorphic T-cell lymphoma a distinct cutaneous lymphoma? *Dermatopathol Pract Concept* 2000;**6**:298–300.
11. Arai E, Okubo H, Tsuchida T, Kitamura K, Katayama I. Pseudolymphomatous folliculitis: a clinicopathologic study of 15 cases of cutaneous pseudolymphoma with follicular invasion. *Am J Surg Pathol* 1999;**23**:1313–1319.
12. Oliver GF, Winkelmann RK. Unilesional mycosis fungoides: a distinct entity. *J Am Acad Dermatol* 1989;**20**:63–70.
13. Rijlaarsdam JU, Willemze R. Cutaneous pseudo-T-cell lymphomas. *Semin Diagn Pathol* 1991;**8**:102–108.
14. Bergman R, Khamaysi Z, Sahar D, Ben-Arieh Y. Cutaneous lymphoid hyperplasia presenting as a solitary facial nodule. *Arch Dermatol* 2006;**142**:1561–1566.
15. Setyadi HG, Nash JW, Duvic M. The solitary lymphomatoid papule, nodule, or tumor. *J Am Acad Dermatol* 2007;**57**:1072–1083.
16. Kazakov DV, Belousova IE, Kacerovska D *et al.* Hyperplasia of hair follicles and other adnexal structures in cutaneous lymphoproliferative disorders. A study of 53 cases, including so-called pseudolymphomatous folliculitis and overt lymphomas. *Am J Surg Pathol* 2008;**32**:1468–1478.
17. Berti E, Tomasini D, Vermeer MH *et al.* Primary cutaneous CD8-positive epidermotropic cytotoxic T-cell lymphomas: a distinct clinicopathological entity with an aggressive clinical behaviour. *Am J Pathol* 1999;**155** 483–492.

18. Nagore E, Ledesma E, Collado C *et al.* Detection of Epstein–Barr virus and human herpesvirus 7 and 8 genomes in primary cutaneous T- and B-cell lymphomas. *Br J Dermatol* 2000;**143**:320–323.

19. Beljaards RC, Meijer CJLM, van der Putte SCJ *et al.* Primary cutaneous T-cell lymphoma: clinicopathological features and prognostic parameters of 35 cases other than mycosis fungoides and CD30-positive large cell lymphoma. *J Pathol* 1994;**172**:53–60.

20. Scarabello A, Leinweber B, Ardigó M *et al.* Cutaneous lymphomas with prominent granulomatous reaction: a potential pitfall in the histopathologic diagnosis of cutaneous T- and B-cell lymphomas. *Am J Surg Pathol* 2002;**26**:1259–1268.

21. Blechet C, Pasquier Y, Maitre F, Esteve E. Lymphome cutane T pleomorphe simulant une sarcoidose. *Les Nouvelles Dermatologiques* 2000;**19**:212–213.

22. Rodriguez-Pinilla SM, Roncador G, Rodriguez-Peralto JJ, *et al.* Primary Cutaneous CD4+ Small/Medium-sized Pleomorphic T-cell Lymphoma Expresses Follicular T-cell Markers. *Am J Surg Pathol* 2009;**33**:81–90.

23. Petrella T, Maubec E, Cornillet-Lefebvre P *et al.* Indolent CD8-positive lymphoid proliferation of the ear. A distinct primary cutaneous T-cell lymphoma? *Am J Surg Pathol* 2007;**31**:1887–1892.

24. Petrella T, Maubec E, Cornillet-Lefebvre P *et al.* Indolent CD8-positive lymphoid proliferation of the face. A distinct primary cutaneous T-cell lymphoma? *J Haematopathol* 2008;**1**:235.

25. Beltraminelli H, Müllegger R, Cerroni L. Indolent CD8+ lymphoid proliferation of the ear: A phenotypic variant of the small-medium pleomorphic cutaneous T-cell lymphoma? Report of three cases. *J Cut Pathol* (in press).

26. Fink-Puches R, Zenahlik P, Bäck B *et al.* Primary cutaneous lymphomas: applicability of current classification schemes (European Organization for Research and Treatment of Cancer, World Health Organization) based on clinicopathologic features observed in a large group of patients. *Blood* 2002;**99**:800–805.

27. Bekkenk MW, Vermeer MH, Jansen PM *et al.* Peripheral T-cell lymphomas unspecified presenting in the skin: analysis of prognostic factors in a group of 82 patients. *Blood* 2003;**102**:2213–2219.

28. Leinweber B, Beltraminelli H, Kerl H, Cerroni L. Solitary small-medium pleomorphic T-cell nodules of undetermined significance: clinical, histopathological, immunohistochemical, and molecular analysis of 26 cases. *Dermatology* (in press).

29. Beltraminelli H, Leinweber B, Kerl H, Cerroni L. Primary cutaneous CD4+ small/medium-sized pleomorphic T cell lymphoma: A cutaneous nodular proliferation of pleomorphic T lymphocytes of undetermined significance? A study of 136 cases. *Am J Dermatopathol* (in press).

9

Other cutaneous T-cell lymphomas

Several other types of T-cell lymphoma have been described at cutaneous sites, including cases arising both primary and secondary in the skin. Clinicopathologic aspects of T-lymphoblastic lymphoma are summarized in Chapter 17, of T-prolymphocytic leukemia in Chapter 20, and of intravascular large NK/T-cell lymphoma in Chapter 14. Other entities will be discussed in this chapter.

PRIMARY CUTANEOUS PERIPHERAL T-CELL LYMPHOMA, NOT OTHERWISE SPECIFIED (NOS)

The World Health Organization (WHO)-European Organization for Research and Treatment of Cancer (EORTC) classification of primary cutaneous lymphomas includes a group of primary cutaneous T-cell lymphomas that do not fit into any of the other categories, giving to this group the name "primary cutaneous peripheral T-cell lymphoma, unspecified" [1]. Similar cases were called in the past "CD30⁻ medium/large pleomorphic T-cell lymphoma" [2–4]. In the new WHO classification of tumors of hematopoietic and lymphoid tissues these cases would be lumped in the category of peripheral T-cell lymphoma, NOS [5]. In our experience, many of the cases classified in this group in the past represented in truth one of the newly characterized aggressive cytotoxic lymphomas of the skin (see Chapter 6) or rarely of blastic plasmacytoid dendritic cell neoplasm (formerly CD4⁺/CD56⁺ hematodermic neoplasm or blastic NK cell lymphoma) (see Chapter 16). However, even after complete phenotypic and genotypic investigations, a small group of cases of cutaneous medium/large T-cell lymphoma that do not fit into one of the well-defined categories can be identified [6]. These patients do not have a history of mycosis fungoides, nor do they have lesions suspicious of mycosis fungoides clinically. The phenotype of the tumor cells is $\beta F1^+$, $CD4^{+/-}$, $CD8^-$, $CD56^-$. Although the WHO-EORTC classification states that a cytotoxic phenotype is uncommon, in our experience one or more cytotoxic proteins (T-cell intracellular antigen (TIA)-1, granzyme-B, perforin) are expressed in the great majority of the cases, including those with a clear-cut $CD4^+$ phenotype. Thus, in our experience many of these cases represent in fact variants of cytotoxic lymphomas that cannot be properly classified into the groups described in Chapter 6.

It is important to emphasize that the diagnosis of primary cutaneous peripheral T-cell lymphoma, NOS, is one of exclusion, and that large cell transformation of mycosis fungoides or Sézary syndrome can show identical features to those observed in these patients, thus implying that an accurate clinical history is crucial for the diagnosis [7]. In the past, some of these cases were designated as mycosis fungoides "a tumeur d'emblee." In addition, the skin may be involved by different types of T-cell lymphoma arising primary in the lymph nodes or in other organs, so complete and accurate staging investigations are mandatory.

Clinical features

Patients are adults of both genders. Clinically they present with solitary, regionally localized or generalized reddish to brown-purplish plaques and tumors, often ulcerated (Fig. 9.1).

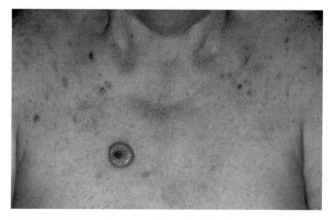

Figure 9.1 Primary cutaneous peripheral T-cell lymphoma, unspecified. Large erythematous tumor on the chest. The small crust in the center represents the site of a punch biopsy.

Skin Lymphoma: The Illustrated Guide. By L. Cerroni, K. Gatter and H. Kerl. Published 2009 Blackwell Publishing. ISBN: 978-1-4051-8554-7.

The clinical features are similar to those observed in other high-grade T-cell lymphomas of the skin.

Histopathology, immunophenotype and molecular genetics

Histopathology
Histology shows nodular or diffuse infiltrates involving the entire dermis and subcutaneous fat, characterized by the predominance of medium-sized and large pleomorphic cells or immunoblasts (Figs. 9.2, 9.3). Epidermotropism is infrequent. There is a high mitotic rate. Prominent necrosis, presence of angiocentricity and/or angiodestruction or predominant involvement of the subcutaneous tissues are uncommon.

Immunophenotype
Immunohistology reveals a characteristic phenotype of the neoplastic cells (βF1$^+$, CD4$^{+/-}$, CD8$^-$, CD56$^-$), commonly with loss of one or more pan-T-cell antigens. CD30 and anaplastic lymphoma kinase (ALK) are negative. Cytotoxic proteins (TIA-1, granzyme B and perforin) are expressed in the great majority of cases, demonstrating that these lesions, too, belong to the group of so-called cutaneous cytotoxic lymphomas [6,8].

There is no association with Epstein–Barr virus (EBV) infection.

Molecular genetics
Molecular analysis of the T-cell receptor (TCR) genes reveals a monoclonal rearrangement in most cases. At present no specific genetic features associated with this type of lymphoma have been detected.

Treatment

The treatment of choice is systemic chemotherapy using regimens for high-grade T-cell non-Hodgkin lymphoma.

Prognosis

The prognosis of cutaneous peripheral T-cell lymphoma, NOS is very poor, and most patients die within a few months from the onset of the disease. The estimated 5-year survival is less than 20% [1,9].

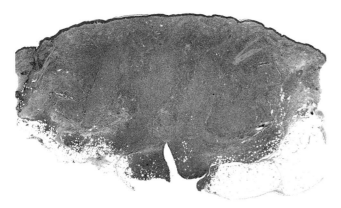

Figure 9.2 Primary cutaneous peripheral T-cell lymphoma, unspecified. Dense nodules of lymphocytes within the entire dermis involving the subcutaneous fat.

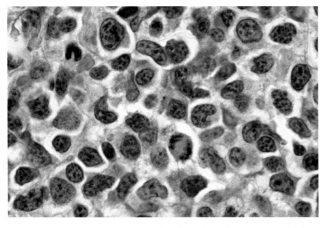

Figure 9.3 Primary cutaneous peripheral T-cell lymphoma, unspecified. Medium- and large-sized pleomorphic lymphocytes.

Résumé	
Primary cutaneous peripheral T-cell lymphoma, NOS	
Clinical	Adults. Solitary, regionally localized or generalized plaques and tumors, sometimes ulcerated. Aggressive course. No previous history of mycosis fungoides.
Morphology	Nodular or diffuse infiltrates characterized by medium-sized and large pleomorphic cells or immunoblasts.
Immunology	CD2, 3, 5, (+) CD4 +(−) βF1 + CD30 − CD8 − TIA-1 +(−)
Genetics	Monoclonal rearrangement of the TCR genes detected in the majority of the cases. No specific genetic alteration.
Treatment guidelines	Systemic chemotherapy.

ANGIO-IMMUNOBLASTIC T-CELL LYMPHOMA

Angio-immunoblastic T-cell lymphoma, formerly called angio-immunoblastic lymphadenopathy, is considered to be a peripheral T-cell lymphoma with a peculiar proliferation of so-called high endothelial venules. It is recognized as a distinct entity in the WHO classification of tumors of hematopoietic and lymphoid tissues [10], but it is not mentioned in the WHO-EORTC classification of primary cutaneous lymphomas. Non-specific skin manifestations have been described in several patients including maculopapular eruptions, purpura and erythroderma. Specific skin involvement is uncommon.

Clinical features, histopathology, immunophenotype and molecular genetics

Patients are elderly adults, though cutaneous involvement in children has been reported [11]. Restriction to the skin is rare but skin lesions may be the first manifestation of the disease [12]. Specific cutaneous involvement in angio-immunoblastic T-cell lymphoma is characterized by erythematous papules, plaques and tumors (Fig. 9.4) consisting of an infiltrate of small- to medium-sized pleomorphic lymphocytes inter-

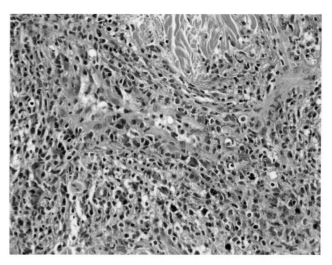

Figure 9.5 Cutaneous angio-immunoblastic T-cell lymphoma. Dense infiltrate of pleomorphic cells of different size and shape; note high endothelial venules. (Courtesy of Dr R. Weenig, Rochester, USA.)

mingled with plasma cells, eosinophils, histiocytes and immunoblasts (Fig. 9.5). Increased numbers of venules with a prominent endothelial lining are typically found ("high endothelial venules") [13,14]. A histopathologic presentation resembling an infectious process has been reported [15].

Clusters of CD21+ follicular dendritic cells can be observed, especially around the high endothelial venules. Immunohistology reveals in the majority of cases a phenotype of neoplastic cells corresponding to follicular helper T-cells (CD3+, CD4+, CD8−, CD10+, chemokine ligand CXCL13+) (Fig. 9.6). CXCL13+ is a chemokine which is expressed by helper T lymphocytes involved in the normal maturation process of germinal center B lymphocytes within lymph nodes. Recent studies have shown that CXCL13+ T lymphocytes can be

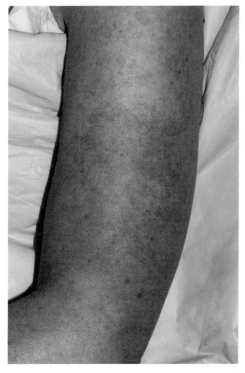

Figure 9.4 Cutaneous angioimmunoblastic T-cell lymphoma. Infiltrated lesions on the arm simulating panniculitis. (Courtesy of Dr R. Weenig, Rochester, USA.)

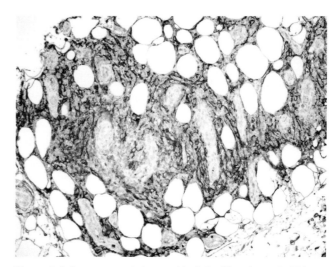

Figure 9.6 Cutaneous angio-immunoblastic T-cell lymphoma. Positivity for CD10. (Courtesy of Dr R. Weenig, Rochester, USA.)

identified in most cutaneous cases of angio-immunoblastic lymphoma, whereas expression of CD10 can be found in a minority of cases only [16–21]. In this context, we must underline that evaluation of CD10 staining in skin biopsies is very difficult because of strong background and positivity of dermal dendritic cells. Clusters of polyclonal B lymphocytes are commonly present. EBV can be demonstrated almost constantly within these B lymphocytes (development of a second, EBV-associated B-cell lymphoma has been observed) [22], but the neoplastic T-cells are constantly negative.

Molecular genetics show a monoclonal rearrangement of TCR genes, and usually a polyclonal pattern of immunoglobulin heavy chain (J_H) genes (a monoclonal rearrangement of the J_H genes can be found in 20–30% of cases). Trisomy 3 and 5 and an additional X chromosome are frequent genetic aberrations in nodal cases. Gains of 22q, 19 and 11q13 and losses of 13q have been shown in some cases by comparative genomic hybridization. In a case with cutaneous involvement, DNA microarrays revealed the expression of secondary lymphoid tissue chemokines, including tumor necrosis factor-β, and an apoptosis-inhibitory protein in the affected lymph nodes [23].

Treatment and prognosis

There are only limited data on the prognosis and treatment of patients with specific skin involvement of angio-immunoblastic T-cell lymphoma. The prognosis is generally poor. Systemic treatment options include glucocorticoids, interferon-α, and chemotherapy. Commencing therapy at an early stage of the disease may give better results in terms of survival.

Résumé

Angio-immunoblastic T-cell lymphoma

Clinical	Elderly adults. Cutaneous lesions may be rarely the first manifestation of the disease.
Morphology	Small- to medium-sized pleomorphic lymphocytes intermingled with plasma cells, eosinophils, histiocytes and immunoblasts.
Immunology	CD3, 4, 5 + CXCL13 + CD10 +/– CD8 – EBV+/CD20 + cells (non-neoplastic) CD21 + cells in clusters (non-neoplastic)
Genetics	Monoclonal rearrangement of the TCR genes.
Treatment guidelines	Glucocorticoids; interferon-α; systemic chemotherapy.

References

1. Willemze R, Jaffe ES, Burg G et al. WHO-EORTC classification for cutaneous lymphomas. *Blood* 2005;**105**:3768–3785.
2. Beljaards RC, Meijer CJLM, van der Putte SCJ et al. Primary cutaneous T cell lymphoma: clinicopathological features and prognostic parameters of 35 cases other than mycosis fungoides and CD30-positive large cell lymphoma. *J Pathol* 1994;**172**:53–60.
3. Joly P, Vasseur E, Esteve E et al. Primary cutaneous medium and large cell lymphomas other than mycosis fungoides. An immunohistological and follow-up study on 54 cases. *Br J Dermatol* 1995;**132**:506–512.
4. Sterry W, Siebel A, Mielke V. HTLV-I-negative pleomorphic T-cell lymphoma of the skin: the clinicopathological correlations and natural history of 15 patients. *Br J Dermatol* 1992;**126**:456–462.
5. Pileri SA, Ralfkiaer E, Weisenburger DD et al. Peripehral T-cell lymphoma, not otherwise specified. In: Swerdlow SH, Campo E, Harris NL et al., eds. *WHO Classification of Tumours of Haematopoietic and Lymphoid Tissues*. Lyon: IARC Press, 2008: 306–308.
6. Massone C, Chott A, Metze D et al. Subcutaneous, blastic natural killer (NK) NK/T-cell and other cytotoxic lymphomas of the skin: a morphologic, immunophenotypic and molecular study of 50 patients. *Am J Surg Pathol* 2004;**28**:719–735.
7. Cerroni L, Rieger E, Hödl S, Kerl H. Clinicopathologic and immunologic features associated with transformation of mycosis fungoides to large-cell lymphoma. *Am J Surg Pathol* 1992;**16**:543–552.
8. Hagiwara M, Takata K, Shimoyama Y et al. Primary cutaneous T-cell lymphoma of unspecified type with cytotoxic phenotype: Clinicopathological analysis of 27 patients. *Cancer Sci* 2009;**100**: 33–41.
9. Fink-Puches R, Zenahlik P, Bäck B, Smolle J, Kerl H, Cerroni L. Primary cutaneous lymphomas: applicability of current classification schemes (European Organization for Research and Treatment of Cancer, World Health Organization) based on clinicopathologic features observed in a large group of patients. *Blood* 2002;**99**: 800–805.
10. Dogan A, Gaulard P, Jaffe ES, Ralfkiaer E, Müller-Hermelink HK. Angio-immunoblastic T-cell lymphoma. In: Swerdlow SH, Campo E, Harris NL et al., eds. *WHO Classification of Tumours of Haematopoietic and Lymphoid Tissues*. Lyon: IARC Press, 2008: 309–311.
11. Schotte U, Megahed M, Jansen T et al. Angio-immunoblastische Lymphadenopathie mit kutanen Manifestationen bei einem 13jährigen Mädchen. *Hautarzt* 1992;**43**:728–734.
12. Suarez-Vilela D, Izquierdo-Garcia FM. Angio-immunoblastic lymphadenopathy-like T-cell lymphoma: cutaneous clinical onset with prominent granulomatous reaction. *Am J Surg Pathol* 2003; **27**:699–700.
13. Martel P, Laroche L, Courville P et al. Cutaneous involvement in patients with angio-immunoblastic lymphadenopathy with dysproteinemia. *Arch Dermatol* 2000;**136**:881–886.
14. Schmuth M, Ramaker J, Trautmann C et al. Cutaneous involvement in prelymphomatous angio-immunoblastic lymphadenopathy. *J Am Acad Dermatol* 1997;**36**:290–295.
15. Jayaraman AG, Cassarino D, Advani R, Kim YH, Tsai E, Kohler S. Cutaneous involvement by angio-immunoblastic T-cell lymphoma: a unique histologic presentation, mimicking an infectious etiology. *J Cut Pathol* 2006;**33**(suppl 2):6–11.

16. Attygalle A, Al-Jehani R, Diss TC *et al.* Neoplastic T cells in angio-immunoblastic T-cell lymphoma express CD10. *Blood* 2002;**99**: 627–633.

17. Grogg KL, Attygalle AD, Macon WR, Remstein ED, Kurtin PJ, Dogan A. Angio-immunoblastic T-cell lymphoma: a neoplasm of germinal-center T-helper cells? *Blood* 2005;**106**:1501–1502.

18. Ortonne N, Dupuis J, Plonquet A *et al.* Characterization of CXCL13+ neoplastic T cells in cutaneous lesions of angio-immunoblastic T-cell lymphoma (AITL). *Am J Surg Pathol* 2007;**31**:1068–1076.

19. de Leval L, Rickman DS, Thielen C *et al.* The gene expression profile of nodal peripheral T-cell lymphoma demonstrates a molecular link between angioimmunoblastic T-cell lymphoma (AITL) and follicular helper T (TFH) cells. *Blood* 2007;**109**:4952–4963.

20. Grogg KL, Attygale AD, Macon WR, Remstein ED, Kurtin PJ, Dogan A. Expression of CXCL13, a chemokine highly upregulated in germinal center T-helper cells, distinguishes angioimmunoblastic T-cell lymphoma from peripheral T-cell lymphoma, unspecified. *Mod Pathol* 2006;**19**:1101–1107.

21. Yu H, Shahsafaei A, Dorfman DM. Germinal-Center T-Helper-Cell Markers PD-1 and CXCL13 are both expressed by neoplastic cells in angioimmunoblastic T-cell lymphoma. *Am J Clin Pathol* 2009;**131**:33–41.

22. Brown HA, Macon WR, Kurtin PJ, Gibson LE. Cutaneous involvement by angio-immunoblastic T-cell lymphoma with remarkable heterogeneous Epstein-Barr virus expression. *J Cutan Pathol* 2001;**28**:432–438.

23. Murakami T, Ohtsuki M, Nakagawa H. Angio-immunoblastic lymphadenopathy-type peripheral T-cell lymphoma with cutaneous infiltration: report of a case and its gene expression profile. *Br J Dermatol* 2001;**144**:878–884.

Section 2: Cutaneous B-cell lymphomas

The classification of cutaneous lymphomas proposed in 2005 by the European Organization for Research and Treatment of Cancer (EORTC) and the World Health Organization (WHO) [1], based mainly on data from the original EORTC classification of cutaneous lymphomas published in 1997 [2], listed three main entities of cutaneous lymphomas: cutaneous marginal zone B-cell lymphoma, cutaneous follicle center lymphoma, and cutaneous diffuse large B-cell lymphoma, leg type. Two of these three categories (cutaneous follicle center lymphoma and cutaneous diffuse large B-cell lymphoma, leg type) have been included as specific entities in the new WHO classification of tumors of hematopoietic and lymphoid tissues published in 2008, whereas the cutaneous marginal zone B-cell lymphoma has been lumped within the group of the extranodal marginal zone lymphoma of mucosal-associated lymphoid tissue (MALT) [3]. Thus, for most cases the long-standing notion among dermatologists and dermatopathologists that cutaneous B-cell lymphomas represent specific entities of extranodal lymphomas [4] has been finally acknowledged within classification schemes used by hematologists and hematopathologists.

A small percentage of primary cutaneous B-cell lymphomas was demonstrated to harbor *Borrelia burgdorferi* DNA sequences within specific skin lesions in studies carried out in different countries, but negative results have also been reported [5–7]. This association may be important in particular for cases classified in the past as "cutaneous immunocytoma" (today classified as cutaneous marginal zone B-cell lymphoma) (see Chapter 11). The presence of *B. burgdorferi* within skin lesions of cutaneous lymphoma underlines the analogies between B-cell lymphomas of the skin and those of the gastric mucosa, where, at least in some cases, infection by *Helicobacter pylori* is considered to be a causative agent. The observation of *B. burgdorferi*-specific DNA within skin lesions of cutaneous B-cell lymphoma also provided the rationale for antibiotic treatment of these patients, and indeed good results have been observed in some cases [8]. Other new treatment modalities include the use of the anti-CD20 antibody (rituximab), which has been applied intralesionally or systemically for the treatment of different types of cutaneous B-cell lymphoma. The knowledge that many patients experience a protracted course with long survival also provided the rationale for a "watchful waiting" strategy, which is now being increasingly used in low-grade cutaneous B-cell lymphomas, especially of the marginal zone type.

References

1. Willemze R, Jaffe ES, Burg G *et al.* WHO-EORTC classification for cutaneous lymphomas. *Blood* 2005;**105**:3768–3785.
2. Willemze R, Kerl H, Sterry W *et al.* EORTC classification for primary cutaneous lymphomas: a proposal from the Cutaneous Lymphoma Study Group of the European Organization for Research and Treatment of Cancer. *Blood* 1997;**90**:354–371.
3. Swerdlow SH, Campo E, Harris NL *et al.*, eds. *WHO Classification of Tumours of Haematopoietic and Lymphoid Tissues.* Lyon: IARC Press, 2008.
4. Kerl H, Rauch HJ, Hödl S. Cutaneous B cell lymphomas. In: Goos M, Christophers E, eds. *Lymphoproliferative Diseases of the Skin.* Berlin: Springer Verlag, 1982: 179–191.
5. Cerroni L, Zöchling N, Pütz B, Kerl H. Infection by *Borrelia burgdorferi* and cutaneous B-cell lymphoma. *J Cutan Pathol* 1997;**24**:457–461.
6. Goodlad JR, Davidson MM, Hollowood K *et al.* Primary cutaneous B-cell lymphoma and *Borrelia burgdorferi* infection in patients from the highlands of Scotland. *Am J Surg Pathol* 2000;**24**:1279–1285.
7. Wood GS, Kamath NV, Guitart J *et al.* Absence of *Borrelia burgdorferi* DNA in cutaneous B-cell lymphomas from the United States. *J Cutan Pathol* 2001;**28**:502–507.
8. Zenahlik P, Fink-Puches R, Kapp KS, Kerl H, Cerroni L. Die Therapie der primären kutanen B-Zell-Lymphome. *Hautarzt* 2000;**51**:19–24.

10

Cutaneous follicle center lymphoma

Cutaneous follicle center lymphoma is defined as the neoplastic proliferation of germinal center cells confined to the skin. The pattern of growth can be purely follicular, purely diffuse or mixed. This lymphoma is listed as a specific entity in both the European Organization for Research and Treatment of Cancer (EORTC)–World Health Organization (WHO) classification of primary cutaneous lymphomas [1] and the new WHO classification of tumous of hematopoietic and lymphoid tissues [2].

The inclusion of primary cutaneous follicle center lymphoma in the new WHO classification is a major change with respect to the recent past. In fact, cutaneous follicle center lymphoma as defined in the EORTC classification of 1997 and nodal follicular lymphoma according to the WHO classification of 2001 differed substantially in their definitions, particularly concerning the diffuse type of cutaneous follicle center lymphoma [3,4]. In fact, this variant of cutaneous follicle center lymphoma was classified as diffuse type follicle center lymphoma in the EORTC classification and as diffuse large B-cell lymphoma in the WHO classification. The different classifications based on morphologic, phenotypic and molecular diversities between the cutaneous and nodal variants [4–23], and were one of the major reasons for misunderstanding between the different diagnostic and therapeutic centers. On the other hand, the EORTC approach had been validated in a large study [24] and has finally been incorporated in the new WHO classification.

Complete staging investigations must be performed in all patients, as the clinicopathologic features alone cannot distinguish with certainty between primary cutaneous follicle center lymphoma and secondary involvement of extracutaneous lymphoma with a similar morphology [25]. Primary cutaneous lymphoma is currently defined by the absence of extracutaneous manifestations after complete staging investigations have been performed (see Chapter 1) [1,24].

Clinical features

Patients are adults of both genders. Onset in children has been reported, but is exceptional [26]. Cutaneous follicle center lymphoma presents clinically with erythematous papules, plaques and tumors, usually non-ulcerated. Lesions are located mostly on the head and neck and on the trunk (Figs 10.1–10.6). A distinct clinical presentation with plaques and tumors on the back surrounded by erythematous macules and papules expanding centrifugally around the central tumors has been described in the past as "reticulohistiocytoma of the dorsum" or "Crosti's lymphoma" (Figs 10.4, 10.6) [27,28].

Lesions are usually clustered at a single site, but may be multiple at different sites. Although there are no clear-cut

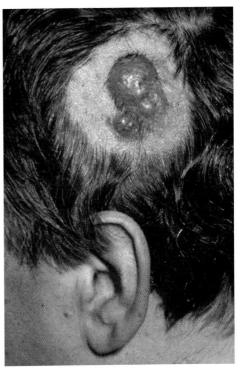

Figure 10.1 Cutaneous follicle center lymphoma. Clustered tumors on the scalp.

Skin Lymphoma: The Illustrated Guide. By L. Cerroni, K. Gatter and H. Kerl. Published 2009 Blackwell Publishing. ISBN: 978-1-4051-8554-7.

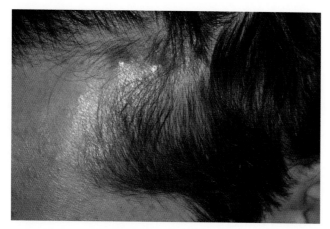

Figure 10.2 Cutaneous follicle center lymphoma (early lesions). Two papular lesions on the scalp.

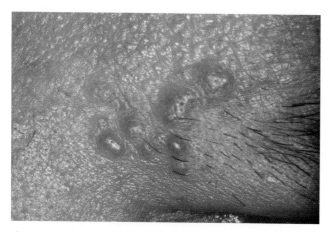

Figure 10.3 Cutaneous follicle center lymphoma (early lesions). Clustered papules on the right eyebrow.

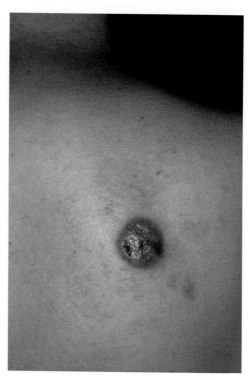

Figure 10.4 Cutaneous follicle center lymphoma. Large erythematous tumor on the shoulder. Note infiltrated erythematous patches and papules in the surroundings.

differences in clinical presentation between the diffuse and follicular variants of cutaneous follicle center lymphoma, cases with a follicular pattern have a predilection for the head and neck region, whereas the so-called Crosti's lymphoma corresponds in the majority of cases to a follicle center lymphoma with a diffuse pattern of growth [19,27].

In some patients with the clinical presentation of Crosti's lymphoma, small erythematous papules located far from the main lesions can be observed (Fig. 10.7). These papules represent early manifestations of the disease and reveal histopathologically specific features of follicle center lymphoma (Fig. 10.8). The question arises as to whether local radiotherapy is the more appropriate treatment modality for these patients, and what the radiation field should be. The relatively high incidence of local recurrences observed in Crosti's lymphoma may be caused, at least in part, by the presence of early lesions far from the main tumor, which had not been identified clinically at the time of treatment planning.

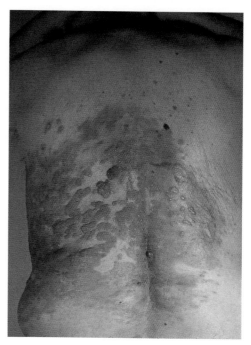

Figure 10.5 Cutaneous follicle center lymphoma. Large erythematous tumors surrounded by plaques and papules covering a large area of the back (so-called "reticulohistiocytoma of the dorsum," "Crosti's lymphoma").

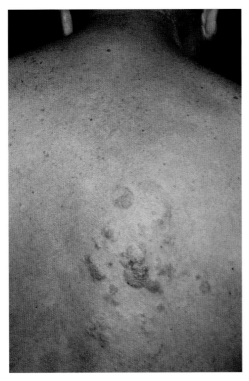

Figure 10.6 Cutaneous follicle center lymphoma. Erythematous papules and plaques on the back (early lesions of "Crosti's lymphoma").

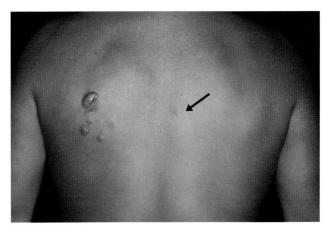

Figure 10.7 Cutaneous follicle center lymphoma. A large tumor on the left side of the back. Note small papules located at the right paravertebral area (*arrow*).

Some patients report that small papular lesions (particularly on the back) undergo spontaneous regression. We have observed this phenomenon in a few cases, but it may be more common than we currently realize.

Association with infections such as *Borrelia burgdorferi*, hepatitis C or human herpesvirus 8 has been described in sporadic patients, but does not seem to be a major etiologic factor for cutaneous follicle center lymphoma [29–32]. In one patient the lesions arose at the site of previous radiotherapy for breast cancer [33].

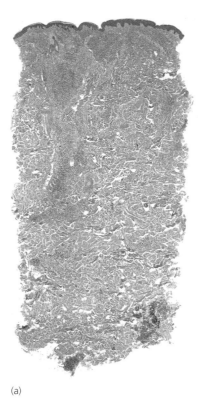

Figure 10.8 Cutaneous follicle center lymphoma, early lesion. (a) Histology reveals small nodular infiltrates throughout the dermis. (b) Cytomorphology shows small lymphocytes admixed with centrocytes and centroblasts.

(a)

(b)

Histopathology, immunophenotype and molecular genetics

Histopathology

Well-developed lesions of cutaneous follicle center lymphoma with a diffuse pattern of growth involve the entire dermis, often extending into the subcutaneous fat. They are characterized by a proliferation of small, medium and large cleaved cells (centrocytes) admixed with variable numbers of large cells with the morphologic features of centroblasts (Figs 10.9, 10.10). Small reactive T lymphocytes are almost invariably admixed with the tumor cells. In contrast, the histopathologic features of cases with a follicular pattern of growth resemble those of follicular lymphomas at extracutaneous sites [20,34]. They consist of nodular infiltrates extending into the entire dermis, usually involving the subcutaneous tissues, characterized by a prominent follicular pattern (Fig. 10.11). The epidermis is spared as a rule. Neoplastic follicles in follicular lymphoma show several morphologic abnormalities, such as reduced or absent mantle zones,

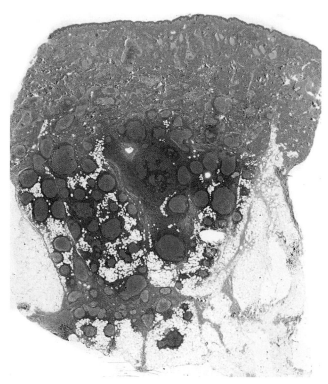

Figure 10.11 Cutaneous follicle center lymphoma, follicular type. Dense infiltrate within the deep dermis and subcutaneous fat. Note prominent lymphoid follicles with reduced or absent mantle.

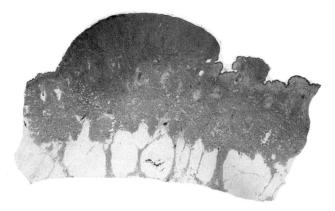

Figure 10.9 Cutaneous follicle center lymphoma, diffuse type. Dense nodular infiltrates within the dermis.

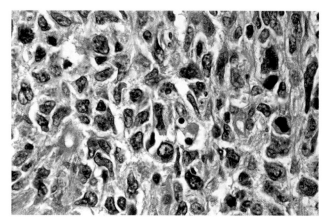

Figure 10.10 Cutaneous follicle center lymphoma, diffuse type. Centrocytes predominate, admixed with some centroblasts (detail of Fig. 10.9).

reduced numbers or complete lack of tingible body macrophages, and monomorphous appearance without a clear-cut distinction between dark and light areas (Fig. 10.12). These features are readily observed at low power and provide valuable clues for the diagnosis. Cytomorphologically, neoplastic follicles consist of small and large centrocytes admixed with centroblasts, often intermingled with reactive small lymphocytes. Small clusters of neoplastic cells can be found in the interfollicular areas as well.

In some cases, both patterns of growth (diffuse and follicular) can be observed in one and the same tumor (Fig. 10.13). In these cases, residual follicles are usually visible at the periphery of the infiltrate with a more diffuse pattern in the middle.

A morphologic variant of cutaneous follicle center lymphoma showing nodules of medium–large centrocytes admixed with some centroblasts without a prominent interfollicular infiltrate has been termed in the past "large cell lymphocytoma" [35,36]. It seems likely that many, if not all, of these cases represent cutaneous follicle center lymphomas. Another peculiar histopathologic variant is characterized by the predominance of spindle and bizarre cells, and has been termed "spindle cell B-cell lymphoma" (Fig. 10.14) [37–43]. The bizarre cells are centrocytes that show different sizes and shapes. Although these cases were previously interpreted as a variant of cutaneous diffuse large B-cell lymphoma, they

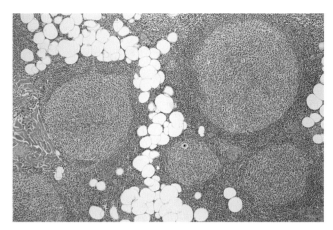

Figure 10.12 Cutaneous follicle center lymphoma, follicular type. Lymphoid follicles reveal several atypical morphologic aspects: reduced mantle zone, monomorphism (lack of dark and light areas), and absence of tingible body macrophages (detail of Fig. 10.11).

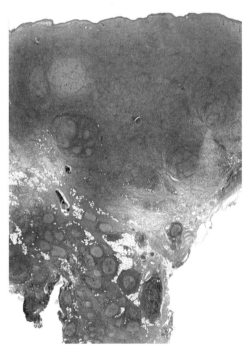

Figure 10.13 Cutaneous follicle center lymphoma, mixed follicular and diffuse type. Dense nodular infiltrates within the dermis and subcutaneous fat. Note neoplastic follicles arranged mainly at the periphery of areas with a diffuse pattern of growth.

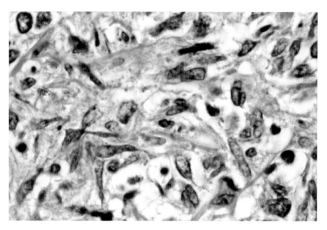

Figure 10.14 Cutaneous follicle center lymphoma, spindle cell type. Note several cells with bizarre elongated nuclei representing morphologic variations of centrocytes.

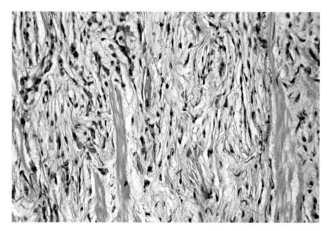

Figure 10.15 Cutaneous follicle center lymphoma, spindle cell variant. Proliferation of spindled lymphocytes within a myxoid stroma.

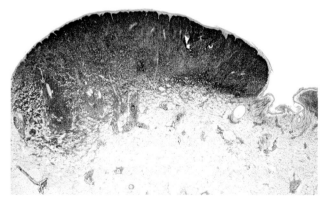

Figure 10.16 Cutaneous follicle center lymphoma, diffuse type. Positive staining for CD10 (same case as Fig. 10.9).

are currently classified in the group of cutaneous follicle center lymphoma, diffuse type. Sclerosis and myxoid areas may also be observed in cases of cutaneous follicle center lymphoma (Fig. 10.15).

Immunophenotype

Neoplastic cells are positive for B-cell markers such as CD20 and CD79a in both the diffuse and follicular variants of cutaneous follicle center lymphoma. Remarkably, most cases

showing a diffuse pattern of growth are usually (but not always! see Fig. 10.16) CD10⁻ and do not show a network of CD21 follicular dendritic cells in the background. In contrast, cases of follicle center lymphoma with a follicular pattern of growth are positive for markers of germinal center cells such

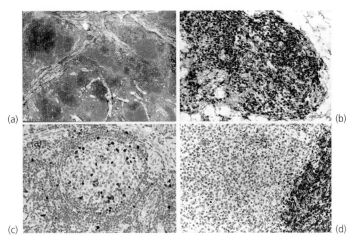

Figure 10.17 Cutaneous follicle center lymphoma, follicular type. Neoplastic follicles stain for (a) CD10 and (b) Bcl-6. (c) Reduced proliferation rate within a neoplastic follicle detected by the antibody MIB-1. (d) Negativity of neoplastic cells for Bcl-2. Note positive small lymphocytes at the edge of the neoplastic aggregate representing positive internal controls.

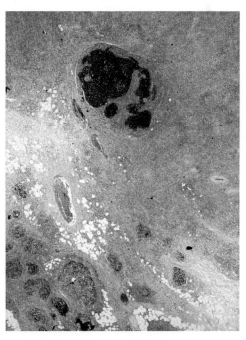

Figure 10.18 Cutaneous follicle center lymphoma, mixed follicular and diffuse type. Note large aggregates of CD21 dendritic follicular cells at the margin of an area with a diffuse pattern of growth (same case as Fig. 10.13).

as CD10 and Bcl-6 (Fig. 10.17a, b) [20,44,45]. The presence of small clusters of CD10+ and/or Bcl-6+ cells outside neoplastic follicles can be observed in a proportion of these cases [20]. This phenomenon, caused by the active "migration" of neoplastic follicular cells from the follicle to the interfollicular area and back, has been described in nodal follicular lymphomas as well, and is not observed as a rule in reactive lymphoid infiltrates, thus being virtually diagnostic of follicular lymphoma [46].

Other markers that can be used in order to confirm germinal center differentiation of neoplastic cells include paired box gene (PAX)-5 and interferon regulatory factor (IRF)8 [47], but other B cells are positive as well. In cases showing both patterns (follicular and diffuse), CD21+ follicular dendritic cells are usually located at the periphery of large areas with a diffuse pattern of growth (Fig. 10.18). A good diagnostic clue for cutaneous follicle center lymphoma with a follicular pattern is provided by the staining for proliferating cells (Ki67/MIB-1). Reactive germinal centers show a high degree of proliferation (more than 90% of cells), whereas neoplastic follicles often show a proliferative fraction of less than 50% of the cells (Fig. 10.17c) [20,44]. A residual network of CD21 follicular dendritic cells is usually found within the neoplastic follicles. There is no aberrant expression of CD5 or CD43 by the neoplastic B lymphocytes.

Although conflicting statements have been proposed, analysis of published reports shows that Bcl-2 expression can be found only in a minority of cases of primary cutaneous follicle center lymphoma [11,20–23,33,48–50]. Bcl-2 expression is present in 10–15% of cases within a small minority of the follicular cells, and only very rarely in the whole neoplastic population (Fig. 10.17d). However, when present,

Bcl-2 positivity in germinal center cells is virtually diagnostic of follicle center lymphoma and is incompatible with a reactive process. The multiple myeloma oncogene-1 (MUM-1) is positive only in a minority of cells (<30%) in cutaneous follicle center lymphoma (Fig. 10.19) [51].

The detection of an immunoglobulin light chain restriction is difficult in paraffin sections, but can be observed more often on snap-frozen tissue sections. However, negativity for both κ and λ seems to be relatively common in cutaneous cases, thus hindering the diagnostic value of immunohistologic staining for immunoglobulin light chains [16,20].

Molecular genetics

Cutaneous follicle center lymphoma shows a monoclonal rearrangement of the J_H gene in the majority of cases, but lack of detection of rearrangement by polymerase chain reaction (PCR) can be observed. This may be caused, at least in part, by the high number of somatic hypermutations that are characteristic of these tumors, thus hindering annealing of the DNA probes to neoplastic DNA.

In a study on cases with a follicular pattern of growth, using a laser beam-based microdissection technique, we demonstrated the presence of the same monoclonal population of B lymphocytes within different follicles from a given tumor, thus proving beyond doubt that these cases represented examples of true follicular lymphoma [20]. Remarkably, in some of the cases a band corresponding to the same monoclonal population of follicular lymphocytes could be observed

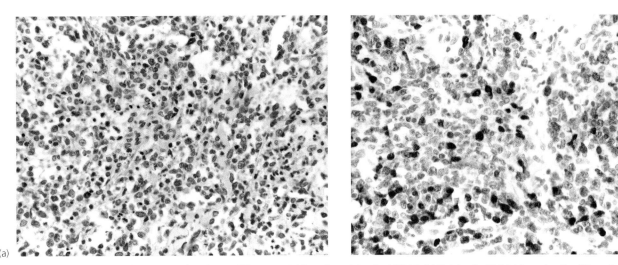

Figure 10.19 Cutaneous follicle center lymphoma, diffuse type. (a) Negative staining for MUM-1. (b) Staining for MUM-1 in a minority of the cells. These staining patterns are commonly seen in cutaneous follicle center lymphoma, in contrast to the strong positivity found in cases of cutaneous diffuse large B-cell lymphoma, leg type (see Fig. 12.9).

in interfollicular areas as well, confirming that neoplastic cells are actively migrating between follicles and interfollicular areas, as already suggested by the pattern of CD10 and Bcl-6 staining described above.

Analysis of data from the literature clearly shows that the interchromosomal (14;18) translocation is extremely uncommon in primary cutaneous follicle center lymphoma, although the frequency varies in different studies (depending also on the method used for detection) [11,12,20–23,52–55]. A t(12;21)(q13;q22) has been detected in one patient [56]. Gene expression studies using cDNA microarrays revealed that cases of cutaneous follicle center lymphoma have a germinal center cell signature [57,58]. A study on genes involved in apoptosis showed that follicle center lymphoma, diffuse type, is characterized by a cellular cytotoxic immune response [59].

A clonal evolution of neoplastic B lymphocytes has been demonstrated by single-cell PCR studies [60]. Differential expression of a group of genes involved in regulation of lymphopoiesis and malignant transformation (Polycomb group) was found in cutaneous B-cell lymphomas arising on the head and trunk as opposed to those located on the legs, confirming that these lymphomas represent distinct entities [61].

Differential diagnosis of cutaneous follicle center lymphoma from cutaneous diffuse large B-cell lymphoma, leg type

Both the diffuse type of cutaneous follicle center lymphoma and the diffuse large B-cell lymphoma, leg type, are characterized by a predominant population of large B lymphocytes,

thus creating problems in the differential diagnosis (problems that were reflected in the different classification of these cases in the previous EORTC and WHO classifications – see beginning of this chapter). Morphologically, the diffuse type of cutaneous follicle center lymphoma shows predominance of large cleaved lymphocytes, in contrast to cutaneous diffuse large B-cell lymphoma, leg type, where large round cells (particularly immunoblasts) are the majority [51]. Immunohistology reveals negativity for Bcl-2, MUM-1 and forkhead box protein 1 (FOX-P1) in cutaneous follicle center lymphoma, as opposed to positivity for these three markers in the vast majority of cases of cutaneous diffuse large B-cell lymphoma, leg type [51]. Markers of germinal center cells such as Bcl-6 and less frequently CD10 are positive in cutaneous follicle center lymphoma, but may be positive in diffuse large B-cell lymphoma, leg type, too, thus not providing helpful clues for the differential diagnosis. Molecular studies showed that neoplastic cells in the two subgroups have different gene signatures (cutaneous follicle center lymphoma: germinal center signature; cutaneous diffuse large B-cell lymphoma, leg type: activated B-lymphocyte signature) [58].

It should be noted that cases of follicle center lymphoma, diffuse type, arising on the legs have a bad prognosis, similar to that of cutaneous diffuse large B-cell lymphoma, leg type [51,62]. The reason for this peculiar behavior is currently unclear; we suspect that, in spite of predominant large cleaved morphology and/or negativity for Bcl-2, MUM-1 and FOX-P1, these rare cases represent in fact morphologic and/or phenotypic variations of diffuse large B-cell lymphoma, leg type. Be that as it may, patients with follicle center lymphoma arising on the legs should be managed with the greatest caution (see also Chapter 12).

Treatment

Patients are mainly treated by local radiotherapy [1,18,63–66]. Solitary tumors can be excised surgically, generally followed by local radiotherapy to the surgical field and surrounding skin. Systemic chemotherapy is usually not necessary in these patients [1]. Interferon-α (either systemically or intralesionally) has been used for treatment of patients with cutaneous follicle center lymphoma, sometimes associated with other treatment regimens [65,67–69]. Other modalities used sporadically include intralesional chemotherapy and antibiotic treatment [65,70].

Recently, a promising new treatment has been introduced with the use of an anti-CD20 monoclonal antibody (rituximab), which can be administered either systemically or intralesionally [71–77]. Rituximab can also be combined with systemic chemotherapy in patients with generalized skin or extracutaneous involvement [78]. The anti-CD20 antibody can also be conjugated with radionuclides, in order to provide selective irradiation of tumor cells. In some patients, we have observed CD20⁻ cutaneous recurrences of follicle center lymphoma after use of rituximab.

Prognosis

The prognosis of patients with primary cutaneous follicle center lymphoma is very good, regardless of the pattern of growth [1,18,20,79,80]. Although local recurrences can be frequently observed, extracutaneous involvement is uncommon. Involvement of the central nervous system has been observed rarely [81]. There is no prognostic difference between cases with a follicular pattern as compared to those with a diffuse pattern of growth [1,24].

Résumé

Clinical	Adults. Solitary or grouped papules, plaques and tumors, often surrounded by erythematous patches. Preferential locations: scalp, back (reticulohistiocytoma of the dorsum).
Morphology	Nodular or diffuse infiltrates characterized by predominance of centroblasts and centrocytes admixed with small lymphocytes. The pattern of growth can be follicular, diffuse or mixed.
Immunology	CD20, 79a + CD10, Bcl-6 + CD5, 43 − Bcl-2 − MUM-1 − MIB-1/Ki67 Reduced proliferation of neoplastic follicles
Genetics	Monoclonal rearrangement of the J_H gene detected in the majority of cases. t(14;18) absent in most cases. Germinal center signature of neoplastic cells.
Treatment guidelines	Radiotherapy; excision of solitary lesions, interferon-α; anti-CD20 antibody. Systemic chemotherapy is reserved for generalized lesions and/or extracutaneous spread.

TEACHING CASE

This 71-year-old woman complained of hair loss for the last few months (Fig. 10.20a). Local treatments were not successful and a biopsy was done. Histology revealed dense lymphoid infiltrates with a nodular pattern (Fig. 10.20b), characterized by predominance of medium and large cleaved cells (Fig. 10.20c). Immunohistology showed strong positivity for CD20 as well as the presence of many clusters of CD21+ follicular dendritic cells. There were also large clusters of Bcl-6+ follicular cells that expressed Bcl-2 as well (Fig. 10.20d, e). Staging investigations disclosed a nodal follicular lymphoma in the abdominal lymph nodes.

Comment: This case shows two pitfalls in the diagnosis of cutaneous follicle center lymphoma: the first is represented by the clinical presentation, which is sometimes uncharacteristic (both in primary cutaneous cases and in secondary involvement by nodal lymphoma); the second concerns positivity of follicular lymphocytes for Bcl-2, which should always be considered suspicious for secondary cutaneous involvement by nodal follicular lymphoma, as in this case. Examples of primary cutaneous follicle center lymphoma with positivity of follicular B lymphocytes for Bcl-2 exist, but are extremely rare.

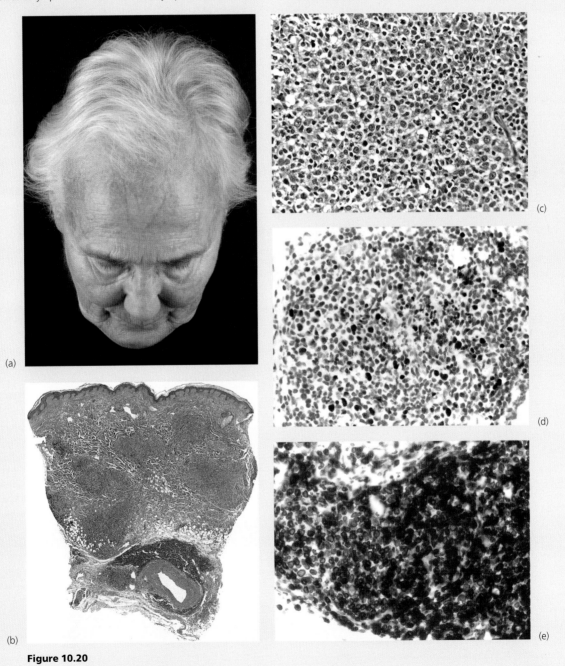

(a)

(b)

(c)

(d)

(e)

Figure 10.20

References

1. Willemze R, Jaffe ES, Burg G et al. WHO-EORTC classification for cutaneous lymphomas. Blood 2005;**105**:3768–3785.
2. Willemze R, Swerdlow SH, Harris NL, Vrgier B. Primary cutaneous follicle centre lymphoma. In: Swerdlow SH, Campo E, Harris NL et al., eds. WHO Classification of Tumours of Haematopoietic and Lymphoid Tissues. Lyon: IARC Press, 2008: 227–228.
3. Willemze R, Kerl H, Sterry W et al. EORTC classification for primary cutaneous lymphomas: a proposal from the Cutaneous Lymphoma Study Group of the European Organization for Research and Treatment of Cancer. Blood 1997;**90**:354–371.
4. Nathwani BN, Harris NL, Weisenburger D et al. Follicular lymphoma. In: Jaffe ES, Harris NL, Stein H, Vardiman JW, eds. World Health Organization Classification of Tumours: Tumours of Haematopoietic and Lymphoid Tissues. Lyon: IARC Press, 2001: 162–167.
5. Dogan A, Bagdi E, Munson P, Isaacson PG. CD10 and Bcl-6 expression in paraffin sections of normal lymphoid tissue and B-cell lymphomas. Am J Surg Pathol 2000;**24**:846–852.
6. Isaacson PG. Malignant lymphomas with a follicular growth pattern. Histopathology 1996;**28**:487–495.
7. Gaulard P, D'Agay MF, Peuchmaur M et al. Expression of the bcl-2 gene product in follicular lymphoma. Am J Surg Pathol 1992;**140**:1089–1095.
8. Tsujimoto Y, Cossman J, Jaffe E, Croce CM. Involvement of the bcl-2 gene in human follicular lymphoma. Science 1985;**228**:1440–1443.
9. Pezzella F, Gatter KC, Mason DY et al. Bcl-2 protein expression in follicular lymphomas in absence of 14;18 translocation. Lancet 1990;**336**:1510–1511.
10. Ngan BY, Chen-Levy Z, Weiss LM, Warnke RA, Cleary ML. Expression in non-Hodgkin's lymphoma of the bcl-2 protein associated with the t(14;18) chromosomal translocation. N Engl J Med 1988;**318**:1638–1644.
11. Cerroni L, Volkenandt M, Rieger E, Soyer HP, Kerl H. Bcl-2 protein expression and correlation with the interchromosomal 14;18 translocation in cutaneous lymphomas and pseudolymphomas. J Invest Dermatol 1994;**102**:231–235.
12. Delia D, Borrello MG, Berti E et al. Clonal immunoglobulin gene rearrangements and normal T-cell receptor, bcl-2, and c-myc genes in primary cutaneous B-cell lymphomas. Cancer Res 1989;**49**:4901–4905.
13. Isaacson PG, Norton AJ. Extranodal Lymphomas, Edinburgh: Churchill Livingstone, 1994: 131–191.
14. Slater DN. Are most primary cutaneous B-cell lymphomas 'marginal cell lymphomas'?: reply. Br J Dermatol 1995;**133**:953–954.
15. Berti E, Gianotti R, Alessi E, Caputo R. Primary cutaneous follicle center cell lymphoma: immunogenotypical and immunophenotypical aspects. In: van Vloten WA, Willemze R, Lange Vejlsgaard G, Thomsen K, eds. Cutaneous Lymphomas and Pseudolymphomas. Basel: Karger, 1990: 196–202.
16. Garcia CF, Weiss LM, Warnke RA, Wood GS. Cutaneous follicular lymphoma. Am J Surg Pathol 1986;**10**:454–463.
17. Kerl H, Kresbach H. Germinal center cell-derived lymphomas of the skin. J Dermatol Surg Oncol 1984;**10**:291–295.
18. Pimpinelli N, Santucci M, Bosi A et al. Primary cutaneous follicular centre-cell lymphoma: a lymphoproliferative disease with favourable prognosis. Clin Exp Dermatol 1989;**14**:12–19.
19. Pimpinelli N, Santucci M, Carli P et al. Primary cutaneous follicular center cell lymphoma: clinical and histological aspects. In: van Vloten WA, Willemze R, Lange Vejlsgaard G, Thomsen K, eds. Cutaneous Lymphomas and Pseudolymphomas. Basel: Karger, 1990: 203–220.
20. Cerroni L, Arzberger E, Pütz B et al. Primary cutaneous follicle center lymphoma with follicular growth pattern. Blood 2000;**95**:3922–3928.
21. Goodlad JR, Krajewski AS, Batstone PJ et al. Primary cutaneous follicular lymphoma: a clinicopathologic and molecular study of 16 cases in support of a distinct entity. Am J Surg Pathol 2002;**26**:733–741.
22. Mirza I, Macpherson N, Paproski S et al. Primary cutaneous follicular lymphoma: an assessment of clinical, histopathologic, immunophenotypic, and molecular features. J Clin Oncol 2002;**20**:647–655.
23. Lawnicki LC, Weisenburger DD, Aoun P et al. The t(14;18) and bcl-2 expression are present in a subset of primary cutaneous follicular lymphoma. Am J Clin Pathol 2002;**118**:765–772.
24. Fink-Puches R, Zenahlik P, Bäck B et al. Primary cutaneous lymphomas: applicability of current classification schemes (European Organization for Research and Treatment of Cancer, World Health Organization) based on clinicopathologic features observed in a large group of patients. Blood 2002;**99**:800–805.
25. Senff NJ, Kluin-Nelemans JC, Willemze R. Results of bone marrow examination in 275 patients with histological features that suggest an indolent type of cutaneous B-cell lymphoma. Br J Haematol 2008;**142**:52–56.
26. Ghislanzoni M, Gambini D, Perrone T, Alessi E, Berti E. Primary cutaneous follicular center cell lymphoma of the nose with maxillary sinus involvement in a pediatric patient. J Am Acad Dermatol 2005;**52**:s73–s75.
27. Crosti A. Micosi fungoide e reticuloistiocitomi cutanei maligni. Min Dermatol 1951;**26**:3–11.
28. Berti E, Alessi E, Caputo R et al. Reticulohistiocytoma of the dorsum. J Am Acad Dermatol 1988;**19**:259–272.
29. Cerroni L, Zöchling N, Pütz B, Kerl H. Infection by Borrelia burgdorferi and cutaneous B-cell lymphoma. J Cutan Pathol 1997;**24**:457–461.
30. Goodlad JR, Davidson MM, Hollowood K et al. Primary cutaneous B-cell lymphoma and Borrelia burgdorferi infection in patients from the highlands of Scotland. Am J Surg Pathol 2000;**24**:1279–1285.
31. Zöchling N, Pütz B, Wolf P, Kerl H, Cerroni L. Human herpesvirus 8–specific DNA sequences in primary cutaneous B-cell lymphomas. Arch Dermatol 1998;**134**:246–247.
32. Viguier M, River J, Agbalika F et al. B-cell lymphomas involving the skin associated with hepatitis C virus infection. Int J Dermatol 2002;**41**:577–582.
33. Bachmeyer C, Khosrotehrani K, Moguelet P, Aractingi S. Primary cutaneous follicular B-cell lymphoma arising at the site of radiotherapy for breast cancer. Br J Dermatol 2006;**156**:198–199.
34. Nathwani BN, Winberg CD, Diamond LW, Bearman RM, Kim H. Morphologic criteria for the differentiation of follicular lymphoma from florid reactive follicular hyperplasia: a study of 80 cases. Cancer 1981;**48**:1794–1806.
35. English JSC, Smith NP, Spaull J, Wilson Jones E, Winkelmann RK. Large cell lymphocytoma: a clinicopathological study. Clin Exp Dermatol 1989;**14**:181–185.

36. Winkelmann RK, Dabski K. Large cell lymphocytoma: follow-up, immunopathology studies, and comparison to cutaneous follicular and Crosti lymphoma. *Arch Dermatol Res* 1987;**279**:S81–87.

37. Cerroni L, El-Shabrawi-Caelen L, Fink-Puches R, LeBoit PE, Kerl H. Cutaneous spindle-cell B-cell lymphoma: a morphologic variant of cutaneous large B-cell lymphoma. *Am J Dermatopathol* 2000;**22**:299–304.

38. Ferrara G, Bevilacqua M, Argenziano G. Cutaneous spindle B-cell lymphoma: a reappraisal. *Am J Dermatopathol* 2002;**24**:526–527.

39. Cerroni L. Reply to cutaneous spindle B-cell lymphoma: a reappraisal. *Am J Dermatopathol* 2002;**24**:527–528.

40. Goodlad JR. Spindle-cell B-cell lymphoma presenting in the skin. *Br J Dermatol* 2001;**145**:313–317.

41. Ries S, Barr R, LeBoit P, McCalmont TH, Waldman J. Cutaneous sarcomatoid B-cell lymphoma. *Am J Dermatopathol* 2007;**29**:96–98.

42. Carbone A, Gloghini A, Libra M *et al.* A spindle cell variant of diffuse large B-cell lymphoma possesses genotypic and phenotypic markers characteristic of a germinal center B-cell origin. *Mod Pathol* 2006;**19**:299–306.

43. Yun SJ, Lee KH, Yang DW, *et al.* Primary cutaneous spindle cell B-cell lymphoma with multiple figurate erythema-like manifestation. *J Cut Pathol* 2009;**36**:49–52.

44. Leinweber B, Colli C, Chott A, Kerl H, Cerroni L. Differential diagnosis of cutaneous infiltrates of B lymphocytes with follicular growth pattern. *Am J Dermatopathol* 2004;**26**:4–13.

45. Hoefnagel JJ, Vermeer MH, Jansen PM *et al.* Bcl-2, Bcl-6 and CD10 expression in cutaneous B-cell lymphoma: further support for a follicle centre cell origin and differential diagnostic significance. *Br J Dermatol* 2003;**149**:1183–1191.

46. Dogan AMQ, Aiello A, Diss TC *et al.* Follicular lymphomas contain a clonally linked but phenotypically distinct neoplastic B-cell population in the interfollicular zone. *Blood* 1988;**91**: 4708–4714.

47. Martinez A, Pittaluga S, Rudelius M *et al.* Expression of the interferon regulatory factor 8/ICSBP-1 in human reactive lymphoid tissues and B-cell lymphomas: a novel germinal center marker. *Am J Surg Pathol* 2008;**32**:1190–1200.

48. De Leval L, Harris NL, Longtine J, Ferry JA, Duncan LM. Cutaneous B-cell lymphomas of follicular and marginal zone types: use of Bcl-6, CD10, Bcl-2 and CD21 in differential diagnosis and classification. *Am J Surg Pathol* 2001;**25**:732–741.

49. Rijlaarsdam JU, Meijer CJLM, Willemze R. Differentiation between lymphadenosis benigna cutis and primary cutaneous follicular center cell lymphomas: a comparative clinicopathologic study of 57 patients. *Cancer* 1990;**65**:2301–2306.

50. Triscott JA, Ritter JH, Swanson PE, Wick MR. Immunoreactivity for bcl-2 protein in cutaneous lymphomas and lymphoid hyperplasias. *J Cutan Pathol* 1995;**22**:2–10.

51. Kodama K, Massone C, Chott A, Metze D, Kerl H, Cerroni L. Primary cutaneous large B-cell lymphomas: clinicopathologic features, classification, and prognostic factors in a large series of patients. *Blood* 2005;**106**:2491–2497.

52. Franco R, Fernandez-Vazquez A, Rodriguez-Peralto JL *et al.* Cutaneous follicular B-cell lymphoma: description of a series of 18 cases. *Am J Surg Pathol* 2001;**25**:875–883.

53. Child FJ, Russell-Jones R, Woolford AJ *et al.* Absence of the t(14;18) chromosomal translocation in primary cutaneous B-cell lymphoma. *Br J Dermatol* 2001;**144**:735–744.

54. Streubel B, Scheucher B, Valencak J *et al.* Molecular cytogenetic evidence of t(14;18)(*IGH;BCL2*) in a substantial proportion of primary cutaneous follicle center lymphomas. *Am J Surg Pathol* 2006;**30**:529–536.

55. Kim BK, Surti U, Pandya A, Cohen J, Rabkin MS, Swerdlow SH. Clinicopathologic, immunophenotypic, and molecular cytogenetic fluorescence in situ hybridization analysis of primary and secondary cutaneous follicular lymphomas. *Am J Surg Pathol* 2005;**29**:69–82.

56. Jetic TM, Berry PK, Jubetirer SJ *et al.* Primary cutaneous follicle center lymphoma of the arm with a novel chromosomal translocation t(12;21)(q13;q22): a case report. *Am J Hematol* 2006;**81**:448–453.

57. Storz MN, van de Rijn M, Kim YH *et al.* Gene expression profiles of cutaneous B cell lymphoma. *J Invest Dermatol* 2003;**120**:865–870.

58. Hoefnagel JJ, Dijkman R, Basso K *et al.* Distinct types of primary cutaneous large B-cell lymphoma identified by gene expression profiling. *Blood* 2005;**105**:3671–3678.

59. van Galen JC, Hoefnagel JJ, Vermeer MH *et al.* Profiling of apoptosis genes identifies distinct types of primary cutaneous large B cell lymphoma. *J Pathol* 2008;**215**:340–346.

60. Golembowsky S, Gellrich S, von Zimmermann M *et al.* Clonal evolution in a primary cutaneous follicle center B cell lymphoma revealed by single cell analysis in sequential biopsies. *Immunobiology* 2000;**201**:631–644.

61. Raaphorst FM, Vermeer M, Fieret E *et al.* Site-specific expression of polycomb-group genes encoding the HPC-HPH/PRC1 complex in clinically defined primary nodal and cutaneous large B-cell lymphomas. *Am J Pathol* 2004;**164**:533–542.

62. Senff NJ, Hoefnagel JJ, Jansen PM *et al.* Reclassification of 300 primary cutaneous B-cell lymphomas according to the new WHO-EORTC classification for cutaneous lymphomas: comparison with previous classifications and identification of prognostic markers. *J Clin Oncol* 2007;**25**:1581–1587.

63. Rijlaarsdam JU, Toonstra J, Meijer CJLM, Noordijk EM, Willemze R. Treatment of primary cutaneous B-cell lymphomas of follicle center cell origin: a clinical follow-up study of 55 patients treated with radiotherapy or polychemotherapy. *J Clin Oncol* 1996;**14**:549–555.

64. Piccinno R, Caccialanza M, Berti E. Dermatologic radiotherapy of primary cutaneous follicle center cell lymphoma. *Eur J Dermatol* 2003;**13**:49–52.

65. Zenahlik P, Fink-Puches R, Kapp KS, Kerl H, Cerroni L. Die Therapie der primären kutanen B-Zell-Lymphome. *Hautarzt* 2000;**51**:19–24.

66. Senff NJ, Noordijk EM, Kim YH *et al.* European Organization for Research and Treatment of Cancer and International Society for Cutaneous Lymphoma consensus recommendations for the management of cutaneous B-cell lymphomas. *Blood* 2008;**112**: 1600–1609.

67. Parodi A, Micalizzi C, Rebora A. Intralesional natural interferon-α in the treatment of Crosti's lymphoma (primary cutaneous B follicular centre-cell lymphoma): report of four cases. *J Dermatol Treatm* 1996;**7**:105–107.

68. Cerroni L, Peris K, Torlone G, Chimenti S. Use of recombinant interferon-α2a in the treatment of cutaneous lymphomas of T- and B-cell lineage. In: Lambert WC, Giannotti B, van Vloten WA, eds. *Basic Mechanisms of Physiologic and Aberrant Lymphoproliferation in the Skin.* New York: Plenum Press, 1994: 545–551.

69. Trent JT, Romanelli P, Kerdel FA. Topical targretin and intralesional interferon-α for cutaneous lymphoma of the scalp. *Arch Dermatol* 2002;**138**:1421–1423.

70. Kempf W, Dummer R, Hess Schmid M *et al.* Intralesional cisplatin for the treatment of cutaneous B-cell lymphoma. *Arch Dermatol* 1998;**134**:1343–1345.

71. Heinzerling LM, Urbanek M, Funk JO *et al.* Reduction of tumor burden and stabilization of disease by systemic therapy with anti-CD20 antibody (rituximab) in patients with primary cutaneous B-cell lymphoma. *Cancer* 2000;**89**:1835–1844.

72. Schmook T, Stockfleth E, Lischner S *et al.* Remarkable remission of a follicular lymphoma treated with rituximab and polychemotherapy (CHOP). *Clin Exp Dermatol* 2003;**28**:31–33.

73. Paul T, Radny P, Kröber SM *et al.* Intralesional rituximab for cutaneous B-cell lymphoma. *Br J Dermatol* 2001;**144**:1239–1243.

74. Gellrich S, Muche JM, Pelzer K, Audring H, Sterry W. Der Anti-CD20-Antikörper bei primär kutanen B-Zell-Lymphomen. *Hautarzt* 2001;**52**:205–210.

75. Heinzerling L, Dummer R, Kempf W, Hess Schmid M, Burg G. Intralesional therapy with anti-CD20 monoclonal antibody rituximab in primary cutaneous B-cell lymphoma. *Arch Dermatol* 2000;**136**:374–378.

76. Kennedy GA, Blum R, McCormack C, Prince HM. Treatment of primary cutaneous follicular centre lymphoma with rituximab: a report of two cases. *Australas J Dermatol* 2004;**45**:54–57.

77. Fink-Puches R, Wolf IH, Zalaudek I, Kerl H, Cerroni L. Treatment of primary cutaneous B-cell lymphoma with rituximab. *J Am Acad Dermatol* 2005;**52**:847–853.

78. Fierro MT, Savoia P, Quaglino P *et al.* Systemic therapy with cyclophosphamide and anti-CD20 antibody (rituximab) in relapsed primary cutaneous B-cell lymphoma: a report of 7 cases. *J Am Acad Dermatol* 2003;**49**:281–287.

79. Willemze R, Meijer CJLM, Sentis HJ *et al.* Primary cutaneous large cell lymphomas of follicular center cell origin: a clinical follow-up study of 19 patients. *J Am Acad Dermatol* 1987;**16**:518–526.

80. Zinzani PL, Quaglino P, Pimpinelli N *et al.* Prognostic factors in primary cutaneous B-cell lymphoma: the Italian Study Group for Cutaneous Lymphomas. *J Clin Oncol* 2006;**24**:1376–1382.

81. Bekkenk MW, Postma TJ, Meijer CJLM, Willemze R. Frequency of central nervous system involvement in primary cutaneous B-cell lymphoma. *Cancer* 2000;**89**:913–919.

11 Cutaneous marginal zone lymphoma and variants

Primary cutaneous marginal zone lymphoma is one of the major subtypes of the low-grade malignant cutaneous B-cell lymphomas. In the World Health Organization (WHO)-European Organization for Research and Treatment of Cancer (EORTC) classification of primary cutaneous lymphomas the group of marginal zone lymphoma includes also lesions that were formerly classified as primary cutaneous immunocytoma and primary cutaneous plasmacytoma [1]. In fact, most authors have agreed that cutaneous marginal zone lymphoma and cutaneous immunocytoma represent two subtypes of a single entity of low-grade malignant cutaneous B-cell lymphoma, and the term "cutaneous marginal zone lymphoma" has been widely used to refer to both [2–9]. Cases reported in the past as "cutaneous follicular lymphoid hyperplasia with monotypic plasma cells" most likely represent examples of marginal zone lymphoma of the skin [10]. A review of cases classified previously as "cutaneous lymphoid hyperplasia" allowed reclassification of at least some of them as true cutaneous marginal zone lymphomas [11].

Recently, the knowledge of cases classified as "primary cutaneous plasmacytoma" that have subsequently recurred as cutaneous marginal zone lymphoma induced the WHO-EORTC panel to include cutaneous plasmacytoma in the same group as well [1].

There is no doubt that these three entities (that is, cutaneous marginal zone lymphoma, cutaneous immunocytoma and cutaneous plasmacytoma) are closely related. However, some differences do exist and in this edition of the book, as well as in the second edition, we dedicate specific sections to all three variants. In fact, we believe that for the moment one should still try to characterize each of them separately, in order to check whether the differences are substantial or not. Unfortunately, in the new WHO classification of tumors of hematopoietic and lymphoid tissues published in 2008 the cutaneous marginal zone B-cell lymphoma has been lumped into the group of extranodal marginal zone lymphoma of the mucosal-associated lymphoid tissue (MALT) [12], thus

rendering the distinction of specific variants of it even more difficult.

As the terms "cutaneous immunocytoma" and "cutaneous plasmacytoma" (used in the second edition of this book) are misleading, we will divide this chapter into three parts:
1 cutaneous marginal zone lymphoma, conventional variant
2 cutaneous marginal zone lymphoma, lymphoplasmacytic variant (formerly cutaneous immunocytoma)
3 cutaneous marginal zone lymphoma, plasmacytic variant (formerly cutaneous plasmacytoma).
In our view, particularly between the conventional and the lymphoplasmacytic variants of cutaneous marginal zone lymphoma there are differences that are worth mentioning, and that can be summarized as follows.
• The conventional variant of cutaneous marginal zone lymphoma is a tumor of younger adults and adults, whereas the lymphoplasmacytic variant is seen more often in the elderly.
• The preferential location differs (trunk and upper extremities for the conventional variant, lower extremities for the lymphoplasmacytic variant).
• Association with *Borrelia burgdorferi* infection is more common in the lymphoplasmacytic variant [13]. We have observed cases of the lymphoplasmacytic variant, but not of conventional marginal zone lymphoma, arising on the background of acrodermatitis chronica atrophicans.
• The histopathologic pattern differs (see below); intranuclear inclusions (Dutcher bodies) are seen only in the lymphoplasmacytic variant.
However, we fully acknowledge that the differences may be just variations on the theme of a single entity of low-grade cutaneous B-cell lymphoma, and have therefore decided to include all variants in a single chapter in this edition of the book. The terminology, notwithstanding the term adopted, is still not correct. Cutaneous marginal zone lymphomas are different from extranodal marginal zone lymphomas (which in turn are different from nodal marginal zone lymphomas and from splenic marginal zone lymphomas). The terminology of the new WHO classification is incorrect as well, as the skin is not a MALT organ. In short, a confusing language is being used and better terms for these entities will have to be found in due course.

Skin Lymphoma: The Illustrated Guide. By L. Cerroni, K. Gatter and H. Kerl. Published 2009 Blackwell Publishing, ISBN: 978-1-4051-8554-7.

In this context, it is interesting to note that in the new WHO classification, lymphoplasmacytic lymphoma is included as a specific entity defined as "a neoplasm of small B lymphocytes, plasmacytoid lymphocytes, and plasma cells, (. . .) which does not fulfil the criteria for any of the other small B-cell lymphoid neoplasms that may also have plasmacytic differentiation" [12]. In the same chapter the following statement is also made: "Because the distinction between lymphoplasmacytic lymphoma and one of these other lymphomas, especially some marginal zone lymphomas, is not always clear-cut, some cases may need to be diagnosed as a small B-cell lymphoma with plasmacytic differentiation and a differential diagnosis provided." In short, at sites other than the skin, too, the distinction between lymphoplasmacytic lymphoma and marginal zone lymphoma is not clear-cut, yet the WHO scheme includes both groups as separate entities.

A relationship between extracutaneous marginal zone lymphoma and extramedullary plasmacytoma had been postulated previously [14], again suggesting that these entities of low-grade B-cell lymphoma may be related. In addition, transformation to pure proliferations of plasma cells has been observed in six cases of extracutaneous marginal zone lymphoma treated with rituximab [15].

Finally, notwithstanding the exact classification of cases formerly diagnosed as "primary cutaneous plasmacytoma," it must be underlined that multiple myeloma can present with specific cutaneous manifestations that have peculiar and repeatable clinicopathologic features, and that should be clearly distinguished from cases of cutaneous marginal zone lymphoma with plasmacytic differentiation. We included a short discussion on specific cutaneous manifestations of multiple myeloma in the chapter on "Other cutaneous B-cell lymphomas" (see Chapter 13).

CUTANEOUS MARGINAL ZONE LYMPHOMA, CONVENTIONAL VARIANT

The conventional variant of primary cutaneous marginal zone lymphoma is by far the most frequent among the three morphologic subtypes. Association with *B. burgdorferi* has been detected in some cases in areas both with and without endemic infection [11,16,17]. However, this association may be regional, as other studies on cutaneous marginal zone lymphoma did not show evidence of infection by *B. burgdorferi* [18–20]. In addition, it seems that association with *B. burgdorferi* is more frequent in the lymphoplasmacytic type of marginal zone lymphoma (see corresponding section). A link with *Helicobacter pylori* infection has been proposed by some and ruled out by others [21,22], and association with hepatitis C virus infection seems unlikely [23,24]. Other micro-organisms have been related to extranodal marginal zone lymphomas of MALT arising at sites other than the skin, including *Chlamydia jejuni* and *psittaci*, suggesting that this

group of lymphomas may be related to different infectious micro-organisms, irrespective of the site of origin [25]. In spite of rare positive cases, there seems to be no involvement of human herpes viruses (HHV) 7 and 8 in the pathogenesis of cutaneous marginal zone lymphoma [26,27]. The knowledge that different examples of cutaneous marginal zone lymphoma recognize similar antigens supports the hypothesis of an antigen-driven disorder [28,29], similar to what happens in MALT lymphoma of the gastric mucosa.

An alternative hypothesis has been proposed by Breza *et al*, who observed a case of cutaneous marginal zone lymphoma in a patient under fluoxetine therapy and suggested that an inhibitory effect on T-suppressor lymphocyte function may lead to excessive antigen-driven B-cell proliferations [30].

In two patients, the onset of cutaneous marginal zone lymphoma followed successful treatment of nodal Hodgkin lymphoma, and one further case has been reported following vaccination [31,32].

Clinical features

Patients are typically younger adults with a male predominance [3,33]. Onset in childhood has been observed [34,35]. They present with red to reddish brown papules, plaques and nodules localized particularly to the upper extremities or the trunk. Lesions are commonly solitary but may be multiple, characterized either by localized clusters of papules and small nodules or by several lesions scattered on the trunk and upper extremities (Figs 11.1–11.3). Cutaneous recurrences are frequent and may be distant from the primary site of involvement. The clinical picture of "Crosti's lymphoma" (see Chapter 10) is not found in patients with cutaneous marginal zone lymphoma, but clustered lesions may be observed.

The onset of anetoderma in some lesions of cutaneous marginal zone lymphoma has been reported [36,37].

Complete staging investigations should be performed, particularly to exclude cutaneous involvement from other types of extranodal marginal zone lymphoma of MALT. It seems that bone marrow involvement is very rare in patients with cutaneous disease [38–40], thus questioning the need for bone marrow biopsy as a standard staging investigation in these patients.

Histopathology, immunophenotype and molecular genetics

Histopathology

Histology shows patchy, nodular or diffuse infiltrates involving the dermis and sometimes the superficial part of the subcutaneous fat. The epidermis is not involved. The infiltrate may be top-heavy (Fig. 11.4) or, more frequently, bottom-heavy

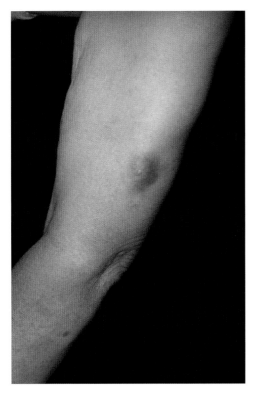

Figure 11.1 Cutaneous marginal zone B-cell lymphoma, conventional variant. Solitary erythematous nodule on the arm.

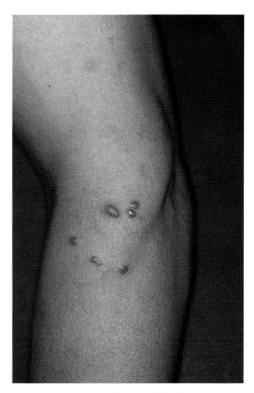

Figure 11.3 Cutaneous marginal zone B-cell lymphoma, conventional variant. Cluster of small erythematous nodules on the arm.

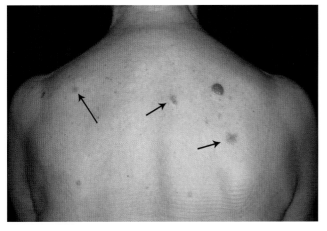

Figure 11.2 Cutaneous marginal zone B-cell lymphoma, conventional variant. Large erythematous nodule on the upper back. Note an earlier lesion on the left shoulder (*long arrow*) and two scars from previous excisions of similar lesions on the back (*short arrows*).

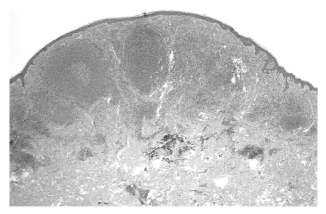

Figure 11.4 Cutaneous marginal zone B-cell lymphoma, conventional variant. Dense nodular infiltrates within the dermis. Note characteristic arrangement of the cells with central nodules of reactive lymphocytes, one with a germinal center, surrounded by small amounts of neoplastic cells (see text).

(Fig. 11.5). A characteristic pattern can be observed at scanning magnification: nodular infiltrates with follicles, sometimes containing reactive germinal centers, are surrounded by a pale-staining peri- and interfollicular population of small- to medium-sized cells with indented nuclei, inconspicuous nucleoli and abundant pale cytoplasm (marginal zone cells, centrocyte-like cells) (Fig. 11.6) [3]. In addition,

plasma cells (at the margins of the infiltrate), lymphoplasmacytoid cells, small lymphocytes and occasional large blasts are observed. The number of neoplastic cells within the infiltrate is variable and can be very low (Fig. 11.7) [41].

In typical cases, the neoplastic population is composed of marginal zone cells, a few lymphoplasmacytoid lymphocytes and several plasma cells, these last arranged at the periphery

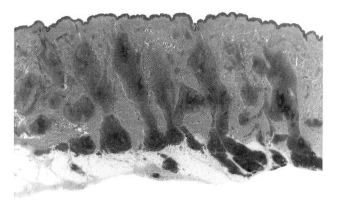

Figure 11.5 Cutaneous marginal zone lymphoma, conventional variant. Dense, "bottom-heavy" lymphoid infiltrates with reactive germinal centers. Note focal "triphasic" pattern characterized by pale cells in the center (corresponding to germinal center cells) surrounded by dark cells of the follicular mantle and by pale neoplastic marginal zone cells (see text).

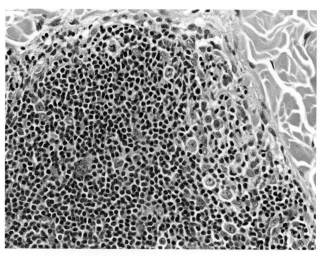

Figure 11.7 Cutaneous marginal zone lymphoma, conventional variant. Nodule of reactive lymphocytes showing at the periphery a proliferation of larger cells (marginal zone cells).

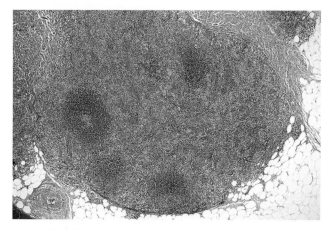

Figure 11.6 Cutaneous marginal zone B-cell lymphoma, conventional variant. Dense nodule within the deep dermis and superficial subcutaneous fat. Note small nodules of reactive lymphocytes (dark), one with a germinal center, surrounded by large numbers of neoplastic cells (pale) (see text).

of the aggregates and/or in small clusters. Usually marginal zone cells represent only a proportion of the neoplastic population (Fig. 11.8a), but in rare cases they predominate, forming sheets without plasma cell differentiation (Fig. 11.8c). In other lesions, neoplastic plasma cells predominate admixed with a few marginal zone cells, resembling the picture of cutaneous plasmacytoma (Fig. 11.8b) [42]. We classify these cases as cutaneous marginal zone lymphoma, plasmacytic variant (see corresponding section). Cases with predominance of blasts are rare (Fig. 11.9) and should be distinguished from examples of follicle center lymphoma by accurate immunophenotyping. Even in cases with predominance of blasts, reactive cells are a prominent component of the infiltrate and neoplastic cells are usually a minority of it. Eosinophils, as well as a granulomatous reaction, can be observed in some cases [3,43].

It should be emphasized that reactive cells (T and B lymphocytes, histiocytes, eosinophils) represent often the majority of the infiltrating cells in lesions of cutaneous marginal zone lymphoma, thus creating diagnostic problems.

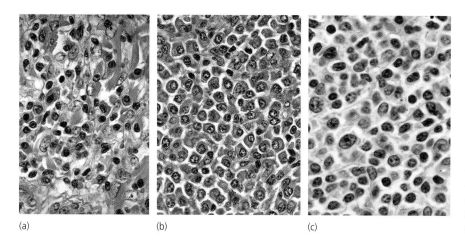

(a)   (b)   (c)

Figure 11.8 Cutaneous marginal zone B-cell lymphoma. (a) Marginal zone cells ("centrocyte-like") with abundant cytoplasm admixed with plasma cells, small lymphocytes and eosinophils. (b) Lymphoplasmacytoid cells and plasma cells predominate, admixed with some blastic cells. (c) Marginal zone cells, some with blastic morphology, predominate.

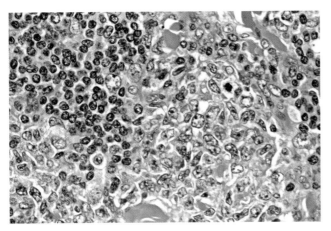

Figure 11.9 Cutaneous marginal zone B-cell lymphoma, conventional variant. Note several blastic cells admixed with small reactive lymphocytes.

Immunophenotype

The marginal zone cells reveal a CD20$^+$, CD79a$^+$, Bcl-2$^+$, CD5$^-$, CD10$^-$ and Bcl-6$^-$ phenotype. Bcl-6 and CD10 antibodies are particularly useful for differentiation of cutaneous marginal zone lymphoma with blastic differentiation from follicle center lymphoma [44–46]. Co-expression of CD20 and CD43 is usually not found [47]. Aberrant nuclear expression of Bcl-10 has been detected, representing a potential pitfall [48]. In approximately 75–85% of cases, intracytoplasmic monotypic expression of immunoglobulin light chains can be observed (Fig. 11.10). *In situ* hybridization for the immunoglobulin light chains is a more sensitive method than immunohistochemistry for detection of clonality (Fig. 11.11a, b).

Staining for Ki67 (MIB-1) shows that the proliferating population of B lymphocytes is characteristically disposed at the periphery of the cellular aggregates.

Interestingly, staining for CD123 shows in some cases clusters of positive plasmacytoid dendritic cells (Fig. 11.12). The role of these cells (if any) in the pathogenesis of cutaneous marginal zone lymphoma is still unclear.

Molecular genetics

A monoclonal rearrangement of the immunoglobulin heavy chain (J$_H$) gene can be observed in approximately 50–60% of cases. The t(11;18) and t(1;14) are not present in cutaneous cases [18,48–50]. A specific interchromosomal 14;18 translocation involving *IGH* and *MALT1* has been described in a subset of cutaneous marginal zone lymphomas as well as marginal zone lymphomas of other organs including the liver, ocular adnexa and salivary glands, indicating the relationship of some cutaneous cases to those arising at extracutaneous sites [49]. It seems that rare cases of cutaneous marginal zone lymphoma may harbor a conventional t(14;18) involving *IGH* and *BCL2* as well [51]. A new t(3;14)(p14;q32) involving *IGH* and *FOXP1* has been detected in a subset of MALT lymphomas arising at different sites, including 2/20 cutaneous cases tested [52]. It seems also that those cases showing a trisomy 3 are characterized by upregulation of *FOXP1* [52]. Gene expression studies using cDNA microarrays revealed that cases of cutaneous marginal zone lymphoma have a plasma cell signature [53].

Hypermethylation of *p15* and/or *p16* and expression of p15 and/or p16 protein have been observed in some patients with cutaneous marginal zone lymphoma [54].

Figure 11.10 Cutaneous marginal zone B-cell lymphoma, conventional variant. Monoclonal lambda expression of plasma cells at the periphery of nodular infiltrates.

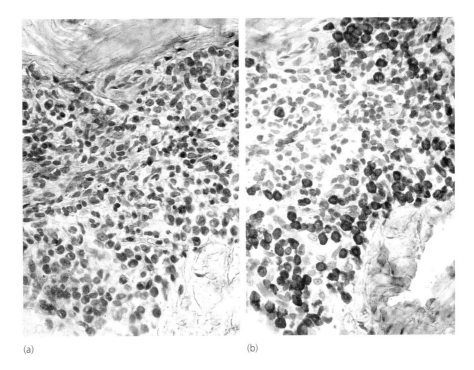

(a)

(b)

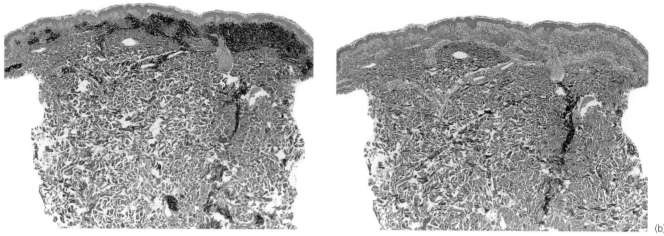

(a) (b)

Figure 11.11 Cutaneous marginal zone lymphoma, conventional variant. (a) Expression of κ immunoglobulin light-chain detected by *in situ* hybridization. (b) *In situ* hybridization for λ is negative.

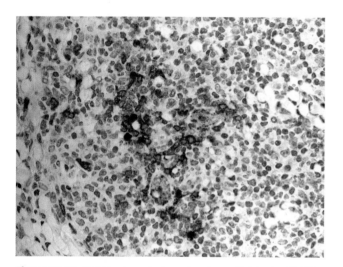

Figure 11.12 Cutaneous marginal zone lymphoma. Staining for CD123 shows a small cluster of positive cells.

A study on class-switched immunoglobulins revealed that cutaneous marginal zone lymphoma deviates from the general profile of extranodal marginal zone lymphoma of MALT [55]. IgM is expressed in most non-cutaneous cases, whereas cutaneous marginal zone lymphomas express IgG, IgA, and IgE and do not show an obvious immunoglobulin repertoire bias. In addition, in contrast to other extranodal marginal zone lymphomas of MALT, the isotype-switched cutaneous marginal zone lymphomas lack the chemokine receptor CXCR3 and seem to arise in a different inflammatory environment.

Recently, a study demonstrated the presence of aberrant somatic hypermutations in cases of cutaneous marginal zone lymphoma, suggesting that they could contribute to the pathogenesis of the disease by mutating regulatory and coding sequences of specific genes including the proto-oncogenes *PAX5*, *RhoH/TTF*, *c-MYC* and *MIM1* [56].

Treatment

Solitary lesions may be excised [57]. Complete responses have also been achieved after administration of systemic steroids. Many patients can be managed with a so-called "watchful waiting" strategy [57]. Patients with multiple lesions can be treated with interferon-α or anti-CD20 antibodies (rituximab) [58–64]. Complete responses after systemic antibiotics have been reported, and this should probably be the primary treatment for patients with evidence of *B. burgdorferi* infection (see also following section on cutaneous marginal zone lymphoma, lymphoplasmacytic variant) [59,65,66]. For patients presenting with multiple lesions requiring treatment, chlorambucil is often used in European centers (but less so in the United States), especially in older patients and for a maximum of 3 months [57]. Radiotherapy is effective, particularly for single tumors; however, recurrences are usually at sites different from those treated initially, so this option is usually not suggested as first-line treatment, particularly for young patients. Systemic multiagent chemotherapy should be reserved for those rare cases with extracutaneous dissemination.

Prognosis

The prognosis is excellent and the estimated 5-year survival is 98% [67–69]. Recurrences can be observed in 40–50% of patients after successful treatment but retain the low-grade features of the primary tumor. At present, the prognostic significance of different histopathologic subtypes (conventional, lymphoplasmacytic and plasmacytic), if any, is unclear. Blastic transformation in recurrent lesions has been associated with a worse prognosis [70]. It has been suggested that cases with Bcl-10 nuclear expression have a locally more aggressive behavior [18]. It seems that detection of specific cells in the bone marrow does not impact on the prognosis of patients with cutaneous marginal zone lymphoma [39,40].

Résumé

Cutaneous marginal zone lymphoma, conventional variant

Clinical	Young adults and adults; cases in children reported. Solitary or grouped papules or small nodules. Preferential locations: upper extremities, trunk.
Morphology	Patchy, nodular or diffuse infiltrates. Characteristic pattern with central nodular dark area composed of small reactive lymphocytes with or without formation of germinal centers, surrounded by a pale area where neoplastic marginal zone cells and plasma cells predominate.
Immunology	CD20, 79a + Bcl-2 + CD5, 10, 43, Bcl-6 – cIg + (monoclonal)
Genetics	Monoclonal rearrangement of the J_H gene detected in 50–60% of cases. t(14;18)(q32;q21) in a minority of cases.
Treatment guidelines	Excision of solitary lesions; systemic steroids; radiotherapy; "watchful waiting". Interferon-α and anti-CD20 antibody (rituximab) are effective. Antibiotic treatment should be used as first-line treatment if evidence of *B. burgdorferi* infection. Systemic chemotherapy reserved for patients with extracutaneous spread.

CUTANEOUS MARGINAL ZONE LYMPHOMA, LYMPHOPLASMACYTIC VARIANT

The lymphoplasmacytic variant of cutaneous marginal zone lymphoma is characterized by a monomorphous proliferation of small lymphocytes, lymphoplasmacytoid cells and plasma cells showing monotypic intracytoplasmic immunoglobulins. Patients do not show the features of Waldenström macroglobulinemia and have an excellent prognosis and response to treatment. Rare reports on cutaneous lymphoplasmacytic lymphoma in patients with Waldenström macroglobulinemia probably represent secondary cutaneous involvement rather than primary cutaneous lymphoplasmacytic lymphoma [71]. Most of the cases reported in the recent past as cutaneous immunocytomas would be classified today as "conventional" marginal zone lymphomas, but some show the peculiar clinicopathologic features analyzed in this section [72,73].

There may be a link between this variant of marginal zone lymphoma and infection by *B. burgdorferi*. In the past, cases of

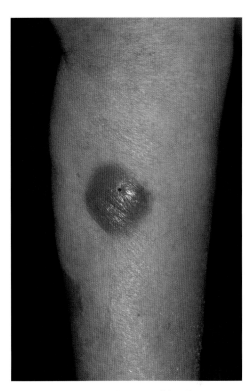

Figure 11.13 Cutaneous marginal zone B-cell lymphoma, lymphoplasmacytic variant. Large dome-shaped tumor on the lower leg.

"cutaneous immunocytoma" have been observed arising within skin lesions of acrodermatitis chronica atrophicans [74]. In a study using the polymerase chain reaction (PCR) technique, 75% of cases classified as cutaneous immunocytoma were positive compared to 10% of cases of marginal zone lymphoma [11].

Clinical features

Patients are typically elderly, of either gender. Clinical examination reveals erythematous, reddish-brown plaques or dome-shaped tumors located especially on the lower extremities (Fig. 11.13). Ulceration is uncommon. Generalized tumors are never encountered; rarely, patients present with miliary lesions restricted to an anatomic area (Fig. 11.14) [75]. Anetoderma may develop within skin lesions of the lymphoplasmacytic variant of cutaneous marginal zone lymphoma (Fig. 11.15) [76].

Histopathology, immunophenotype and molecular genetics

Histopathology

The architectural pattern is characterized by dense, monomorphous, nodular or diffuse infiltrates with involvement of the

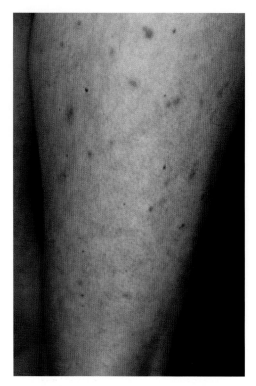

Figure 11.14 Cutaneous marginal zone B-cell lymphoma, lymphoplasmacytic variant. Miliary lesions on the upper leg.

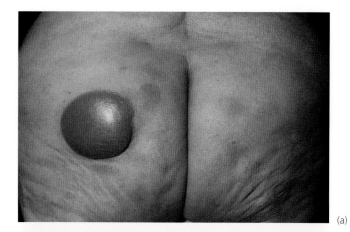

(a)

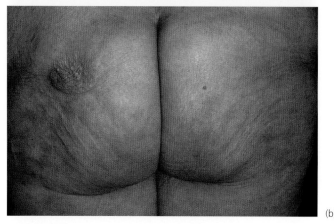

(b)

Figure 11.15 Cutaneous marginal zone B-cell lymphoma, lymphoplasmacytic variant. (a) Large dome-shaped tumor on the buttock. (b) Note resolution with anetoderma after radiotherapy.

dermis and subcutis (Fig. 11.16). The epidermis is usually spared. At scanning power, the "peripheral" pattern observed in conventional cases of cutaneous marginal zone lymphoma is not seen because the infiltrate is monomorphous. In addition, the neoplastic cells do not possess the abundant clear cytoplasm of marginal zone cells, giving the tumor a "darker" appearance compared to cutaneous marginal zone lymphoma, conventional variant.

The predominating cell types are lymphoplasmacytoid cells and small lymphocytes (Fig. 11.17a). In addition, plasma cells are usually present, often located at the periphery of the infiltrates. Periodic acid-Schiff (PAS)-positive intranuclear inclusions (Dutcher bodies) are observed as a rule and represent a valuable diagnostic clue (Fig. 11.17b). Reactive lymphoid follicles and germinal centers are rare.

In contrast to the conventional variant of cutaneous marginal zone lymphoma, neoplastic cells in the lymphoplasmacytic variant represent the great majority of the infiltrate, and reactive T and B lymphocytes and histiocytes are only a minority. Eosinophils and a granulomatous reaction are absent.

Immunophenotype

The neoplastic cells express monoclonal cytoplasmic immunoglobulins, more often IgG. B-cell-associated markers are positive, and CD5, CD10 and Bcl-6 are negative. Staining for CD43 reveals positivity of neoplastic cells in some cases.

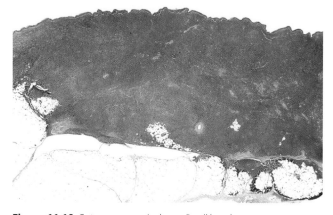

Figure 11.16 Cutaneous marginal zone B-cell lymphoma, lymphoplasmacytic variant. Dense diffuse infiltrates within the dermis and the subcutaneous fat.

Molecular genetics

Molecular analysis reveals monoclonal rearrangement of the J_H gene in most cases. The evaluation of specific genetic abnormalities is difficult, as cases are lumped together with those of the conventional variant of marginal zone lymphoma.

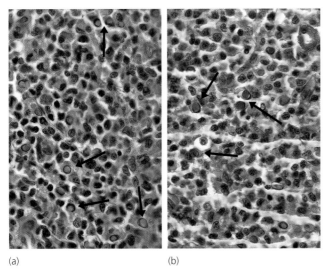

(a)   (b)

Figure 11.17 Cutaneous marginal zone B-cell lymphoma, lymphoplasmacytic variant. (a) Lymphoplasmacytoid lymphocytes predominate. Note several eosinophilic intranuclear inclusions ("Dutcher bodies") (*arrows*). (b) Intranuclear inclusions ("Dutcher bodies") stain bright purple–red with periodic acid–Schiff (PAS) (*arrows*).

Treatment

Small solitary nodules can be surgically excised. Larger lesions can be treated by local radiotherapy. As for other types of low-grade lymphoma, a "watchful waiting" strategy may be appropriate in some patients. Systemic chemotherapy usually is not used.

Cases with proven association with *B. burgdorferi* infection should be managed with systemic antibiotics first. At present this is the first-line treatment in cases of the lymphoplasmacytic variant of cutaneous marginal zone lymphoma treated in Graz (Austria), even when association with *B. burgdorferi* cannot be demonstrated with certainty. It should be underlined, however, that Graz lies in an endemic area of *B. burgdorferi* infection, thus lending a rationale to this approach that may be missing in non-endemic regions. On the other hand, our experience compared to that of other centers shows that this particular variant of marginal zone lymphoma arises more frequently, if not exclusively, in areas with endemic *B. burgdorferi* infection.

Prognosis

The prognosis of the lymphoplasmacytic variant of cutaneous marginal zone lymphoma is excellent, with only a few patients experiencing a more aggressive course [77]. Recurrences can be observed after treatment, usually at the same site. Cutaneous recurrences (without extracutaneous disease) have also been observed after systemic chemotherapy [78].

Résumé

Cutaneous marginal zone lymphoma, lymphoplasmacytic variant

Clinical	Adults and elderly. Solitary or grouped plaques or dome-shaped tumors. Preferential location: lower extremities. Frequent association with *B. burgdorferi* infection.
Morphology	Monomorphous, nodular or diffuse infiltrates characterized by predominance of lymphoplasmacytoid lymphocytes, small lymphocytes and plasma cells. Often Dutcher bodies.
Immunology	CD20, 79a + Bcl-2 + CD5, 10, Bcl-6 – CD43 +/– cIg + (monoclonal)
Genetics	Monoclonal rearrangement of the J_H gene detected in the majority of cases.
Treatment guidelines	Radiotherapy; surgical excision of small solitary lesions; "watchful waiting." Antibiotic treatment may be effective and is used as first-line treatment in some countries with endemic *B. burgdorferi* infection.

CUTANEOUS MARGINAL ZONE LYMPHOMA, PLASMACYTIC VARIANT

The plasmacytic variant of cutaneous marginal zone lymphoma is characterized by an almost exclusive proliferation of neoplastic plasma cells, hence the former classification as "cutaneous plasmacytoma" [79–86]. This variant of cutaneous marginal zone lymphoma is exceedingly rare, and should be distinguished from secondary skin involvement by multiple myeloma (see Chapter 13) [87].

In the second edition of this book we mentioned that probably most cases of so-called "primary cutaneous plasmacytoma" are in fact examples of cutaneous marginal zone lymphoma with a prominent plasma cell differentiation, and this view has been adopted also in the WHO-EORTC classification of cutaneous lymphomas [1]. In fact, we have observed patients with "cutaneous plasmacytoma" who, after successful treatment, relapsed with skin lesions showing histopathologic and phenotypical features of cutaneous marginal zone lymphoma. In addition, in a workshop on cutaneous plasmacytoma organized by the EORTC–Cutaneous Lymphomas Task Force in Bilbao in

2001, no clear-cut cases of primary cutaneous plasmacytoma could be identified. We believe that the literature on primary cutaneous plasmacytoma should be analyzed with a critical mind; it would also be interesting to have long-term follow-up data from cases published in the past.

Clinical features

The clinical presentation is similar to that of the conventional variant of cutaneous marginal zone lymphoma, with papules and small nodules, often solitary, located mostly on the upper extremities and the trunk.

Histopathology, immunophenotype and molecular genetics

Histopathology

Lesions consist of dense nodules and/or sheets of cells within the entire dermis and subcutis (Fig. 11.18), predominantly composed of mature plasma cells (Fig. 11.19). Dutcher bodies and Russell bodies are found occasionally. Small reactive lymphocytes are few or absent.

Amyloid deposits are almost never found in cutaneous marginal zone lymphoma, plasmacytic variant. Crystalloid intracytoplasmic inclusions within histiocytes and macrophages are also a feature of secondary cutaneous involvement by multiple myeloma rather than of primary cutaneous marginal zone lymphoma, plasmacytic variant (see Chapter 13).

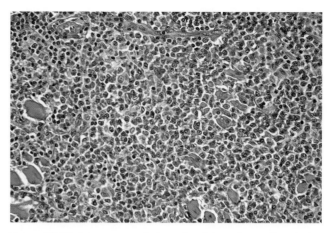

Figure 11.19 Cutaneous marginal zone lymphoma, plasmacytic variant. Predominance of mature plasma cells.

Immunophenotype

Neoplastic plasma cells show monoclonal expression of one immunoglobulin light chain, which is usually easy to detect in routine specimens (Fig. 11.20). Most B-cell-associated markers are negative, but cells can be stained by antibodies specific for CD38 or CD138 in most cases, and for CD79a in some cases. Immunohistochemical expression of cytokeratins, HMB45 and CD30 can be observed within neoplastic plasma cells, representing a source of diagnostic error.

Molecular genetics

Molecular analysis usually reveals a monoclonal rearrangement of the J_H gene. As already mentioned for the lymphoplasmacytic variant, also for the plasmacytic variant of cutaneous marginal zone lymphoma the evaluation of

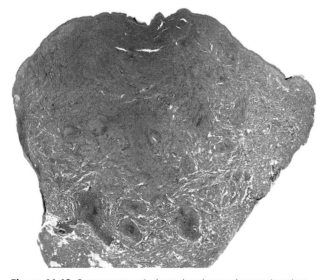

Figure 11.18 Cutaneous marginal zone lymphoma, plasmacytic variant. Dense infiltrate within the entire dermis.

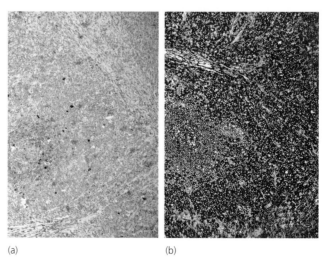

(a)   (b)

Figure 11.20 Cutaneous marginal zone lymphoma, plasmacytic variant. (a) Negative staining for λ and (b) positive staining for κ immunoglobulin light-chain.

specific genetic abnormalities is difficult, as cases are lumped together with those of the conventional variant.

Treatment and prognosis

Analysis of data published in the past on treatment of this variant of cutaneous marginal zone lymphoma is hindered by the fact that some cases reported as cutaneous plasmacytoma may have represented in truth examples of specific skin manifestations of multiple myeloma. The prognosis and treatment of choice seem to be the same as for the conventional variant of cutaneous marginal zone lymphoma.

Résumé

Cutaneous marginal zone lymphoma, plasmacytic variant

Clinical	Same features as the conventional variant of cutaneous marginal zone lymphoma.
Morphology	Nodular or diffuse infiltrates characterized by predominance of plasma cells.
Immunology	CD20 − CD38, 138 + CD79a +/− CIg + (monoclonal)
Genetics	Monoclonal rearrangement of the J_H gene detected in the majority of cases.
Treatment guidelines	Same as for the conventional variant of cutaneous marginal zone lymphoma.

TEACHING CASE

This 12-year-old girl presented with a small nodule on the right arm for some months (Fig. 11.21a). Although the clinical impression was not particularly suspicious, a biopsy revealed dense, bottom-heavy lymphoid infiltrates within the entire dermis and superficial subcutis (Fig. 11.21b). Cytomorphology was characterized by nodules of reactive small lymphocytes with a peripheral population of marginal zone cells, lymphoplasmacytoid cells and plasma cells (Fig. 11.21c). The proliferation rate was high at the periphery of the nodules (Fig. 11.21d), and there was a monoclonal expression of the immunoglobulin light chain κ. A diagnosis of cutaneous marginal zone lymphoma was made.

A PCR investigation of *Borrelia burgdorferi* DNA yielded a positive result, and the patient was treated with ceftriaxone for 3 weeks. Complete resolution was achieved within a few months of treatment completion.

Comment: This case illustrates the "iceberg" phenomenon of many cutaneous marginal zone lymphomas, that despite a clinically innocuous appearance they contain dense, bottom-heavy lymphoid infiltrates. It also shows that neoplastic cells in many cases of marginal zone lymphoma are only a minority, confined to the periphery of the nodules. Treatment with antibiotic led to complete remission and should be considered the first-line strategy in patients with proven *B. burgdorferi* infection. Finally, it should be remembered that cutaneous marginal zone lymphoma can be observed in pediatric patients [88].

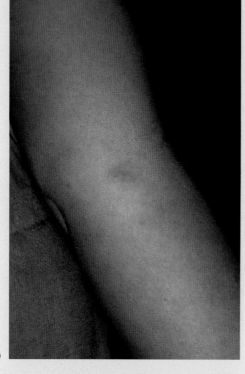

(a)

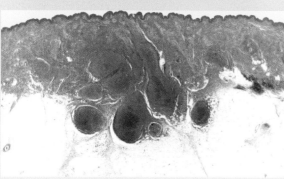

(b)

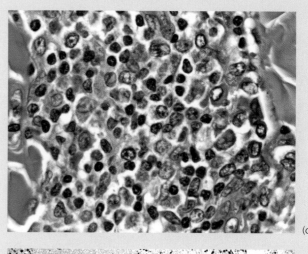

(c)

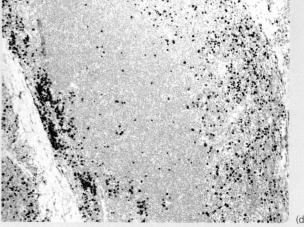

(d)

Figure 11.21

References

1. Willemze R, Jaffe ES, Burg G *et al.* WHO-EORTC classification for cutaneous lymphomas. *Blood* 2005;**105**:3768–3785.

2. Bailey EM, Ferry JA, Harris NL *et al.* Marginal zone lymphoma (low-grade B-cell lymphoma of mucosa-associated lymphoid tissue type) of skin and subcutaneous tissue: a study of 15 patients. *Am J Surg Pathol* 1996;**20**:1011–1023.

3. Cerroni L, Signoretti S, Höfler G *et al.* Primary cutaneous marginal zone B-cell lymphoma: a recently described entity of low-grade malignant cutaneous B-cell lymphoma. *Am J Surg Pathol* 1997;**21**:1307–1315.

4. de la Fouchardiére A, Balme B, Chouvet B *et al.* Primary cutaneous marginal zone B-cell lymphoma: a report of 9 cases. *J Am Acad Dermatol* 1999;**41**:181–188.

5. Duncan LN, LeBoit PE. Are primary cutaneous immunocytoma and marginal zone lymphoma the same disease? *Am J Surg Pathol* 1997;**21**:1368–1372.

6. Sander CA, Kaudewitz P, Schirren CG, Jaffe ES, Kind P. Immunocytoma and marginal zone B-cell lymphoma (MALT lymphoma), presenting in skin: different entities or a spectrum of disease? *J Cutan Pathol* 1996;**23**:59.

7. Servitje O, Gallardo F, Estrach T *et al.* Primary cutaneous marginal zone B-cell lymphoma: a clinical, histopathological, immunophenotypic and molecular genetic study of 22 cases. *Br J Dermatol* 2002;**147**:1147–1158.

8. Tomaszewski MM, Abbondanzo SL, Lupton GP. Extranodal marginal zone B-cell lymphoma of the skin: a morphologic and immunophenotypic study of 11 cases. *Am J Dermatopathol* 2000;**22**:205–211.

9. Yang B, Tubbs RR, Finn W *et al.* Clinicopathologic reassessment of primary cutaneous B-cell lymphomas with immunophenotypic and molecular genetic characterization. *Am J Surg Pathol* 2000;**24**:694–702.

10. Schmid U, Eckert F, Griesser H *et al.* Cutaneous follicular lymphoid hyperplasia with monotypic plasma cells: a clinico-pathologic study of 18 patients. *Am J Surg Pathol* 1995;**19**:12–20.

11. Arai E, Shimizu M, Hirose T. A review of 55 cases of cutaneous lymphoid hyperplasia: reassessment of the histopathologic findings leading to reclassification of 4 lesions as cutaneous marginal zone lymphoma and 19 as pseudolymphomatous folliculitis. *Hum Pathol* 2005;**36**:505–511.

12. Isaacson PG, Chott A, Nakamura S, Müller-Hermelink HK, Harris NL, Swerdlow SH. Extranodal marginal zone lymphoma of mucosa-associated lymphoid tissue (MALT lymphoma). In: Swerdlow SH, Campo E, Harris NL *et al.*, eds. *WHO Classification of Tumours of Haematopoietic and Lymphoid Tissues.* Lyon: IARC Press, 2008: 214–217.

13. Cerroni L, Zöchling N, Pütz B, Kerl H. Infection by *Borrelia burgdorferi* and cutaneous B-cell lymphoma. *J Cutan Pathol* 1997;**24**:457–461.

14. Hussong JW, Perkins SL, Schnitzer B, Hargreaves H, Frizzera G. Extramedullary plasmacytoma: a form of marginal zone cell lymphoma? *Am J Clin Pathol* 1999;**111**:111–116.

15. Dimosthenous K, Papanikolaou A, Athanasiadou I *et al.* Transformation of marginal zone lymphomas to pure plasma cell histology following treatment with the anti-CD20 antibody rituximab. *J Haematopathol* 2008;**1**:170–171.

16. Goodlad JR, Davidson MM, Hollowood K *et al.* Primary cutaneous B-cell lymphoma and *Borrelia burgdorferi* infection in patients from the highlands of Scotland. *Am J Surg Pathol* 2000;**24**:1279–1285.

17. de la Fouchardiére A, Vandenesch F, Berger F. *Borrelia*-associated primary cutaneous MALT lymphoma in a non-endemic region. *Am J Surg Pathol* 2003;**27**:702–703.

18. Li C, Inagaki H, Kuo TT *et al.* Primary cutaneous marginal zone B-cell lymphoma: a molecular and clinicopathologic study of 24 Asian cases. *Am J Surg Pathol* 2003;**27**:1061–1069.

19. Wood GS, Kamath NV, Guitart J *et al.* Absence of *Borrelia burgdorferi* DNA in cutaneous B-cell lymphomas from the United States. *J Cutan Pathol* 2001;**28**:502–507.

20. Goteri G, Ranaldi R, Simonetti O *et al.* Clinicopathological features of primary cutaneous B-cell lymphomas from an academic regional hospital in central Italy: no evidence of *Borrelia burgdorferi* association. *Leukem Lymph* 2007;**48**:2184–2188.

21. Mandekou-Lefaki I, Delli FS, Kountouras I, Athanasiou E, Mattheou-Vakali G. Primary cutaneous MALT-type lymphoma and Helicobacter pylori: a possible relationship. *J Eur Acad Dermatol Venereol* 2006;**18**:606–608.

22. Yazdi AS, Puchta U, Flaig MJ, Sander CA. *Helicobacter pylori* not detected in cutaneous mucosa-associated lymphoid tissue (MALT) lymphomas. *Arch Dermatol Res* 2003;**294**:447–448.

23. Viguier M, River J, Agbalika F *et al.* B-cell lymphomas involving the skin associated with hepatitis C virus infection. *Int J Dermatol* 2002;**41**:577–582.

24. Prati D, Zanella A, De Mattei C *et al.* Chronic hepatitis C virus infection and primary cutaneous B-cell lymphoma. *Br J Haematol* 1999;**105**:841.

25. Suarez F, Lortholary O, Hermine O, Lecuit M. Infection-associated lymphomas derived from marginal zone B cells: a model of antigen-driven lymphoproliferation. *Blood* 2006;**107**:3034–3044.

26. Zöchling N, Pütz B, Wolf P, Kerl H, Cerroni L. Human herpesvirus 8-specific DNA sequences in primary cutaneous B-cell lymphomas. *Arch Dermatol* 1998;**134**:246–247.

27. Nagore E, Ledesma E, Collado C *et al.* Detection of Epstein–Barr virus and human herpesvirus 7 and 8 genomes in primary cutaneous T- and B-cell lymphomas. *Br J Dermatol* 2000;**143**: 320–323.

28. Bahler DW, Kim BK, Gao A, Swerdlow SH. Analysis of immunoglobulin VH genes suggests cutaneous marginal zone B-cell lymphomas recognise similar antigens. *Br J Haematol* 2006;**132**: 571–575.

29. Lenze D, Berg E, Volkmer-Engert R *et al.* Influence of antigen on the development of MALT lymphoma. *Blood* 2006;**107**:1141–1148.

30. Breza TS Jr, Zheng P, Porcu P, Magro CM. Cutaneous marginal zone B-cell lymphoma in the setting of fluoxetine therapy: a hypothesis regarding pathogenesis based on in vitro suppression of T-cell-proliferative response. *J Cutan Pathol* 2006;**33**: 522–528.

31. Servitje O, Marti RM, Estrach T *et al.* Occurrence of Hodgkin's disease and cutaneous B cell lymphoma in the same patient: a report of two cases. *Eur J Dermatol* 2000;**10**:43–46.

32. May SA, Netto G, Domiati-Saad R, Kasper C. Cutaneous lymphoid hyperplasia and marginal zone B-cell lymphoma following vaccination. *J Am Acad Dermatol* 2005;**53**:512–516.

33. Hoefnagel JJ, Vermeer MH, Jansen PM *et al*. Primary cutaneous marginal zone B-cell lymphoma. Clinical and therapeutic features in 50 cases. *Arch Dermatol* 2005;**141**:1139–1145.

34. Fink-Puches R, Chott A, Ardigo M *et al*. The spectrum of cutaneous lymphomas in patients less than 20 years of age. *Ped Dermatol* 2004;**21**:525–533.

35. Taddesse-Heath L, Pittaluga S, Sorbara L *et al*. Marginal zone B-cell lymphoma in children and young adults. *Am J Surg Pathol* 2003;**27**:522–531.

36. Kasper RC, Wood GS, Nihal M, LeBoit PE. Anetoderma arising in cutaneous B-cell lymphoproliferative disease. *Am J Dermatopathol* 2001;**23**:124–132.

37. Child FJ, Woollons A, Price ML, Calonje E, Russell-Jones R. Multiple cutaneous immunocytoma with secondary anetoderma: a report of two cases. *Br J Dermatol* 2000;**143**:165–170.

38. Senff NJ, Kluin-Nelemans JC, Willemze R. Results of bone marrow examination in 275 patients with histological features that suggest an indolent type of cutaneous B-cell lymphoma. *Br J Haematol* 2008;**142**:52–56.

39. Bathelier E, Thomas L, Balme B *et al*. Asymptomatic bone marrow involvement in patients presenting with cutaneous marginal zone B-cell lymphoma. *Br J Dermatol* 2008;**159**:498–500.

40. Zucca E, Conconi A, Pedrinis E *et al*. Nongastric marginal zone B-cell lymphoma of mucosa-associated lymphoid tissue. *Blood* 2003;**101**:2489–2495.

41. Cerroni L. Lymphoproliferative lesions of the skin. *J Clin Pathol* 2006;**59**:813–826.

42. Kiyohara T, Kumakiri M, Kobayashi H, Nakamura H, Ohkawara A. Cutaneous marginal zone B-cell lymphoma: a case accompanied by massive plasmacytoid cells. *J Am Acad Dermatol* 2003;**48**:s82–s85.

43. Cerroni L. Cutaneous granulomas and malignant lymphomas. *Dermatology* 2003;**206**:78–80.

44. Leinweber B, Colli C, Chott A, Kerl H, Cerroni L. Differential diagnosis of cutaneous infiltrates of B lymphocytes with follicular growth pattern. *Am J Dermatopathol* 2004;**26**:4–13.

45. de Leval L, Harris NL, Longtine J, Ferry JA, Duncan LM. Cutaneous B-cell lymphomas of follicular and marginal zone types: use of Bcl-6, CD10, Bcl-2, and CD21 in differential diagnosis and classification. *Am J Surg Pathol* 2001;**25**:732–741.

46. Cerroni L, Kerl H. Diagnostic immunohistology: cutaneous lymphomas and pseudolymphomas. *Semin Cutan Med Surg* 1999;**18**:64–70.

47. Baldassano MF, Bailey EM, Ferry JA, Harris NL, Duncan LM. Cutaneous lymphoid hyperplasia and cutaneous marginal zone lymphoma: comparison of morphologic and immunophenotypic features. *Am J Surg Pathol* 1999;**23**:88–96.

48. Gallardo F, Bellosillo B, Espinet B *et al*. Aberrant nuclear BCL10 expression and lack of t(11;18)(q21;q21) in primary cutaneous marginal zone B-cell lymphoma. *Hum Pathol* 2006;**37**:867–873.

49. Streubel B, Lamprecht A, Dierlamm J *et al*. T(14;18)(q32;q21) involving *IGH* and *MALT1* is a frequent chromosomal aberration in MALT lymphoma. *Blood* 2003;**101**:2335–2339.

50. Schreuder MI, Hoefnagel JJ, Jansen PM, van Krieken JHJM, Willemze R, Hebeda KM. FISH analysis of MALT lymphoma-specific translocations and aneuploidy in primary cutaneous marginal zone lymphoma. *J Pathol* 2005;**205**:302–310.

51. Palmedo G, Hantschke M, Rütten A *et al*. Primary cutaneous marginal zone B-cell lymphoma may exhibit both the t(14;18)(q32;q21) *IGH/BCL2* and the t(14;18)(q;32;q21) *IGH/MALT1* translocation: an indicator for clonal transformation towards higher-grade B-cell lymphoma? *Am J Dermatopathol* 2007;**29**:231–236.

52. Streubel B, Vinatzer U, Lamprecht A, Raderer M, Chott A. t(3;14)(p14.1;q32) involving IgH and FOXP1 is a novel recurrent chromosomal aberration in MALT lymphoma. *Leukemia* 2005;**19**:652–658.

53. Storz MN, van de Rijn M, Kim YH *et al*. Gene expression profiles of cutaneous B cell lymphoma. *J Invest Dermatol* 2003;**120**:865–870.

54. Child FJ, Scarisbrick JJ, Calonje E *et al*. Inactivation of tumor suppressor genes p15[INK4b] and p16[INK4a] in primary cutaneous B cell lymphoma. *J Invest Dermatol* 2002;**118**:941–948.

55. van Maldegem F, van Dijk R, Wormhoudt TA *et al*. The majority of cutaneous marginal zone B-cell lymphomas expresses class-switched immunoglobulins and develops in a T-helper type 2 inflammatory environment. *Blood* 2008;**112**:3355–3361.

56. Deutsch AJA, Frühwirth M, Aigelsreiter A, Cerroni L, Neumeister P. Primary cutaneous marginal zone B-cell lymphomas are targeted by aberrant somatic hypermutation. *J Invest Dermatol* 2009;**129**:476–479.

57. Senff NJ, Noordijk EM, Kim YH *et al*. European Organization for Research and Treatment of Cancer and International Society for Cutaneous Lymphoma consensus recommendations for the management of cutaneous B-cell lymphomas. *Blood* 2008;**112**:1600–1609.

58. Soda R, Costanzo A, Cantonetti M *et al*. Systemic therapy of primary cutaneous B-cell lymphoma, marginal zone type, with rituximab, a chimeric anti-CD20 monoclonal antibody. *Acta Derm Venereol (Stockh)* 2001;**81**:207–208.

59. Zenahlik P, Fink-Puches R, Kapp KS, Kerl H, Cerroni L. Die Therapie der primären kutanen B-Zell-Lymphome. *Hautarzt* 2000;**51**:19–24.

60. Wollina U, Hahnfeld S, Kosmehl H. Primary cutaneous marginal center lymphoma: complete remission induced by interferon-α2a. *J Cancer Res Clin Oncol* 1999;**125**:305–308.

61. Massengale WT, McBurney E, Gurtler J. CD20-negative relapse of cutaneous B-cell lymphoma after anti-CD20 monoclonal antibody therapy. *J Am Acad Dermatol* 2002;**46**:441–443.

62. Fink-Puches R, Wolf IH, Zalaudek I, Kerl H, Cerroni L. Treatment of primary cutaneous B-cell lymphoma with rituximab. *J Am Acad Dermatol* 2005;**52**:847–853.

63. Kyrtsonis MC, Siakarantis MP, Kalpadakis C *et al*. Favorable outcome of primary cutaneous marginal zone lymphoma treated with intralesional rituximab. *Eur J Haematol* 2006;**77**:300–303.

64. Cozzio A, Kempf W, Schmid-Meyer R *et al*. Intra-lesional low-dose interferon a2a therapy for primary cutaneous marginal zone B-cell lymphoma. *Leukem Lymph* 2006;**47**:865–869.

65. Roggero E, Zucca E, Mainetti C *et al*. Eradication of *Borrelia burgdorferi* infection in primary marginal zone B-cell lymphoma of the skin. *Hum Pathol* 2000;**31**:263–268.

66. Kütting B, Bonsmann G, Metze D, Luger TA, Cerroni L. *Borrelia burgdorferi*-associated primary cutaneous B cell lymphoma: complete clearing of skin lesions after antibiotic pulse therapy or intralesional injection of interferon-α2a. *J Am Acad Dermatol* 1997;**36**:311–314.

67. Fink-Puches R, Zenahlik P, Bäck B *et al*. Primary cutaneous lymphomas: applicability of current classification schemes (European Organization for Research and Treatment of Cancer, World Health Organization) based on clinicopathologic features observed in a large group of patients. *Blood* 2002;**99**:800–805.
68. Bouaziz JD, Bastuji-Garin S, Poszepczynska-Guigne E, Wechsler J, Bagot M. Relative frequency and survival of patients with primary cutaneous lymphomas: data from a single-centre study of 203 patients. *Br J Dermatol* 2006;**154**:1206–1207.
69. Zinzani PL, Quaglino P, Pimpinelli N *et al*. Prognostic factors in primary cutaneous B-cell lymphoma: The Italian Study Group for Cutaneous Lymphomas. *J Clin Oncol* 2006;**24**:1376–1382.
70. Gronbaeck K, Moller PH, Nedergaard T *et al*. Primary cutaneous B-cell lymphoma: a clinical, histological, phenotypic and genotypic study of 21 cases. *Br J Dermatol* 2000;**142**:913–923.
71. Lin P, Bueso-Ramos C, Wilson CS, Mansoor A, Medeiros LJ. Waldenström macroglobulinemia involving extramedullary sites: morphologic and immunophenotypic findings in 44 patients. *Am J Surg Pathol* 2003;**27**:1104–1113.
72. LeBoit PE, McNutt NS, Reed JA, Jacobson M, Weiss LM. Primary cutaneous immunocytoma: a B-cell lymphoma that can easily be mistaken for cutaneous lymphoid hyperplasia. *Am J Surg Pathol* 1994;**18**:969–978.
73. Rijlaarsdam JU, van der Putte SCJ, Berti E *et al*. Cutaneous immunocytomas: a clinicopathologic study of 26 cases. *Histopathology* 1993;**23**:117–125.
74. Goos N. Acrodermatitis chronica atrophicans and malignant lymphoma. *Acta Derm Venereol (Stockh)* 1971;**51**:457–459.
75. Aberer E, Cerroni L, Kerl H. Cutaneous immunocytoma presenting with multiple infiltrated macules and papules. *J Am Acad Dermatol* 2001;**44**:324–329.
76. Machet MC, Machet L, Vaillant L *et al*. Acquired localized cutis laxa due to cutaneous lymphoplasmacytoid lymphoma. *Arch Dermatol* 1995;**131**:110–111.
77. Sangueza OP, Burket JM, Sacks Y. Primary cutaneous immunocytoma: report of an unusual case with secondary spreading to the gastrointestinal tract. *J Cutan Pathol* 1997;**24**:43–46.
78. Allbritton JI, Horn TD. Cutaneous lymphoplasmacytic lymphoma. *J Am Acad Dermatol* 1998;**38**:820–824.
79. Torne R, Su WPD, Winkelmann RK, Smolle J, Kerl H. Clinicopathologic study of cutaneous plasmacytoma. *Int J Dermatol* 1990;**29**:562–566.
80. Wong KF, Chan JKC, Li LPK, Yau TK, Lee AWM. Primary cutaneous plasmacytoma: report of two cases and review of the literature. *Am J Dermatopathol* 1994;**16**:392–397.
81. Tüting T, Bork K. Primary plasmacytoma of the skin. *J Am Acad Dermatol* 1996;**34**:386–390.
82. Muscardin LM, Pulsoni A, Cerroni L. Primary cutaneous plasmacytoma: report of a case with review of the literature. *J Am Acad Dermatol* 2000;**43**:962–965.
83. Chang YT, Wong CK. Primary cutaneous plasmacytomas. *Clin Exp Dermatol* 1994;**19**:177–180.
84. Llamas-Martin R, Postigo-Iorente C, Vanaclocha-Sebastian F, Gil-Martin R, Iglesias-Diez L. Primary cutaneous extramedullary plasmacytoma secreting lambda IgG. *Clin Exp Dermatol* 1993;**18**:351–355.
85. Miyamoto T, Kobayashi T, Hagari Y, Mihara M. The value of genotypic analysis in the assessment of cutaneous plasmacytomas. *Br J Dermatol* 1997;**137**:418–421.
86. Müller RPA, Krausse S, Rahlf G. Primär kutanes Plasmozytom: Fallbericht und Literaturübersicht. *Hautarzt* 1990;**41**:232–235.
87. Requena L, Kutzner H, Palmedo G *et al*. Cutaneous involvement in multiple myeloma: a clinicopathologic, immunohistochemical, and cytogenetic study of 8 cases. *Arch Dermatol* 2003;**139**:475–486.
88. Sharon V, Mecca PS, Steinherz PG, Trippett TM, Myskowski PL. Two Pediatric Cases of Primary Cutaneous B-cell Lymphoma and Review of the Literature. *Ped Dermatol* 2009;**26**:34–39.

12 Cutaneous diffuse large B-cell lymphoma, leg type

Cutaneous diffuse large B-cell lymphoma, leg type, is a malignant lymphoma of intermediate behavior, occurring mostly on the leg(s) in elderly patients [1–4]. The terminology of this entity has been the basis of a long controversy, but the term cutaneous diffuse large B-cell lymphoma, leg type, is now widely accepted, and this lymphoma is listed as a specific entity in the World Health Organization (WHO)-European Organization for Research and Treatment of Cancer (EORTC) classification of primary cutaneous lymphomas and in the new WHO classification of tumors of hematopoietic and lymphoid tissues [5,6].

It is important to distinguish cutaneous diffuse large B-cell lymphoma, leg type, from follicle center lymphoma with a predominance of centroblasts and large centrocytes (cutaneous follicle centre lymphoma, diffuse type) (see Chapter 10). The latter has clinical and prognostic features similar to other types of cutaneous follicle center lymphoma. Cleaved cells predominate in the diffuse type of follicle center lymphoma, whereas round cells are in the majority in diffuse large B-cell lymphoma, leg type. Differentiation between the two may be difficult in some cases. For a complete discussion of differential diagnostic features see Chapter 10.

Cutaneous diffuse large B-cell lymphoma, leg type, can be seen in immunocompromised patients and has been observed in association with Kaposi sarcoma, but does not seem to be specifically linked to infection by human herpesvirus (HHV) 8 [7–10]. The presence of specific sequences of *Borrelia burgdorferi* DNA has been demonstrated in rare cases from countries with endemic infection [11,12].

We have observed cases with a positive nuclear signal for Epstein–Barr virus (EBV) detected by *in situ* hybridization, and similar cases have been rarely reported in the literature [13,14]. These rare examples should be better classified as cutaneous EBV+ diffuse large B-cell lymphoma of the elderly (see Chapter 13).

Clinical features

The disease predominantly affects elderly patients (over 70 years of age), especially females. Patients present with solitary or clustered erythematous or reddish-brown tumors, mostly located on the distal extremity of one leg (Fig. 12.1). Sometimes both legs are involved. Early lesions may be difficult to diagnose clinically (Fig. 12.2). Ulceration is common. Small erythematous papules can be seen adjacent to larger nodules in some cases. Large ulcers may lead to the misdiagnosis of chronic venous ulceration (Fig. 12.3) [15,16]. Cutaneous diffuse large B-cell lymphoma, leg type, has been observed on the background of chronic lymphedema [17].

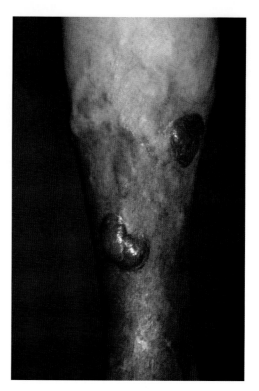

Figure 12.1 Cutaneous diffuse large B-cell lymphoma, leg type. Large tumors on the lower extremity. Note features of chronic venous insufficiency with marked hyperpigmentation.

Skin Lymphoma: The Illustrated Guide. By L. Cerroni, K. Gatter and H. Kerl. Published 2009 Blackwell Publishing. ISBN: 978-1-4051-8554-7.

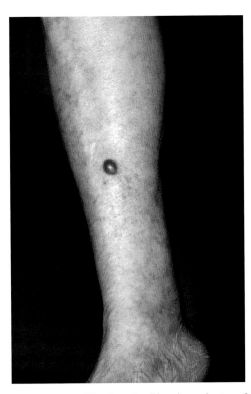

Figure 12.2 Cutaneous diffuse large B-cell lymphoma, leg type. Solitary tumor on the right lower extremity.

We and others have observed patients presenting with annular lesions that resembled erythema chronicum migrans clinically [18]; in these cases, due to the innocuous clinical presentation and the histopathologic features characterized by relatively sparse perivascular aggregates of cells, the correct diagnosis may be missed, thus delaying proper treatment.

It is important to stress that lesions with similar histopathologic and phenotypical features can arise at cutaneous sites other than the legs (diffuse large B-cell lymphoma, leg type, occurs in approximately 80–85% of cases on the leg(s) only) [19]. Rarely, patients present with typical tumors on the legs and concomitant lesions at other body sites.

Histopathology, immunophenotype and molecular genetics

Histopathology

There is a dense, diffuse infiltrate within the entire dermis and subcutis (Fig. 12.4). Involvement of the epidermis by large neoplastic cells, simulating a T-cell lymphoma, is possible (Fig. 12.5). Rare cases may even show band-like infiltrates in the superficial and mid-dermis, simulating the pattern of mycosis fungoides [20]. Tiny perivascular collections of large cells may be observed in early lesions, and may be the source of diagnostic problems. The neoplastic infiltrate consists

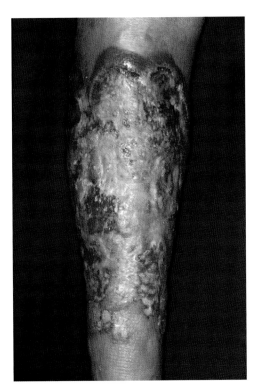

Figure 12.3 Cutaneous diffuse large B-cell lymphoma, leg type. Large ulcerated lesion with infiltrated margins involving the entire lower leg.

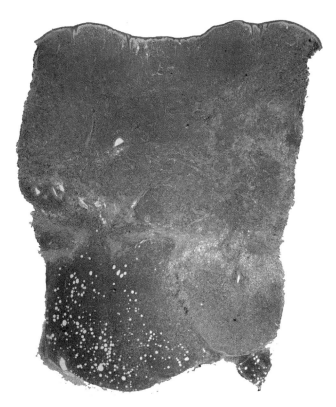

Figure 12.4 Cutaneous diffuse large B-cell lymphoma, leg type. Dense diffuse infiltrate involving the entire dermis and subcutaneous fat.

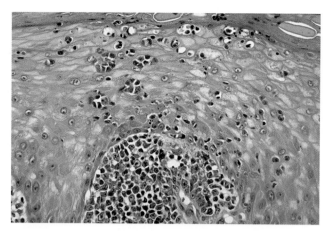

Figure 12.5 Cutaneous diffuse large B-cell lymphoma, leg type. Epidermotropism of neoplastic B lymphocytes.

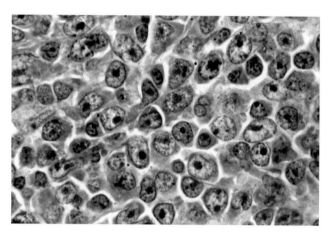

Figure 12.6 Cutaneous diffuse large B-cell lymphoma, leg type. Immunoblasts predominate in this case.

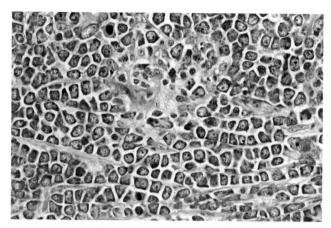

Figure 12.7 Cutaneous diffuse large B-cell lymphoma, leg type. "Mosaic stone"-like arrangement of neoplastic cells resembling features of Burkitt lymphoma or lymphoblastic lymphoma.

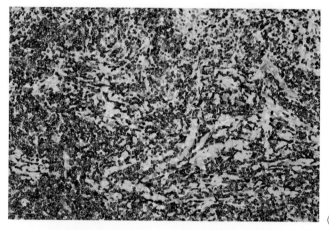

(a)

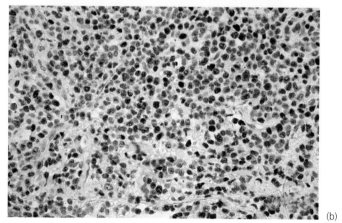

(b)

Figure 12.8 Cutaneous diffuse large B-cell lymphoma, leg type. (a) Positive staining for Bcl-2. (b) Positive nuclear staining for Bcl-6.

predominantly of large cells with round nuclei (immunoblasts and centroblasts) (Fig. 12.6). Cases with predominance of large cleaved cells (large centrocytes) should be classified as cutaneous follicle centre lymphoma, diffuse type (for a complete discussion see Chapter 10). Reactive small lymphocytes are usually only sparse. Mitoses are frequent.

A rare histopathologic variant of diffuse large B-cell lymphoma, leg type, shows a starry sky and/or mosaic stone-like pattern similar to that of Burkitt-like lymphoma (Fig. 12.7), but is characterized by other typical clinical and phenotypic features that allow a correct diagnosis to be made. In rare instances, diffuse large B-cell lymphoma, leg type, may relapse with the clinicopathologic features of intravascular large B-cell lymphoma [21].

Immunophenotype

Neoplastic cells express B-cell markers (CD20, CD79a), but there can be (partial) loss of antigen expression. Bcl-2 protein, multiple myeloma oncogene-1 (MUM-1), and forkhead box protein 1 (FOX-P1) are positive in the great majority of cases (Figs 12.8a, 12.9) [22,23]. Bcl-2⁻ cases that otherwise

fit into this group should not be classified as follicle center lymphoma. The proliferation markers usually stain a large proportion of the cells. In the majority of cases, neoplastic cells express Bcl-6 or rarely CD10, demonstrating a derivation from germinal center cells (Fig. 12.8b) [24–28]. Markers of

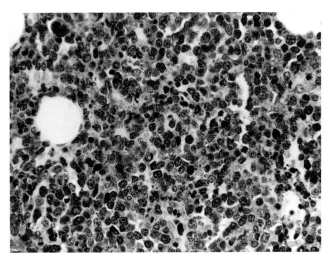

Figure 12.9 Cutaneous diffuse large B-cell lymphoma, leg type. Strong positivity for MUM-1 in the neoplastic cells. This pattern contrasts with the negativity or focal positivity observed in cutaneous follicle center lymphoma, diffuse type (see Fig. 10.19).

plasma cell differentiation (CD138) are negative as a rule, allowing the differentiation from plasmablastic lymphoma (see also Chapter 15).

Some cases of cutaneous diffuse large B-cell lymphoma, leg type, show an anaplastic morphology histopathologically, and expression of CD30 phenotypically (Fig. 12.10) [29]. Similar cases arising in the lymph nodes belong to the group of diffuse large B-cell lymphoma not otherwise specified, and are classified as the "anaplastic variant" of it [30]. In a similar way, primary cutaneous cases should not be classified separately, but within the group of cutaneous diffuse large B-cell lymphoma, leg type.

There are no convincing data supporting a different biologic behavior or prognosis between CD30$^+$ and CD30$^-$ cases of cutaneous diffuse large cell lymphoma, B-cell type. However, reports are only sporadic and some cases may have

been questionably classified [31]. Staging investigations are mandatory, keeping in mind that cases presenting with such peculiar morphologic and phenotypic features may represent secondary skin manifestations of a primary extracutaneous lymphoma.

Molecular genetics

The tumors reveal monoclonal rearrangement of the immunoglobulin heavy chain (J$_H$) gene. Analysis of single cells by micromanipulation and polymerase chain reaction (PCR) revealed that cutaneous diffuse large B-cell lymphoma, leg type, is characterized by a proliferation of postgerminal center cells [32,33]. Hypermethylation of *p15* and/or *p16* and expression of p15 and/or p16 protein have been observed in some patients [34]. 9p21 deletions, possibly resulting in the inactivation of *p16*, may have a prognostic meaning in cutaneous diffuse large B-cell lymphoma, leg type [35,36]. Other genetic alterations described include overexpression of genes associated with cell proliferation, overexpression of the protooncogenes *PIM1*, *PIM2*, and *cMYC*, and overexpression of the transcription factors MUM-1/IRF4 and Oct-2 [37]. A study on apoptosis-related genes showed that cutaneous diffuse large B-cell lymphoma, leg type, is characterized by constitutive activation and concomitant downstream inhibition of the intrinsic mediated apoptosis pathway [38].

In nodal diffuse large B-cell lymphomas, analysis of gene expression profiles by DNA microarray revealed the presence of distinct subgroups with prognostic differences [39]. In the skin, there is now a considerable body of evidence showing that cutaneous diffuse large B-cell lymphoma, leg type, has a molecular profile different from that of cutaneous follicle center lymphoma, diffuse type, thus supporting the classification of these morphologic forms of large B-cell lymphomas into separate categories [35,37,38,40]. These studies showed that cutaneous diffuse large B-cell lymphoma, leg type, has the gene signature of activated B lymphocytes [37,41]. In addition, a site-specific expression pattern has

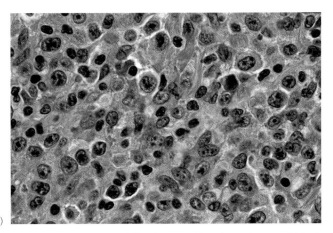

(a)

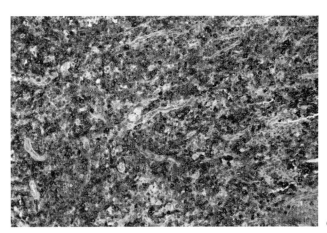

(b)

Figure 12.10 Cutaneous diffuse large B-cell lymphoma, leg-type. (a) Predominance of large anaplastic cells that (b) are positive for CD30.

been observed in cases of cutaneous B-cell lymphomas with large cell morphology arising on the head and neck or on the trunk, as opposed to those located on the leg, confirming that these tumors represent distinct subtypes of cutaneous B-cell lymphoma (see also Chapter 10) [42].

The t(14;18) involving the *BCL-2* und *IGH* genes is not present. A t(14;18)(q32;q21) involving the *IGH* and *MALT1* genes has been detected in one case of cutaneous diffuse large B-cell lymphoma, leg type, but the case may have represented in truth secondary cutaneous spread from an extracutaneous B-cell lymphoma [43]. Recently, differences in expression of polycomb-group genes, which are involved in regulation of lymphopoiesis and malignant transformation, have been detected between cutaneous and extracutaneous diffuse large B-cell lymphomas, supporting the concept that cutaneous cases represent a distinct entity [42].

Treatment

If possible, the therapy of choice should be systemic chemotherapy, but this treatment can be difficult to administer because of the advanced age of most patients (often over 80 years) [44]. Anti-CD20 antibody (rituximab) may also be used, either alone or in combination with systemic chemotherapy [15,45–51]. Recently, it has been suggested that the prognosis could be improved by combining anthracycline-containing chemotherapies and rituximab [52].

Solitary lesions may be treated by radiotherapy [53]. Intralesional administration of interferon-α has been used with a complete response reported in one patient [54]. Short-term response to antibiotic treatment has also been observed [55]. However, these non-aggressive options should be chosen only if more appropriate modalities cannot be used.

Prognosis

Cutaneous diffuse large B-cell lymphoma, leg type, has an intermediate behavior and the estimated disease-specific 5-year survival is less than 60% [5,56]. Relapse after treatment is common, and extracutaneous spread often occurs a few years after the onset of the disease. Involvement of the central nervous system can be observed in some cases [57].

Analysis of prognostic factors is hindered by the fact that in the past cases of cutaneous B-cell lymphomas with large cell morphology belonging to different diagnostic groups were lumped together. In this context, reports on a better prognosis of cases with predominance of cleaved cells over cases with predominance of round cells are due to the inclusion in the same study of examples of cutaneous diffuse large B-cell lymphoma, leg type, and of cutaneous follicle center lymphoma, diffuse type [26,58]. In a similar way, the prognostic

value of Bcl-2 expression observed in the past was due to the fact that Bcl-2 is expressed by cases of cutaneous diffuse large B-cell lymphoma, leg type, but not by those of cutaneous follicle center lymphoma, diffuse type. Other markers discriminating between the two types of lymphoma (e.g. MUM-1) do not have independent prognostic value [19,52,59,60]. Thus, all these parameters have no prognostic meaning if cases are classified correctly [19].

It should be noted that cases classified as follicle center lymphoma, diffuse type, according to the criteria proposed in the WHO-EORTC classification, but arising on the legs, have a bad prognosis, similar to that of cutaneous diffuse large B-cell lymphoma, leg type [19,44]. Thus, patients with follicle center lymphoma arising on the legs should be managed with the greatest caution, as the behavior may be more aggressive than that of the conventional variant arising on the head and neck area or the trunk.

The number of lesions at presentation seems to be related to prognosis in cases of cutaneous diffuse large B-cell lymphoma, leg type [19,26,52,58]. As already mentioned, cases with deletion of 9p21 seem to be characterized by a more aggressive course, but the number of cases observed is still very small [36,40,61].

Histopathologic evaluation of the sentinel lymph node has been proposed for the assessment of extracutaneous spread of cutaneous diffuse large B-cell lymphoma, leg type [62]. However, in our centers we do not use this method and lymph nodes are evaluated histopathologically only if they are involved clinically and/or radiologically.

Résumé

Clinical	Elderly; female to male ratio 3:1. Solitary or clustered tumors, often ulcerated. Preferential locations: distal portion of one leg.
Morphology	Dense diffuse infiltrates characterized by predominance of large cells with round nuclei (centroblasts, immunoblasts). Occasionally shows epidermotropism.
Immunology	CD20, 79a + sIg (cIg) + (monoclonal) Bcl-2 + MUM-1 + FOX-P1 + Bcl-6 +(−)
Genetics	Monoclonal rearrangement of the J_H gene detected in the majority of cases. Deletion of 9p21 bears a worse prognosis.
Treatment guidelines	Systemic chemotherapy; rituximab. Solitary lesions may be treated by radiotherapy if chemotherapy not possible.

TEACHING CASE

This 62-year-old woman had a slowly enlarging, annular erythematous lesion on the lower part of the leg for the last few weeks (Fig. 12.11a). She was treated for erythema migrans without success. A biopsy revealed perivascular lymphoid infiltrates characterized by predominance of large lymphocytes (Fig. 12.11b, c). Immunohistology demonstrated that these cells were positive for CD20, Bcl-2 (Fig. 12.11f), MUM-1 (Fig. 12.11d), focally Bcl-6, and showed a high proliferation (Fig. 12.11e), confirming the diagnosis of cutaneous diffuse large B-cell lymphoma, leg type (Figs 12.11d–f). Molecular analyses confirmed the presence of a monoclonal rearrangement of the J_H genes, and absence of *Borrelia burgdorferi* DNA. Staging investigations did not disclose additional sites of involvement.

Eight months after successful chemotherapy associated with rituximab, the patient experienced recurrent lesions near the site of previous involvement. A biopsy revealed a specific manifestation of the disease, this time with an unusual band-like pattern (Fig. 12.11g, h). The cells had the same phenotype as in the original biopsy, but CD20 was mostly negative (CD79a was positive). A PET scan showed pathologic involvement of an inguinal lymph node.

Comment: This case illustrates the early clinicopathologic features of cutaneous large B-cell lymphoma, leg type, and at the same time the morphologic variations of this lymphoma. A band-like pattern simulating T-cell lymphoma, sometimes with epidermotropism, has been described rarely.

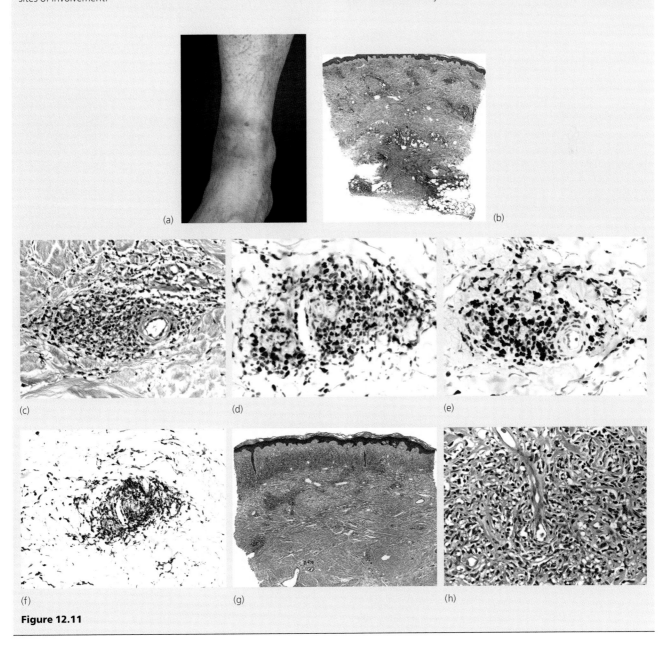

(a)

(b)

(c)

(d)

(e)

(f)

(g)

(h)

Figure 12.11

References

1. Vermeer MH, Geelen FAMJ, van Haselen CW *et al.* Primary cutaneous large B-cell lymphomas of the legs: a distinct type of cutaneous B-cell lymphoma with an intermediate prognosis. *Arch Dermatol* 1996;**132**:1304–1308.

2. Paulli M, Viglio A, Vivenza D *et al.* Primary cutaneous large B-cell lymphoma of the leg: histogenetic analysis of a controversial entity. *Hum Pathol* 2002;**33**:937–943.

3. Cerroni L. B-cell lymphomas of the skin. In: Bolognia JL, Jorizzo JL, Rapini RP, eds. *Dermatology*, 2nd edn. London: Mosby-Elsevier, 2008: 1855–1865.

4. Cerroni L. Lymphoproliferative lesions of the skin. *J Clin Pathol* 2006;**59**:813–826.

5. Willemze R, Jaffe ES, Burg G *et al.* WHO-EORTC classification for cutaneous lymphomas. *Blood* 2005;**105**:3768–3785.

6. Meijer CJLM, Vergier B, Duncan LM, Willemze R. Primary cutaneous diffuse large B-cell lymphoma, leg-type. In: Swerdlow SH, Campo E, Harris NL *et al.*, eds. *WHO Classification of Tumours of Haematopoietic and Lymphoid Tissues*. Lyon: IARC Press, 2008: 242.

7. Berti E, Marzano AV, Decleva I *et al.* Simultaneous onset of primary cutaneous B-cell lymphoma and human herpesvirus 8-associated Kaposi's sarcoma. *Br J Dermatol* 1997;**136**:924–949.

8. Beylot-Barry M, Vergier B, Masquelier B *et al.* The spectrum of cutaneous lymphomas in HIV infection: a study of 21 cases. *Am J Surg Pathol* 1999;**23**:1208–1216.

9. Engels EA, Pittaluga S, Whitby D *et al.* Immunoblastic lymphoma in persons with AIDS-associated Kaposi's sarcoma: a role for Kaposi's sarcoma-associated herpesvirus. *Mod Pathol* 2003;**16**:424–429.

10. Zöchling N, Pütz B, Wolf P, Kerl H, Cerroni L. Human herpesvirus 8-specific DNA sequences in primary cutaneous B-cell lymphomas. *Arch Dermatol* 1998;**134**:246–247.

11. Cerroni L, Zöchling N, Pütz B, Kerl H. Infection by *Borrelia burgdorferi* and cutaneous B-cell lymphoma. *J Cutan Pathol* 1997;**24**:457–461.

12. Goodlad JR, Davidson MM, Hollowood K *et al.* Primary cutaneous B-cell lymphoma and *Borrelia burgdorferi* infection in patients from the highlands of Scotland. *Am J Surg Pathol* 2000;**24**:1279–1285.

13. Tokuda Y, Fukushima M, Nakazawa K *et al.* A case of primary Epstein-Barr virus associated cutaneous diffuse large B-cell lymphoma unassociated with iatrogenic or endogenous immune dysregulation. *J Cutan Pathol* 2008;**35**:666–671.

14. Gaitonde S, Kavuri S, Alagiozian-Angelova V, Peace D, Worobec S. EBV positivity in primary cutaneous large B-cell lymphoma with immunophenotypic features of leg type: an isolated incidence or something more significant? *Acta Oncol* 2008;**47**:461–464.

15. Garbea A, Dippel E, Hildenbrand R *et al.* Cutaneous large B-cell lymphoma of the leg masquerading as a chronic venous ulcer. *Br J Dermatol* 2002;**146**:144–147.

16. Süß A, Simon JC, Sticherling M. Primary cutaneous diffuse large B-cell lymphoma, leg type, with the clinical picture of chronic venous ulceration. *Acta Derm Venereol (Stockh)* 2007;**87**:169–170.

17. Torres-Paoli D, Sanchez JL. Primary cutaneous B-cell lymphoma of the leg in a chronic lymphoedematous extremity. *Am J Dermatopathol* 2000;**22**:257–260.

18. Ekmekci TR, Koslu A, Sakiz D, Barutcuoglu B. Primary cutaneous large B-cell lymphoma, leg type, presented with a migratory lesion. *J Eur Acad Dermatol Venereol* 2007;**21**:1000–1001.

19. Kodama K, Massone C, Chott A, Metze D, Kerl H, Cerroni L. Primary cutaneous large B-cell lymphomas: clinicopathologic features, classification, and prognostic factors in a large series of patients. *Blood* 2005;**106**:2491–2497.

20. Cerroni L, Peris K, Amantea A *et al.* Primary cutaneous B-cell lymphoma with histopathologic features of mycosis fungoides. *Am J Dermatopathol* 1992;**14**:82.

21. Kamath NV, Gilliam AC, Nihal M, Spiro TP, Wood GS. Primary cutaneous large B-cell lymphoma of the leg relapsing as cutaneous intravascular large B-cell lymphoma. *Arch Dermatol* 2001;**137**:1637–1638.

22. Geelen FAMJ, Vermeer MH, Meijer CJLM *et al.* Bcl-2 protein expression in primary cutaneous large B-cell lymphoma is site-related. *J Clin Oncol* 1998;**16**:2080–2085.

23. Gronbaeck K, Moller PH, Nedergaard T *et al.* Primary cutaneous B-cell lymphoma: a clinical, histological, phenotypic and genotypic study of 21 cases. *Br J Dermatol* 2000;**142**:913–923.

24. Kim BK, Surti U, Pandya A, Swerdlow SH. Primary and secondary cutaneous diffuse large B-cell lymphomas: a multiparameter analysis of 25 cases including fluorescence *in situ* hybridization for t(14;18) translocation. *Am J Surg Pathol* 2003;**27**:356–364.

25. Fernandez-Vazquez A, Rodriguez-Peralto JL, Martinez MA *et al.* Primary cutaneous large B-cell lymphoma: the relation between morphology, clinical presentation, immunohistochemical markers, and survival. *Am J Surg Pathol* 2001;**25**:307–315.

26. Goodlad JR, Krajewski AS, Batstone PJ *et al.* Primary cutaneous diffuse large B-cell lymphoma: Prognostic significance of clinicopathological subtypes. *Am J Surg Pathol* 2003;**27**:1538–1545.

27. Hoefnagel JJ, Vermeer MH, Jansen PM *et al.* Bcl-2, Bcl-6 and CD10 expression in cutaneous B-cell lymphoma: further support for a follicle centre cell origin and differential diagnostic significance. *Br J Dermatol* 2003;**149**:1183–1191.

28. Xie X, Sundram U, Natkunam Y *et al.* Expression of HGAL in primary cutaneous large B-cell lymphomas: evidence for germinal center derivation of primary cutaneous follicular lymphoma. *Mod Pathol* 2008;**21**:653–659.

29. Herrera E, Gallardo M, Bosch R *et al.* Primary cutaneous CD30 (Ki-1)-positive non-anaplastic B-cell lymphoma. *J Cutan Pathol* 2002;**29**:181–184.

30. Stein H, Chan JKC, Warnke RA *et al.* Diffuse large B-cell lymphoma, not otherwise specified. In: Swerdlow SH, Campo E, Harris NL *et al.*, eds. *WHO Classification of Tumours of Haematopoietic and Lymphoid Tissues*. Lyon: IARC Press, 2008: 233–237.

31. Magro CM, Nash JW, Werling RW, Porcu P, Crowson AN. Primary cutaneous CD30+ large cell B-cell lymphoma: a series of 10 cases. *Appl Immunhistochem Molec Morphol* 2006;**14**:7–11.

32. Gellrich S, Golembowski S, Audring H, Jahn S, Sterry W. Molecular analysis of the immunoglobulin VH gene rearrangement in a primary cutaneous immunoblastic B-cell lymphoma by micromanipulation and single-cell PCR. *J Invest Dermatol* 1997;**109**:541–545.

33. Gellrich S, Rutz S, Golembowski S *et al.* Primary cutaneous follicle center cell lymphomas and large B cell lymphomas of the leg descend from germinal center cells: a single cell polymerase chain reaction analysis. *J Invest Dermatol* 2001;**117**:1512–1520.

34. Child FJ, Scarisbrick JJ, Calonje E *et al.* Inactivation of tumor suppressor genes p15^{INK4b} and p16^{INK4a} in primary cutaneous B cell lymphoma. *J Invest Dermatol* 2002;**118**:941–948.

35. Wiesner T, Streubel B, Huber D, Kerl H, Chott A, Cerroni L. Genetic aberrations in primary cutaneous large-B-cell lymphoma. A fluorescence in situ hybridization study of 25 cases. *Am J Surg Pathol* 2005;**29**:666–673.

36. Belaud-Rotureau MA, Marietta V, Vergier B *et al.* Inactivation of p16INK4a/CDKN2A gene may be a diagnostic feature of large B cell lymphoma leg type among cutaneous B cell lymphomas. *Virch Arch* 2008;**452**:607–620.

37. Hoefnagel JJ, Dijkman R, Basso K *et al.* Distinct types of primary cutaneous large B-cell lymphoma identified by gene expression profiling. *Blood* 2005;**105**:3671–3678.

38. van Galen JC, Hoefnagel JJ, Vermeer MH *et al.* Profiling of apoptosis genes identifies distinct types of primary cutaneous large B cell lymphoma. *J Pathol* 2008;**215**:340–346.

39. Alizadeh AA, Eisen MB, Davis RE *et al.* Distinct types of diffuse large B-cell lymphoma identified by gene expression profiling. *Nature* 2000;**403**:503–511.

40. Dijkman R, Tensen CP, Jordanova ES *et al.* Array-based comparative genomic hybridization analysis reveals recurrent chromosomal alterations and prognostic parameters in primary cutaneous large B-cell lymphoma. *J Clin Oncol* 2006;**24**:296–305.

41. Storz MN, van de Rijn M, Kim YH *et al.* Gene expression profiles of cutaneous B cell lymphoma. *J Invest Dermatol* 2003;**120**:865–870.

42. Raaphorst FM, Vermeer M, Fieret E *et al.* Site-specific expression of polycomb-group genes encoding the HPC-HPH/PRC1 complex in clinically defined primary nodal and cutaneous large B-cell lymphomas. *Am J Pathol* 2004;**164**:533–542.

43. Cook JR, Sherer M, Craig FE, Shekhter-Levin S, Swerdlow SH. t(14;18)(q32;q21) involving *MALT1* and *IGH* genes in an extranodal diffuse large B-cell lymphoma. *Hum Pathol* 2003;**34**:1212–1215.

44. Senff NJ, Noordijk EM, Kim YH *et al.* European Organization for Research and Treatment of Cancer and International Society for Cutaneous Lymphoma consensus recommendations for the management of cutaneous B-cell lymphomas. *Blood* 2008;**112**:1600–1609.

45. Aboulafia DM. Primary cutaneous large B-cell lymphoma of the legs: a distinct clinical pathologic entity treated with CD20 monoclonal antibody (rituximab). *Am J Clin Oncol* 2001;**24**:237–240.

46. Bonnekoh B, Schulz M, Franke I, Gollnick H. Complete remission of a primary cutaneous B-cell lymphoma of the lower leg by first-line monotherapy with the CD20–antibody rituximab. *J Cancer Res Clin Oncol* 2002;**128**:161–166.

47. Heinzerling LM, Urbanek M, Funk JO *et al.* Reduction of tumor burden and stabilization of disease by systemic therapy with anti-CD20 antibody (rituximab) in patients with primary cutaneous B-cell lymphoma. *Cancer* 2000;**89**:1835–1844.

48. Sabroe RA, Child FJ, Woolford AJ, Spittle MF, Russell-Jones R. Rituximab in cutaneous B-cell lymphoma: a report of two cases. *Br J Dermatol* 2000;**143**:157–161.

49. Viguier M, Bachelez H, Brice P, Rivet J, Dubertret L. Lymphomes cutanes B traites par rituximab: deux cas. *Ann Dermatol Vénéréol* 2002;**129**:1152–1155.

50. Fierro MT, Savoia P, Quaglino P *et al.* Systemic therapy with cyclophosphamide and anti-CD20 antibody (rituximab) in relapsed primary cutaneous B-cell lymphoma: a report of 7 cases. *J Am Acad Dermatol* 2003;**49**:281–287.

51. Brogan BL, Zic JA, Kinney MC *et al.* Large B-cell lymphoma of the leg: clinical and pathologic characteristics in a North American series. *J Am Acad Dermatol* 2003;**49**:223–228.

52. Grange F, Beylot-Barry M, Courville P *et al.* Primary cutaneous diffuse large B-cell lymphoma, leg type. Clinicopathologic features and prognostic analysis in 60 cases. *Arch Dermatol* 2007;**143**:1144–1150.

53. Zenahlik P, Fink-Puches R, Kapp KS, Kerl H, Cerroni L. Die Therapie der primären kutanen B-Zell-Lymphome. *Hautarzt* 2000;**51**:19–24.

54. Wollina U, Mentzel T, Graefe T. Large B-cell lymphoma of the leg: complete remission with perilesional interferon-α. *Dermatology* 2001;**203**:165–167.

55. Hofbauer GFL, Kessler B, Kempf W *et al.* Multilesional primary cutaneous diffuse large B-cell lymphoma responsive to antibiotic treatment. *Dermatology* 2001;**203**:168–170.

56. Fink-Puches R, Zenahlik P, Bäck B *et al.* Primary cutaneous lymphomas: applicability of current classification schemes (European Organization for Research and Treatment of Cancer, World Health Organization) based on clinicopathologic features observed in a large group of patients. *Blood* 2002;**99**:800–805.

57. Bekkenk MW, Postma TJ, Meijer CJLM, Willemze R. Frequency of central nervous system involvement in primary cutaneous B-cell lymphoma. *Cancer* 2000;**89**:913–919.

58. Grange F, Bekkenk MW, Wechsler J *et al.* Prognostic factors in primary cutaneous large B-cell lymphomas: a European multicenter study. *J Clin Oncol* 2001;**19**:3602–3610.

59. Hallermann C, Niermann C, Fischer RJ, Schulze HJ. New prognostic relevant factors in primary cutaneous diffuse large B-cell lymphomas. *J Am Acad Dermatol* 2007;**56**:588–597.

60. Sundram U, Kim Y, Mraz-Gernhard S, Hoppe R, Natkunam Y, Kohler S. Expression of the bcl-6 and MUM1/IRF4 proteins correlate with overall and disease-specific survival in patients with primary cutaneous large B-cell lymphoma: a tissue microarray study. *J Cutan Pathol* 2005;**32**:227–234.

61. Wiesner T, Obenauf AC, Geigl JB *et al.* 9p21 deletion in primary cutaneous large B-cell lymphoma, leg type, may escape detection by standard FISH assays. *J Invest Dermatol* 2009;**129**:238–240.

62. Starz H, Balda BR, Bachter D, Büchels H, Vogt H. Secondary lymph node involvement from primary cutaneous large B-cell lymphoma of the leg: sentinel lymph nodectomy as a new strategy for staging circumscribed cutaneous lymphoma. *Cancer* 1999;**85**:199–207.

13   Other cutaneous B-cell lymphomas

There are a few reports on other entities of B-cell lymphoma arising primary in the skin. In addition, most malignant B-cell lymphomas observed at extracutaneous sites may secondarily involve the skin, especially in their later stages. The text below summarizes the clinicopathologic aspects of skin manifestations in the most important of these cases.

T-CELL/HISTIOCYTE-RICH B-CELL LYMPHOMA

T-cell/histiocyte-rich B-cell lymphoma is characterized by the malignant proliferation of B lymphocytes admixed with a predominant population of reactive histiocytes and/or T lymphocytes. For a diagnosis of T-cell/histiocyte-rich B-cell lymphoma, neoplastic large B cells should not exceed 10% of the infiltrate. Nodal T-cell/histiocyte-rich B-cell lymphoma is considered to be a variant of the diffuse large B-cell lymphomas and is included as such in the new World Health Organization (WHO) classification of tumors of hematopoietic and lymphoid tissues [1]. Cutaneous involvement seems to be extremely uncommon, but rare cases arising primarily in the skin have been reported [2–6]. Most cases reported in the past were described under the term "T-cell-rich B-cell lymphoma."

In our experience, we have never encountered convincing examples of primary cutaneous T-cell/histiocyte-rich B-cell lymphoma. On the other hand, we have observed rarely cases of cutaneous follicle center lymphoma, diffuse type, that in one of the biopsies or, more frequently, in part of a biopsy showed histopathologic features similar to those of T-cell/histiocyte-rich B-cell lymphoma. In this context, we believe that in the skin this morphologic presentation represents a variation of the follicle center lymphoma, diffuse type.

Clinical features

Patients with T-cell/histiocyte-rich B-cell lymphoma are adults of either gender. Clinically, they present with erythematous papules, plaques or nodules usually on the face and trunk. As mentioned before, cases presenting in the skin probably represent variations of follicle center lymphoma, diffuse type, sharing similar clinical features with lymphomas of this group.

The occurrence of cutaneous T-cell/histiocyte-rich B-cell lymphoma followed by nodal Hodgkin lymphoma has been observed in a patient with Gardner syndrome [7].

Histopathology, immunophenotype and molecular genetics

Histology shows large blasts admixed with a predominant population of small lymphocytes (Fig. 13.1a). In a few patients, a biphasic pattern has been observed, suggesting that cutaneous T-cell/histiocyte-rich B-cell lymphoma represents a morphologic variation of a pre-existing low-grade (follicle center) B-cell lymphoma of the skin. Angiocentricity may be observed rarely [8].

Immunohistology reveals the B-cell phenotype of the large cells (CD20+, CD30−), often with positivity for markers of germinal center derivation such as Bcl-6 (Fig. 13.1b). The small reactive lymphocytes express a T-helper phenotype (CD3+, CD4+, CD8−). Molecular genetics shows a polyclonal pattern of T-cell receptor (TCR) genes, and in most cases a monoclonal rearrangement of the immunoglobulin heavy chain (J_H) gene. In cases showing no evidence of monoclonal rearrangement of the J_H gene, the negativity is probably due to the small number of neoplastic cells admixed with a high number of reactive lymphocytes. Polymerase chain reaction (PCR) analysis after microdissection of large cells may be a useful tool for confirmation of monoclonality in such cases.

Treatment and prognosis

As in other cases of primary cutaneous follicle center lym-

Skin Lymphoma: The Illustrated Guide. By L. Cerroni, K. Gatter and H. Kerl. Published 2009 Blackwell Publishing. ISBN: 978-1-4051-8554-7.

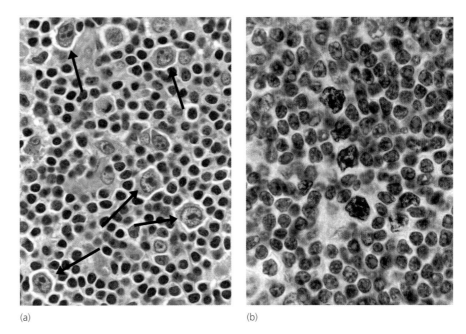

Figure 13.1 Cutaneous "T-cell/histiocyte-rich" large B-cell lymphoma. (a) Large blasts (arrows) scattered among a predominant population of small T lymphocytes and histiocytes. (b) Nuclear positivity of the large cells for Bcl-6.

(a)　　　　　　　　　　　　　　(b)

phoma, therapy of cases confined to the skin should not be aggressive (surgical excision and/or local radiotherapy), at least as first-line treatment strategy. An indolent behavior has been described in a small number of cases arising primarily in the skin, confirming that they belong to the group of the low-grade cutaneous B-cell lymphomas.

Résumé

T-cell/histiocyte-rich B-cell lymphoma

Clinical	Adults. Erythematous papules, plaques and nodules. Preferential locations: face, trunk. Primary cutaneous cases are probably variants of the follicle center B-cell lymphoma, diffuse type.
Morphology	<10% of large B cells in the background of a predominant T-cell population.
Immunology	CD20, 79a + Bcl-6 + CD30 −
Genetics	Monoclonal rearrangement of the J_H gene.
Treatment guidelines	Primary cutaneous cases should be treated as cases of follicle center lymphoma.

MANTLE CELL LYMPHOMA

Mantle cell lymphoma is a rare B-cell lymphoma deriving from the inner mantle zone of lymphoid follicles [9]. Cutaneous involvement is uncommon, but in rare cases specific skin lesions may be the first manifestation of the disease [10–13].

A few examples of mantle cell lymphoma arising primary in the skin have been reported, but the uniform good prognosis observed in these patients casts doubt on the classification of these cases [14]. In our experience, we have never encountered primary cutaneous mantle cell lymphoma.

Clinical features

Patients are middle-aged or older individuals, with a predominance of males. Clinically, the lesions are characterized by solitary or, more commonly, multiple reddish tumors. We have observed one patient with a solitary tumor on the navel presenting clinically with the picture of so-called Sister Mary Joseph's nodule as recurrence of mantle cell lymphoma with diffuse peritoneal involvement and ascites.

Histopathology, immunophenotype and molecular genetics

Histology shows diffuse monomorphous infiltrates throughout the entire dermis and subcutis, composed of small- to medium-sized lymphocytes with irregular nuclei (Fig. 13.2). It has been reported that the blastoid variant, with either lymphoblast-like or large cleaved cells, is frequently found in cutaneous infiltrates. This may reflect a propensity to skin involvement by tumors that undergo progression.

Immunohistology is characterized by positivity for CD20 and CD5 (Fig. 13.3a, b) and negativity for other T-cell markers. In contrast to cases of B-cell chronic lymphocytic leukemia (B-CLL), CD23 is negative or only weakly expressed in neoplastic cells of mantle cell lymphoma. Nuclear staining

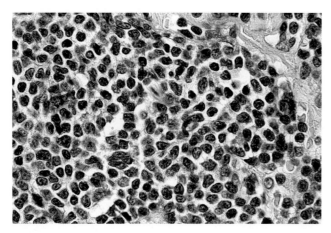

Figure 13.2 Cutaneous mantle cell lymphoma. Monomorphous infiltrate of medium-sized cells with irregular nuclei.

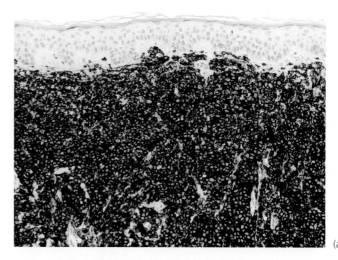

(a)

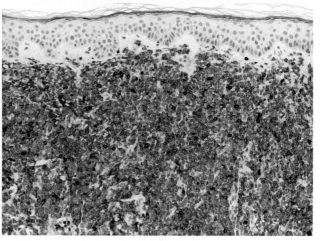

(b)

for cyclin-D1 is a helpful tool for the differentiation of cutaneous mantle cell lymphoma from other malignant B-cell lymphomas, especially B-CLL and B-lymphoblastic lymphoma (Fig. 13.3c) [15]. Molecular analyses reveal a monoclonal rearrangement of the J_H gene in the majority of cases. The typical t(11;14)(q13;q32) can be demonstrated by conventional cytogenetics, fluorescence *in situ* hybridization (FISH) or polymerase chain reaction (PCR).

Treatment and prognosis

The treatment of choice is systemic chemotherapy, often followed by bone marrow transplantation. The prognosis is poor and the median survival is less than 5 years.

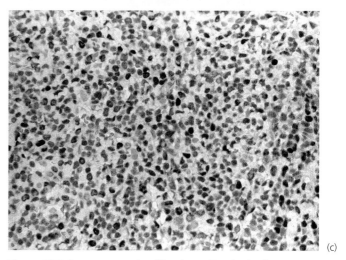

(c)

Figure 13.3 Cutaneous mantle cell lymphoma. Neoplastic cells are positive for (a) CD20, (b) CD5, and (c) cyclin D1.

Résumé

Mantle cell lymphoma

Clinical	Adults. Usually multiple tumors as secondary skin involvement. Existence of true primary cases questionable.
Morphology	Monomorphous proliferation of small- to medium-sized lymphocytes with irregular nuclei.
Immunology	CD20 + CD5 + CD23 – Cyclin-D1 +
Genetics	Monoclonal rearrangement of the J_H gene. t(11;14)(q13;q32).
Treatment guidelines	Systemic chemotherapy; bone marrow transplantation.

LYMPHOMATOID GRANULOMATOSIS

Lymphomatoid granulomatosis is a B-cell lymphoproliferative disorder associated with Epstein–Barr virus (EBV) infection. The disease has a spectrum of presentations and may progress to an overt diffuse large B-cell lymphoma. Lymphomatoid granulomatosis was described first by Liebow *et al* in 1972 as an angiocentric and angiodestructive lymphoproliferative process in the lungs [16]. It is currently divided into three grades according to the proportion of EBV[+] B cells in relation to the reactive infiltrate [17]. Cases characterized by a diffuse proliferation of large B cells should no longer be classified as lymphomatoid granulomatosis but rather as diffuse large B-cell lymphoma [17].

Clinical features

The skin is often involved although the most common site affected is the lungs [18–22]. Patients are usually adults, but skin lesions have been observed in children [23]. The clinical presentation usually is characterized by multiple erythematous papules, plaques or tumors, commonly ulcerated. Sites of predilection are the trunk and extremities. Pulmonary and/or constitutional symptoms are almost invariably present. Cutaneous lesions may precede the onset of pulmonary symptoms but true primary cases have not been observed.

Histopathology, immunophenotype and molecular genetics

The histopathologic features of cutaneous manifestations of lymphomatoid granulomatosis depend on the grade of disease and type of lesions. In some cases, only a non-specific perivascular and periadnexal infiltrate of small- to medium-sized cells can be seen. Cutaneous tumors of lymphomatoid granulomatosis are characterized usually by the presence of an angiocentric/angiodestructive infiltrate with variable numbers of large B lymphocytes (Fig. 13.4a, b). Granulomatous features are often present.

The three histolopathologic grades of lymphomatoid granulomatosis are defined as follows. *Grade 1* lesions are characterized by a polymorphous lymphoid infiltrate without cytologic atypia. Large cells are infrequent. EBER-1[+] cells as detected by *in situ* hybridization techniques are few as well or may even be absent in rare cases. *Grade 2* lesions are characterized by a polymorphous inflammatory background with scattered large cells, sometimes organized in small clusters. EBER-1[+] cells are more numerous than in grade 1 lesions but do not form sheets. In *grade 3* lesions the polymorphous, inflammatory background is still detectable, but sheets of large

B lymphocytes are present as well. The large B lymphocytes may show prominent pleomorphism and/or Hodgkin-like morphology. EBER-1[+] *in situ* hybridization shows many positive cells. The amount of necrosis increases in the three grades from absent or focal in grade 1 to prominent in grade 3. As already mentioned, cases with diffuse infiltrates of large B cells should be classified as diffuse large B-cell lymphoma and not as lymphomatoid granulomatosis.

Immunohistology shows that the large cells have a B-cell phenotype (Fig. 13.4c). It is important to remember that reactive small- to medium-sized lymphocytes with a T-helper phenotype are the predominant cells within the infiltrates, particularly in grades 1 and 2. As discussed before, most neoplastic B lymphocytes show a positive hybridization signal for EBV (Fig. 13.4d). Molecular analyses reveal in some cases a monoclonal rearrangement of the J_H gene.

In the absence of a previous or concomitant diagnosis of typical lymphomatoid granulomatosis in the respiratory tract, a diagnosis of cutaneous lymphomatoid granulomatosis should be made only when all the features described above are present.

Treatment and prognosis

Different treatment modalities have been used for patients with cutaneous lesions of lymphomatoid granulomatosis (e.g. interferon-α, systemic chemotherapy), depending mainly on the grade of lesions at extracutaneous sites. The prognosis, too, depends on the grade and extent of extracutaneous involvement.

Résumé	
Lymphomatoid granulomatosis	
Clinical	Adults. Usually multiple tumors. Lungs usually involved.
Morphology	Depending on grade of lesions; grade 3 lesions show angiocentric/angiodestructive infiltrates with presence of variably large sheets of large B lymphocytes. Reactive T lymphocytes predominate.
Immunology	CD20 + (large B lymphocytes)
	CD3, 4 + (reactive small lymphocytes)
	EBER-1 + (large B lymphocytes)
Genetics	Monoclonal rearrangement of the J_H gene.
Treatment guidelines	Systemic chemotherapy; interferon-α.

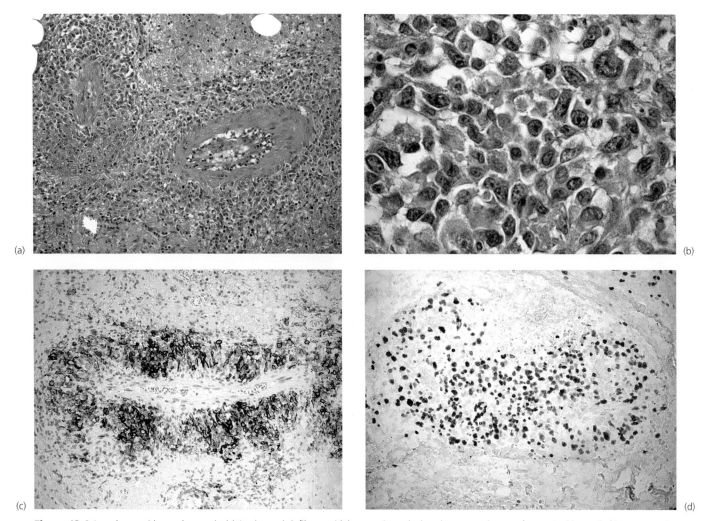

Figure 13.4 Lymphomatoid granulomatosis. (a) Angiocentric infiltrate with large perivascular lymphocytes and areas of necrosis. (b) Detail of large atypical cells. (c) Expression of CD20 by perivascular large lymphocytes. (d) The large B lymphocytes reveal a positive signal after *in situ* hybridization for Epstein–Barr virus (EBER-1).

CUTANEOUS EBV+ DIFFUSE LARGE B-CELL LYMPHOMA OF THE ELDERLY

This type of lymphoma is defined as an EBV-associated diffuse large B-cell lymphoma occurring in patients without known immunosuppression [24,25]. The disease seems to be more common in Asian countries [26]. It is believed that the condition is linked to aging and decreased competence of the immune system. This entity has been included in the new WHO classification of tumors of hematopoietic and lymphoid tissues [27], but is not listed in the WHO-EORTC classification of primary cutaneous lymphomas.

The skin is frequently affected, mostly showing the clinico-pathologic picture of a diffuse large B-cell lymphoma, leg type, with strong positivity for EBV [28,29]. Histopathology may show either a polymorphous or a monomorphic picture (Fig. 13.5a). The histopathologic pattern does not have any prognostic meaning.

Cutaneous cases usually show predominance of large rounded B cells. In contrast to conventional diffuse large B-cell lymphoma, leg type, cases of EBV+ diffuse large B-cell lymphoma of the elderly may show loss of CD20 expression and focal CD30 positivity, thus representing a pitfall in the diagnosis. CD79a is usually positive on neoplastic cells, as well as MUM-1 (Fig. 13.5b, c). Detection of EBV by *in situ* hybridization is a prerequisite for the diagnosis (Fig. 13.5d).

EBV+ diffuse large B-cell lymphoma of the elderly is a very aggressive lymphoma with a median survival of about 2 years. The treatment is often complicated by the advanced age of patients.

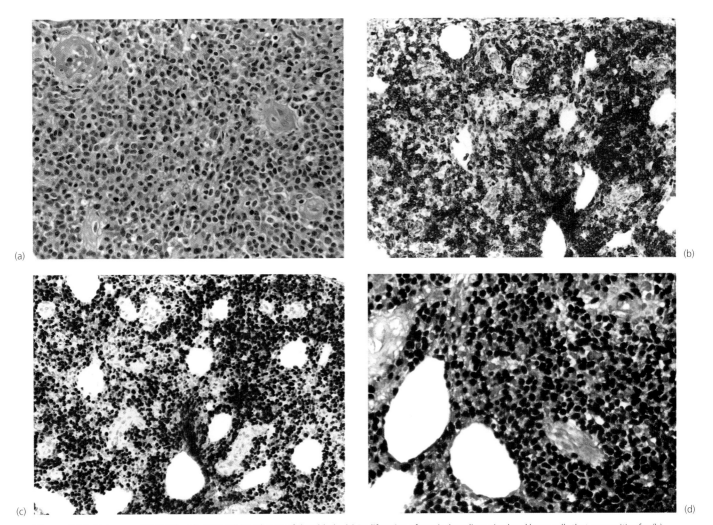

Figure 13.5 Cutaneous EBV⁺ diffuse large B-cell lymphoma of the elderly. (a) Proliferation of atypical medium-sized and large cells that are positive for (b) CD79a and (c) MUM-1, and that show (d) a positive signal upon *in situ* hybridization for EBV (EBER-1).

Résumé

EBV⁺ diffuse large B-cell lymphoma of the elderly

Clinical	Elderly patients. Skin is a relatively common site of presentation.
Morphology	Polymorphous or monomorphic picture. Monomorphic infiltrates show features of diffuse large B-cell lymphoma.
Immunology	CD20 +(–)
	CD79a +
	MUM-1 +
	CD3, 5 –
	CD30 +/–
	EBER-1 +
Genetics	Monoclonal rearrangement of the J_H genes.
Treatment guidelines	Systemic chemotherapy.

SPECIFIC CUTANEOUS MANIFESTATIONS IN MULTIPLE MYELOMA

In the WHO-EORTC classification of cutaneous lymphomas, cases of "cutaneous plasmacytoma" have been reclassified as variants of marginal zone lymphoma with predominant plasmacytic differentiation (see Chapter 11) [30]. Cases of genuine cutaneous plasmacytoma are considered almost invariably as secondary skin manifestations of multiple myeloma [31–39].

Clinical features

Patients present clinically with solitary, clustered or generalized erythematous, reddish brown or violaceous cutaneous or subcutaneous plaques or tumors.

Histopathology, immunophenotype and molecular genetics

Cutaneous manifestations of plasmacytoma consist of dense nodules and/or sheets of cells within the entire dermis and subcutis. Mature and immature plasma cells with varying degrees of atypia predominate (Fig. 13.6). Dutcher bodies and Russell bodies are found occasionally. Small reactive lymphocytes are few or absent. Amyloid deposits may be observed within and/or surrounding the neoplastic infiltrates, particularly around blood vessels (Fig. 13.7). Crystalloid intracytoplasmic inclusions within histiocytes and macrophages may also occur [40,41].

Neoplastic plasma cells contain cytoplasmic immunoglobulin (usually IgA) and show monoclonal expression of one immunoglobulin light chain. Leukocyte common antigen (CD45) and most B-cell-associated markers are negative, but cells can be stained by CD38 or CD138 in most cases, and by CD79a in some cases. Immunohistochemical expression of cytokeratins, HMB45 and CD30 can be observed within neoplastic plasma cells, representing a source of diagnostic error.

Molecular analysis usually reveals a monoclonal rearrangement of the J_H gene.

Treatment and prognosis

The treatment is related to the systemic manifestations. Radiotherapy may be administered for cutaneous tumors.

The prognosis of cutaneous manifestations of multiple myeloma is poor. Analysis of data concerning cases of cutaneous plasmacytoma published in the literature, however, is hindered by the inclusion of cases that today would be classified as cutaneous marginal zone lymphoma, plasmacytic variant (see Chapter 11).

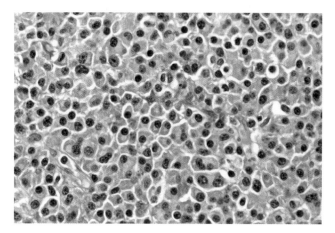

Figure 13.6 Specific cutaneous manifestations of multiple myeloma. The nodule is composed mainly of typical and atypical plasma cells.

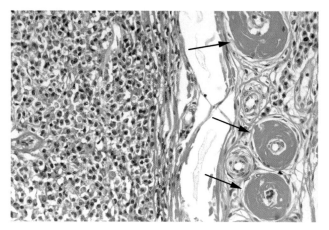

Figure 13.7 Specific cutaneous manifestations of multiple myeloma. Note proliferation of atypical plasma cells and prominent amyloid deposits within the walls of three vessels (*arrows*).

Résumé

Specific cutaneous manifestations in multiple myeloma

Clinical	Solitary, grouped or generalized (sub)cutaneous plaques and tumors.
Morphology	Nodular or diffuse infiltrates characterized by predominance of mature and immature plasma cells.
Immunology	CD45(LCA), CD20 – CD38, 138 + CD79a +/– CIg + (monoclonal)
Genetics	Monoclonal rearrangement of the J_H gene detected in the majority of cases.
Treatment guidelines	Treatment tailored to systemic manifestations of the disease.

References

1. De Wolf-Peeters C, Delabie J, Campo E, Jaffe ES, Delsol G. T cell/histiocyte-rich large B-cell lymphoma. In: Swerdlow SH, Campo E, Harris NL *et al.*, eds. *WHO Classification of Tumours of Haematopoietic and Lymphoid Tissues*. Lyon: IARC Press, 2008: 238–239.

2. Arai E, Sakurai M, Nakayama H, Morinaga S, Katayama I. Primary cutaneous T-cell-rich B-cell lymphoma. *Br J Dermatol* 1993;**129**:196–200.

3. Dommann SN, Dommann-Scherrer CC, Zimmerman D *et al.* Primary cutaneous T-cell-rich B-cell lymphoma: a case report with a 13–year follow-up. *Am J Dermatopathol* 1995;**17**:618–624.

4. Dunphy CH, Nahass GT. Primary cutaneous T-cell-rich B-cell lymphomas with flow cytometric immunophenotypic findings: report of 3 cases and review of the literature. *Arch Pathol Lab Med* 1999;**123**:1236–1240.

5. Li S, Griffin CA, Mann RB, Borowitz MJ. Primary cutaneous T-cell-rich B-cell lymphoma: clinically distinct from its nodal counterpart? *Mod Pathol* 2001;**14**:10–13.

6. Sander CA, Kaudewitz P, Kutzner H *et al.* T-cell-rich B-cell lymphoma presenting in skin: a clinicopathologic analysis of six cases. *J Cutan Pathol* 1996;**23**:101–108.

7. Kamarashev J, Dummer R, Hess Schmid M *et al.* Primary cutaneous T-cell-rich B-cell lymphoma and Hodgkin's disease in a patient with Gardner's syndrome. *Dermatology* 2000;**201**:362–365.

8. Gogstetter D, Brown M, Seab J, Scott G. Angiocentric primary cutaneous T-cell-rich B-cell lymphoma: a case report and review of the literature. *J Cutan Pathol* 2000;**27**:516–525.

9. Swerdlow SH, Campo E, Seto M, Müller-Hermelink HK. Mantle cell lymphoma. In: Swerdlow SH, Campo E, Harris NL *et al.*, eds. *WHO Classification of Tumours of Haematopoietic and Lymphoid Tissues.* Lyon: IARC Press, 2008: 229–232.

10. Sen F, Medeiros LJ, Lu D *et al.* Mantle cell lymphoma involving skin: cutaneous lesions may be the first manifestation of disease and tumors often have blastoid cytologic features. *Am J Surg Pathol* 2002;**26**:1312–1318.

11. Dubus P, Young P, Beylot-Barry M *et al.* Value of interphase FISH for the diagnosis of t(11;14)(q13;q32) on skin lesions of mantle cell lymphoma. *Am J Clin Pathol* 2002;**118**:832–841.

12. Marti RM, Campo E, Bosch F, Palou J, Estrach T. Cutaneous lymphocyte-associated antigen (CLA) expression in a lymphoblastoid mantle cell lymphoma presenting with skin lesions: comparison with other clinicopathologic presentations of mantle cell lymphoma. *J Cutan Pathol* 2001;**28**:256–264.

13. Geerts ML, Busschots AM. Mantle-cell lymphomas of the skin. *Dermatol Clin* 1994;**12**:409–417.

14. Bertero M, Novelli M, Fierro MT, Bernengo MG. Mantle zone lymphoma: an immunohistologic study of skin lesions. *J Am Acad Dermatol* 1994;**30**:23–30.

15. Moody BR, Bartlett NL, George DW *et al.* Cyclin D1 as an aid in the diagnosis of mantle cell lymphoma in skin biopsies: a case report. *Am J Dermatopathol* 2001;**23**:470–476.

16. Liebow AA, Carrington CR, Friedman PJ. Lymphomatoid granulomatosis. *Hum Pathol* 1972;**3**:457–558.

17. Pittaluga S, Wilson WH, Jaffe ES. Lymphomatoid granulomatosis. In: Swerdlow SH, Campo E, Harris NL *et al.*, eds. *WHO Classification of Tumours of Haematopoietic and Lymphoid Tissues.* Lyon: IARC Press, 2008: 247–249.

18. Beaty MW, Toro J, Sorbara L *et al.* Cutaneous lymphomatoid granulomatosis: correlation of clinical and biologic features. *Am J Surg Pathol* 2001;**25**:1111–1120.

19. Carlson KC, Gibson LE. Cutaneous signs of lymphomatoid granulomatosis. *Arch Dermatol* 1991;**127**:1693–1698.

20. Katzenstein ALA, Carrington CB, Liebow AA. Lymphomatoid granulomatosis: a clinicopathologic study of 152 cases. *Cancer* 1979;**43**:360–373.

21. McNiff JM, Cooper D, Howe G *et al.* Lymphomatoid granulomatosis of the skin and lung: an angiocentric T-cell-rich B-cell lymphoproliferative disorder. *Arch Dermatol* 1996;**132**:1464–1470.

22. Tong MM, Cooke B, Barnetson RSC. Lymphomatoid granulomatosis. *J Am Acad Dermatol* 1992;**27**:872–876.

23. LeSueur BW, Ellsworth L, Bangert JL, Hansen RC. Lymphomatoid granulomatosis in a 4-year-old boy. *Pediatr Dermatol* 2000;**17**:369–372.

24. Oyama T, Ichimura K, Suzuki R, *et al.* Senile EBV+ B-Cell Lymphoproliferative Disorders A Clinicopathologic Study of 22 Patients. *Am J Surg Pathol* 2003;**27**:16–26.

25. Wong HH, Wang J, Epstein-Barr virus positive diffuse large B-cell lymphoma of the elderly. *Leuk Lymphoma*; **Mar 2**: [Epub ahead of print].

26. Oyama T, Yamamoto K, Asano N *et al.* Age-related EBV-associated B-cell lymphoproliferative disorders constitute a distinct clinicopathologic group: a study of 96 patients. *Clin Cancer Res* 2007;**13**:5124–5132.

27. Nakamura S, Jaffe ES, Swerdlow SH. EBV positive diffuse large B-cell lymphoma of the elderly. In: Swerdlow SH, Campo E, Harris NL *et al.*, eds. *WHO Classification of Tumours of Haematopoietic and Lymphoid Tissues.* Lyon: IARC Press, 2008: 243–244.

28. Gaitonde S, Kavuri S, Alagiozian-Angelova V, Peace D, Worobec S. EBV positivity in primary cutaneous large B-cell lymphoma with immunophenotypic features of leg type: an isolated incidence or something more significant? *Acta Oncol* 2008;**47**:461–464.

29. Tokuda Y, Fukushima M, Nakazawa K *et al.* A case of primary Epstein–Barr virus associated cutaneous diffuse large B-cell lymphoma unassociated with iatrogenic or endogenous immune dysregulation. *J Cutan Pathol* 2008;**35**:666–671.

30. Willemze R, Jaffe ES, Burg G *et al.* WHO-EORTC classification for cutaneous lymphomas. *Blood* 2005;**105**:3768–3785.

31. Torne R, Su WPD, Winkelmann RK, Smolle J, Kerl H. Clinicopathologic study of cutaneous plasmacytoma. *Int J Dermatol* 1990;**29**:562–566.

32. Wong KF, Chan JKC, Li LPK, Yau TK, Lee AWM. Primary cutaneous plasmacytoma: report of two cases and review of the literature. *Am J Dermatopathol* 1994;**16**:392–397.

33. Tüting T, Bork K. Primary plasmacytoma of the skin. *J Am Acad Dermatol* 1996;**34**:386–390.

34. Muscardin LM, Pulsoni A, Cerroni L. Primary cutaneous plasmacytoma: report of a case with review of the literature. *J Am Acad Dermatol* 2000;**43**:962–965.

35. Chang YT, Wong CK. Primary cutaneous plasmacytomas. *Clin Exp Dermatol* 1994;**19**:177–180.

36. Llamas-Martin R, Postigo-Iorente C, Vanaclocha-Sebastian F, Gil-Martin R, Iglesias-Diez L. Primary cutaneous extramedullary plasmacytoma secreting lambda IgG. *Clin Exp Dermatol* 1993;**18**:351–355.

37. Miyamoto T, Kobayashi T, Hagari Y, Mihara M. The value of genotypic analysis in the assessment of cutaneous plasmacytomas. *Br J Dermatol* 1997;**137**:418–421.

38. Müller RPA, Krausse S, Rahlf G. Primär kutanes Plasmozytom: Fallbericht und Literaturübersicht. *Hautarzt* 1990;**41**:232–235.

39. Requena L, Kutzner H, Palmedo G *et al.* Cutaneous involvement in multiple myeloma: a clinicopathologic, immunohistochemical, and cytogenetic study of 8 cases. *Arch Dermatol* 2003;**139**:475–486.

40. Jenkins RE, Calonje E, Fawcett H, Greaves MW, Wilson-Jones E. Cutaneous crystalline deposits in myeloma. *Arch Dermatol* 1994;**130**:484–488.

41. El-Shabrawi-Caelen L, Cerroni L, Kerl H. Crystal storing histiocytosis. *Dermatopathol Pract Concept* 2001;**7**:305–306.

Section 3: Other cutaneous lymphomas

14 Intravascular large cell lymphoma

In previous editions of this book intravascular lymphomas of B- and T-cell origin were included in separate chapters of other cutaneous B-cell lymphomas and T-cell lymphomas, respectively. However, it seems that intravascular lymphoma represents probably the only example of a lymphoma type where phenotypic considerations play a marginal role, and exact classification is achieved mainly based on the peculiar morphology – that is, intravascular location of the neoplastic cells [1]. In fact, clinicopathologic presentation, prognosis, and treatment are similar for both subtypes, whereas the main differences seem to be related to the presence or absence of an associated hemophagocytic syndrome [2,3].

Intravascular large B-cell lymphoma is considered as a provisional entity in the World Health Organization (WHO)-European Organization for Research and Treatment of Cancer (EORTC) classification of primary cutaneous lymphomas [4], and as a distinct entity in the new WHO classification of tumors of hematopoietic and lymphoid tissues [5]. By contrast, the T-cell variant is probably the only lymphoma type that is not covered by any classification; the WHO classification mentions it only with the following words: "Anecdotal cases of intravascular T-cell or NK-cell lymphoma have been reported, but they should be considered a different entity (than intravascular large B-cell lymphoma);" further details are not provided [5].

The skin may be the only affected site, but more frequently the disease presents with generalized lesions and common neurologic symptoms due to involvement of the central nervous system.

Intravascular large cell lymphoma presents with lesions where neoplastic cells are confined almost exclusively to the lumina of vessels, and it was formerly misinterpreted as a vascular neoplasm (malignant angio-endotheliomatosis) [6]. It is still unclear whether cases classified in the past as large B-cell lymphoma recurring as intravascular lymphoma [7,8]

or as "mixed" intravascular and diffuse large B-cell lymphoma [9] should be included in this category [10]. In addition, recently exceptional cases of a "benign" intravascular proliferation of lymphoid blasts was reported as a simulator of intravascular lymphoma, but the exact classification is unclear (see Chapter 22) [11,12].

The reason(s) why neoplastic cells in intravascular large cell lymphoma are confined within the vessels is unclear. Absence of molecules crucial for adhesion of lymphocytes to endothelial cells and migration out of the vessels (CD29, CD54) has been observed in some cases with B phenotype, leading to the hypothesis that neoplastic lymphocytes in intravascular large B-cell lymphoma are unable to escape outside the vessel walls [13].

Colonization of capillaries of cutaneous hemangiomas by large B-cells of intravascular large B-cell lymphoma has been observed in more cases than pure chance would justify, suggesting that these cells have a special tropism for neoplastic blood vessels [14–16]. Sometimes this is the only manifestation of the lymphoma and no other sites are involved [17–19]. In a similar fashion, neoplastic cells have been detected in the vessels of Kaposi sarcoma and of solid tumors. This is probably one of the most intriguing features of this rare lymphoma, and investigation of such variants may provide some clues concerning the disease.

It should be remembered that in a distinct proportion of the reported cases, particularly in the NK/T-cell variant of the disease, the diagnosis of intravascular large cell lymphoma was a retrospective one made first at autopsy.

INTRAVASCULAR LARGE B-CELL LYMPHOMA

Intravascular large B-cell lymphoma is a malignant proliferation of large B lymphocytes within blood vessels. In rare cases the skin may be the only affected site, though more often the lymphoma is disseminated, with involvement of the central nervous system being common. As already mentioned, cases of intravascular large B-cell lymphoma have been reported in patients with pre-existing cutaneous or, more often, nodal large B-cell lymphoma, probably representing recurrence of

Skin Lymphoma: The Illustrated Guide. By L. Cerroni, K. Gatter and H. Kerl. Published 2009 Blackwell Publishing, ISBN: 978-1-4051-8554-7.

the original disease rather than a genuine intravascular large B-cell lymphoma [7,8].

Clinical features

Patients present with indurated, erythematous or violaceous patches and plaques, preferentially located on the trunk and thighs (Fig. 14.1). The clinical appearance is not typical of lymphoma and may sometimes suggest a diagnosis of panniculitis or purpura [20–24]. Generalized telangiectasia has been observed in one patient [25]. Neurologic symptoms as a sign of involvement of the central nervous system are commonly present[26]. Other organs that are frequently involved are the liver and kidney.

Hemophagocytosis was reported in the majority of Japanese patients [27], but not in European patients [2,28]. It has been suggested that hemophagocytosis-associated cases represent

a distinct variant of the disease with significantly different clinical features, characterized by higher frequency of systemic symptoms (fever, fatigue) and hepatic, splenic and bone marrow involvement, and lower frequency of neurologic and cutaneous involvement [2]. B symptoms, anemia, thrombocytopenia, hepatosplenomegaly, and bone marrow involvement are frequently observed in patients with associated hemophagocytic syndrome.

As already mentioned, intravascular large B-cell lymphoma may arise within the vessels of pre-existent capillary hemangiomas (Fig. 14.2).

Histopathology, immunophenotype and molecular genetics

Histology reveals a proliferation of large lymphocytes filling dilated blood vessels within the dermis and subcutaneous tissues (Fig. 14.3). A perivascular infiltrate of large atypical

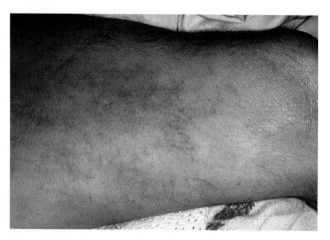

Figure 14.1 Erythematous, infiltrated lesions of intravascular large B-cell lymphoma on the thigh. (Courtesy of Professor Alain Townsend, Oxford, UK.)

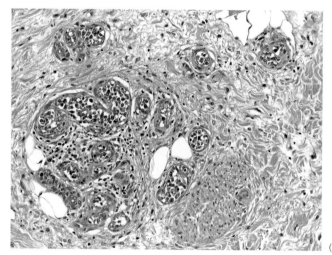

(a)

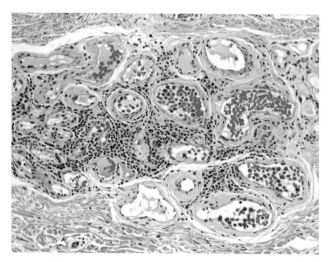

Figure 14.2 Intravascular large B-cell lymphoma colonizing the vessels of a cherry hemangioma.

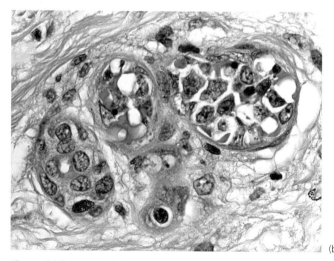

(b)

Figure 14.3 Intravascular large B-cell lymphoma. (a) Several vessels filled with large lymphoma cells. (b) Detail of large atypical cells within the vessels.

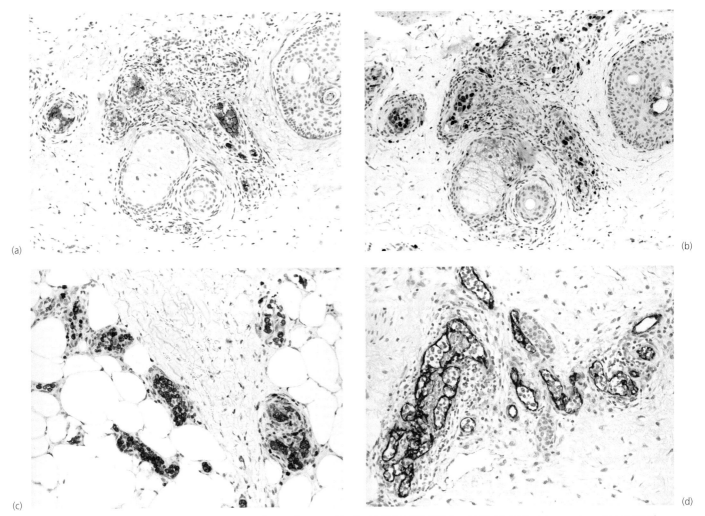

Figure 14.4 Intravascular large B-cell lymphoma. Neoplastic cells are positive for (a) CD20, (b) MUM-1 and (c) Bcl-2; (d) the intravascular arrangement of neoplastic cells is highlighted by the staining for CD31.

cells is present in some cases. The malignant cells are large with scanty cytoplasm, often with prominent nucleoli (immunoblasts).

Neoplastic cells are positive for B-cell-associated markers (CD20, CD79a) (Fig. 14.4a), and in a subset of cases show aberrant CD5 expression [29]. Monoclonal expression of either κ or λ light chain can be demonstrated in the majority of cases on frozen sections of tissue, but detection is usually not possible on routinely fixed material. Positivity for Bcl-2 and multiple myeloma oncogene 1 (MUM-1) is observed in the vast majority of cases, highlighting the similarities with other diffuse large B-cell lymphomas (Fig. 14.4b, c). Bcl-6 and CD10 are positive only in a small minority of cases, whereas cyclin D1 is consistently negative. Positivity for prostatic acid phosphatase has been reported in a small series [30]. Staining with endothelial cell-related antibodies (i.e. CD31, CD34) highlights the characteristic intravascular location of the cells (Fig. 14.4d), which are located in blood vessels (podoplanine-positive lymphatic vessels do not harbor neoplastic cells).

In situ hybridization studies for Epstein–Barr virus (EBV) were negative in a large study [27], but positive cases have been reported. Molecular analysis shows monoclonal rearrangement of the immunoglobulin heavy chain (J_H) gene. Fluorescent *in situ* hybridization (FISH) studies revealed karyotype abnormalities in cases of intravascular large B-cell lymphoma, but observations are limited to small numbers of cases [31]. A t(14;18) was observed in one case [32].

Intravascular large B-cell lymphoma should be distinguished from reactive angio-endotheliomatosis which is a benign skin condition characterized by an intravascular proliferation of either endothelial or histiocytic cells (intravascular histiocytosis) (see Chapter 22) [33].

Treatment and prognosis

The treatment of choice of intravascular large B-cell lymphoma is anthracycline-based systemic chemotherapy [34]. Recently, the efficacy of adding anti-CD20 antibody (rituximab) to the treatment scheme was demonstrated. It has also been suggested to add drugs with a higher bio-availability in the central nervous system, such as methotrexate or cytarabine [10]. Autologous peripheral blood stem cell transplantation has been used in occasional patients with encouraging results [35], but data on large numbers of patients are lacking, and age may be a limiting factor for such a treatment.

The prognosis of cases limited to the skin seems to be better than that of the generalized (multisystem) disease [36]. Unfavorable prognostic factors are lack of anthracycline-based chemotherapy, age older than 60 years, and thrombocytopenia less than 100×10^9/L [27]. Positivity for CD5 does not influence prognosis.

Résumé

Intravascular large B-cell lymphoma

Clinical	Adults. Solitary or multiple indurated patches and plaques, sometimes resembling panniculitis or telangiectatic erythema. Preferential locations: trunk, thighs.
Morphology	Intravascular (blood vessels) proliferation of large atypical lymphoid cells.
Immunology	CD20, 79a + CD5 +/− Bcl-2, MUM-1 + Bcl-6, CD10 −(+) sIg + (monoclonal)
Genetics	Monoclonal rearrangement of the J_H gene. No specific genetic alterations described.
Treatment guidelines	Anthracycline-based systemic chemotherapy, eventually associated with rituximab. Role of peripheral blood stem cell or bone marrow transplantation should be evaluated.

INTRAVASCULAR LARGE NK/T-CELL LYMPHOMA

Rarely, cases of cutaneous intravascular large cell lymphoma may show a T-cell or NK cell phenotype [1]. This is probably the rarest form of lymphoma (not only cutaneous), as less than 50 cases have been reported in the literature. Besides the phenotype, the most striking difference from cases with a B phenotype seems to be the much more common association with EBV infection [37]. Intravascular large T-cell lymphoma is not covered in the WHO classification of tumors of hematopoietic and lymphoid tissues, where there is only a brief remark on it within the chapter on the B-cell counterpart (see first paragraph of this chapter) [5].

Patients are usually elderly adults though a congenital case has been reported [38]. The clinical presentation and histopathologic picture are similar to those seen in the more common B-cell variant. The histopathologic features also are indistinguishable from those of the B-cell variant.

Neoplastic cells in intravascular large NK/T-cell lymphoma express CD2 and CD3, but are commonly negative for CD5 (Fig. 14.5a). Recent studies demonstrated that the vast majority of cases of intravascular large NK/T-cell lymphoma have a NK/T cytotoxic phenotype and are associated with EBV, thus showing some similarities to extranodal NK/T cell lymphoma, nasal type (Fig. 14.5b–d) [1,39,40]. However, rarely cases are characterized by a T-helper or CD30+ phenotype, and at present it seems clear that intravascular large NK/T-cell lymphoma represents a relatively heterogeneous phenotypic entity [1]. CD56 is expressed by neoplastic cells in the majority of cases (Fig. 14.5b), whereas βF1, a marker of α/β T lymphocytes, was negative in all cases tested [1,41]. A summary of cases with sufficient phenotypic data published in the literature is presented in Table 14.1.

Molecular analysis of the T-cell receptor (TCR) gene rearrangement by polymerase chain reaction (PCR) was conducted only in a few instances, revealing monoclonality in approximately one-third of cases (the negative cases possibly representing those with a genuine NK cell phenotype).

Prognosis and treatment of intravascular large NK/T-cell lymphoma do not seem to differ from those of the B-cell type of the disease, but of course anti-CD20 antibodies do not have efficacy in the NK/T-cell variant. At present, data on treatment are available only for a handful of patients and there are no clear-cut guidelines. The prognosis is very poor; data on cases published in the literature reveal a better prognosis for patients with disease limited to one organ only, as compared to those with disease detected in two or more organs.

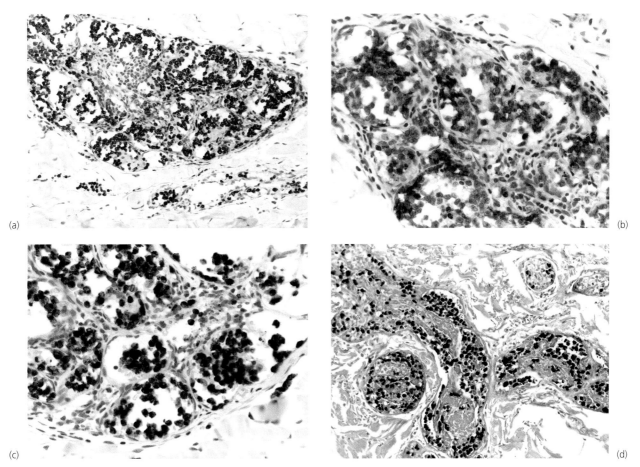

Figure 14.5 Intravascular large NK/T-cell lymphoma. Intravascular large lymphocytes positive for (a) CD3, (b) CD56, and (c) TIA-1, and (d) revealing a positive signal upon *in situ* hybridization for EBV (EBER-1).

Table 14.1 Phenotype of neoplastic cells in cases of intravascular NK/T-cell lymphoma reported in the literature with sufficient immunohistochemical data

Case (reference)	Gender /age	Site of presentation	CD3	CD4	CD5	CD8	CD30	CD56	TIA-1	ßF1	EBER-1	PCR-TCR
Kaluza et al.[42]	M/53	Brain	+	nd	nd	nd	nd	+	nd (§)	nd	+	G
Kuo et al.[43]	F/71	Skin	+	–	–	–	–	+	+	nd	+	G
Merchant et al.[44]	M/37	Autopsy (kidney, brain, liver, lung, adrenal gland)	+	–	–	+	–	–	+	nd	+	M
Santucci et al.[41]	M/54	Skin	+	–	nd	–	+	+	+	nd	+	nd
Song et al.[45]	F/40	Skin, brain	+	–	nd	–	nd	+	+	nd	+	G
Takahashi et al.[46]	M/72	Autopsy (liver, spleen, kidney, lung, bone marrow)	–	+	–	–	+	–	+	–	–	nd
Wu et al.[47]	F/47	Autopsy (brain, pituitary gland, bone marrow, kidney, ovary, cervix)	+	–	–	–	–	+	+	nd	–	G
Wu et al.[47]	M/41	Skin	+	–	–	–	–	+	+	–	+	G
Nakamichi et al.[37]	F/23	Skin, ileum	+	nd	nd	nd	nd	+	+	nd	+	nd
Cerroni et al.[1]	F/67	Skin, brain	+	–	nd	+	+/–	–	+	nd	nd	M
Cerroni et al.[1]	M/63	Skin	+	–	–	–	nd	+	+	–	+	G
Cerroni et al.[1]	M/63	Skin	+	–	–	–	nd	–	+	–	–	G
Cerroni et al.[1]	M/87	Skin (*)	+	–	–	–	–	–	–	–	+	M
Gleason et al.[40]	M/62	Skin	+	–	–	–	–	+	+	–	–	M

Gender: M, male; F, female.
(*) Further studies were not carried out.
nd, not done; (§), positive for granzyme B.
PCR-TCR, polymerase chain reaction analysis of the T-cell receptor gene; G, germline; M, monoclonal.

Résumé

Intravascular large NK/T-cell lymphoma

Clinical	Very rare variant of intravascular large cell lymphoma. Adults. Solitary or multiple indurated patches and plaques; sometimes telangiectasia.	
Morphology	Intravascular proliferation of large atypical lymphoid cells.	
Immunology	CD2, 3	+
	CD5	−
	βF1	−
	CD20, 79a	−
	CD56	+(−)
	TIA-1, granzyme B	+
	CD30	−(+)
	EBER-1	+(−)
Genetics	Monoclonal rearrangement of the TCR genes in approximately one-third of cases.	
Treatment guidelines	Systemic chemotherapy (value of anthracycline-based systemic chemotherapy not tested in cases with NK/T-cell phenotype).	

References

1. Cerroni L, Massone C, Kutzner H, Mentzel T, Umbert P, Kerl H. Intravascular large T-cell or NK-cell lymphoma. A rare variant of intravascular large cell lymphoma with frequent cytotoxic phenotype and association with Epstein-Barr virus infection. *Am J Surg Pathol* 2008;**32**:891–898.

2. Ferreri AJM, Dognini GP, Campo E *et al.* Variations in clinical presentation, frequency of hemophagocytosis and clinical behavior of intravascular lymphoma diagnosed in different geographical regions. *Haematologica* 2007;**92**:486–492.

3. Nakamura S, Murase T, Kinoshita T. Intravascular large B-cell lymphoma: the heterogeneous clinical manifestations of its classical and hemophagocytosis-related forms. *Haematologica* 2007;**92**:434–436.

4. Willemze R, Jaffe ES, Burg G *et al.* WHO-EORTC classification for cutaneous lymphomas. *Blood* 2005;**105**:3768–3785.

5. Nakamura S, Ponzoni M, Campo E. Intravascular large B-cell lymphoma. In: Swerdlow SH, Campo E, Harris NL *et al.*, eds. *WHO Classification of Tumours of Haematopoietic and Lymphoid Tissues*. Lyon: IARC Press, 2008: 252–253.

6. Sheibani K, Battifora H, Winberg CD *et al.* Further evidence that "malignant angioendotheliomatosis" is an angiotropic large-cell lymphoma. *N Engl J Med* 1986;**314**:943–948.

7. Asagoe K, Fujimoto W, Yoshino T *et al.* Intravascular lymphomatosis of the skin as a manifestation of recurrent B-cell lymphoma. *J Am Acad Dermatol* 2003;**48**:S1–4.

8. Kamath NV, Gilliam AC, Nihal M, Spiro TP, Wood GS. Primary cutaneous large B-cell lymphoma of the leg relapsing as cutaneous intravascular large B-cell lymphoma. *Arch Dermatol* 2001;**137**: 1637–1638.

9. Sukpanichnant S, Visuthisakchai S. Intravascular lymphomatosis: a study of 20 cases in Thailand and a review of the literature. *Clin Lymphoma Myeloma* 2006;**6**:319–328.

10. Ponzoni M, Ferreri AJM, Campo E *et al.* Definition, diagnosis, and management of intravascular large B-cell lymphoma: Proposals and perspectives from an international consensus meeting. *J Clin Oncol* 2007;**25**:3168–3173.

11. Bryant A, Lawton H, Al-Talib R, Wright DH, Theaker JM. Intravascular proliferation of reactive lymphoid blasts mimicking intravascular lymphoma – a diagnostic pitfall. *Histopathology* 2007;**51**:401–402.

12. Baum CL, Stone MS, Liu V. Atypical intravascular CD30+ T-cell proliferation following trauma in a healthy 17-year-old male: first reported case of a potential diagnostic pitfall and literature review. *J Cut Pathol* 2009;**36**:350–354.

13. Ponzoni M, Arrigoni G, Gould VE *et al.* Lack of CD29 (beta1 integrin) and CD54 (ICAM-1) adhesion molecules in intravascular lymphomatosis. *Hum Pathol* 2000;**31**:220–226.

14. Kobayashi T, Munakata S, Sugiura H *et al.* Angiotropic lymphoma: proliferation of B cells in the capillaries of cutaneous angiomas. *Br J Dermatol* 2000;**143**:162–164.

15. Rubin MA, Cossman J, Freter CE, Azumi N. Intravascular large cell lymphoma coexisting within hemangiomas of the skin. *Am J Surg Pathol* 1997;**21**:860–864.

16. Nixon BK, Kussick SJ, Carlon MJ, Rubin BP. Intravascular large B-cell lymphoma involving hemangiomas: an unusual presentation of a rare neoplasm. *Mod Pathol* 2005;**18**:1121–1126.

17. Satoh S, Yamazaki M, Yahikozawa H *et al.* Intravascular large B cell lymphoma diagnosed by senile angioma biopsy. *Intern Med* 2003;**42**:117–120.

18. Cerroni L, Zalaudek I, Kerl H. Intravascular large B-cell lymphoma colonizing cutaneous hemangiomas. *Dermatology* 2004; **209**:132–134.

19. Cerroni L. Hemangiomas with (bad) surprise. *Dermatology* 2004; **209**:79–80.

20. Chang A, Zic JA, Boyd AS. Intravascular large cell lymphoma: a patient with asymptomatic purpuric patches and a chronic clinical course. *J Am Acad Dermatol* 1998;**39**:318–321.

21. Di Giuseppe JA, Nelson WG, Seifter EJ, Boitnott JK, Mann RB. Intravascular lymphomatosis: a clinicopathologic study of 10 cases and assessment of response to chemotherapy. *J Clin Oncol* 1994;**12**:2573–2579.

22. Kiyohara T, Kumakiri M, Kobayashi H *et al.* A case of intravascular large B-cell lymphoma mimicking erythema nodosum: the importance of multiple skin biopsies. *J Cutan Pathol* 2000;**27**: 413–418.

23. Stroup RM, Sheibani K, Moncada A, Purdy LJ, Battifora H. Angiotropic (intravascular) lymphoma: a clinicopathologic study of seven cases with unique clinical presentations. *Cancer* 1990; **66**:1781–1788.

24. Yegappan S, Coupland R, Arber DA *et al.* Angiotropic lymphoma: an immunophenotypically and clinically heterogeneous lymphoma. *Mod Pathol* 2001;**14**:1147–1156.

25. Özgüroglu E, Büyülbabani N, Ögzüroglu M, Baykal C. Generalized telangiectasia as the major manifestation of angiotropic (intravascular) lymphoma. *Br J Dermatol* 1997;**137**:422–425.

26. Glass J, Hochberg FH, Miller DC. Intravascular lymphomatosis: a systemic disease with neurologic manifestations. *Cancer* 1993; **71**:3156–3164.

27. Murase T, Yamaguchi M, Suzuki R *et al*. Intravascular large B-cell lymphoma (IVLBCL): a clinicopathologic study of 96 cases with special reference to the immunophenotypic heterogeneity of CD5. *Blood* 2007;**109**:478–485.

28. Terrier B, Aouba A, Vasiliu V *et al*. Intravascular lymphoma associated with haemophagocytic syndrome: a very rare entity in western countries. *Eur J Haematol* 2005;**75**:341–345.

29. Khalidi HS, Brynes RK, Browne P, Koo CH, Battifora H, Medeiros LJ. Intravascular large B-cell lymphoma: the CD5 antigen is expressed by a subset of cases. *Mod Pathol* 1998;**11**:983–988.

30. Seki K, Miyakoshi S, Lee GH *et al*. Prostatic acid phosphatase is a possible tumor marker for intravascular large B-cell lymphoma. *Am J Surg Pathol* 2004;**28**:1384–1388.

31. Khoury H, Lestou VS, Gascoyne RD *et al*. Multicolor karyotyping and clinicopathologic analysis of three intravascular lymphoma cases. *Mod Pathol* 2003;**16**:716–724.

32. Vieites B, Fraga M, Lopez-Presas E, Pintos E, Garcia-Rivero A, Forteza J. Detection of t(14;18) translocation in a case of intravascular large B-cell lymphoma: a germinal centre cell origin in a subset of these lymphomas? *Histopathology* 2005;**46**:466–468.

33. Wick MR, Rocamora A. Reactive and malignant "angioendotheliomatosis": a discriminant clinicopathological study. *J Cutan Pathol* 1988;**15**:260–271.

34. Ferreri AJM, Dognini GP, Bairey O, *et al*. The addition of rituximab to anthracycline-based chemotherapy significantly improves outcome in 'Western' patients with intravascular large B-cell lymphoma. *Br J Haematol* 2008;**143**:253–257.

35. Koizumi M, Nishimura M, Yokota A, Munekata S, Kobayashi T, Saito Y. Successful treatment of intravascular malignant lymphomatosis with high-dose chemotherapy and autologous peripheral blood stem cell transplantation. *Bone Marrow Transplant* 2001;**27**:1101–1103.

36. Ferreri AJM, Campo E, Seymour JF *et al*. Intravascular lymphoma: clinical presentation, natural history, management and prognostic factors in a series of 38 cases, with special emphasis on the "cutaneous variant". *Br J Haematol* 2004;**127**:173–183.

37. Nakamichi N, Fukuhara S, Aozasa K, Morii E. NK-cell intravascular lymphomatosis – a mini-review. *Eur J Haematol* 2008;**81**:1–7.

38. Tateyama H, Eimoto T, Tada T *et al*. Congenital angiotropic lymphoma (intravascular lymphomatosis) of the T-cell type. *Cancer* 1991;**67**:2131–2136.

39. Au WY, Shek WH, Nicholls J *et al*. T-cell intravascular lymphomatosis (angiotropic large cell lymphoma): association with Epstein–Barr viral infection. *Histopathology* 1997;**31**:563–567.

40. Gleason BC, Brinster NK, Granter SR, Pinkus GS, Lindeman NI, Miller DM. Intravascular cytotoxic T-cell lymphoma: a case report and review of the literature. *J Am Acad Dermatol* 2008;**58**:290–294.

41. Santucci M, Pimpinelli N, Massi D *et al*. Cytotoxic/natural killer cell cutaneous lymphomas. Report of the EORTC cutaneous lymphoma task force workshop. *Cancer* 2003;**97**:610–627.

42. Kaluza V, Rao DS, Said JW *et al*. Primary extranodal nasal-type natural killer/T-cell lymphoma of the brain: a case report. *Hum Pathol* 2006;**37**:769–772.

43. Kuo TT, Chen MJ, Kuo M. Cutaneous intravascular NK-cell lymphoma: report of a rare variant associated with Epstein–Barr virus. *Am J Surg Pathol* 2006;**30**:1197–1201.

44. Merchant SH, Viswanatha DS, Zumwalt RE *et al*. Epstein-Barr virus-associated intravascular large T-cell lymphoma presenting as acute renal failure in a patient with acquired immune deficiency syndrome. *Hum Pathol* 2003;**34**:950–954.

45. Song DE, Lee MW, Ryu MH *et al*. Intravascular large cell lymphoma of the natural killer cell type. *J Clin Oncol* 2007;**25**:1279–1282.

46. Takahashi E, Kajimoto K, Fukatsu T *et al*. Intravascular large T-cell lymphoma: a case report of CD30-positive and ALK-negative anaplastic type with cytotoxic molecule expression. *Virchows Arch* 2005;**447**:1000–1006.

47. Wu H, Said JW, Ames ED *et al*. First reported cases of intravascular large cell lymphoma of the NK cell type. Clinical, histologic, immunophenotypic, and molecular features. *Am J Clin Pathol* 2005;**123**:603–611.

Cutaneous lymphomas in immunosuppressed individuals

Individuals who are immunosuppressed, due to a congenital immunodeficiency disorder, or as a consequence of disease (e.g. human immunodeficiency virus (HIV) infection) or specific immunosuppressive treatment, are at higher risk of cutaneous and extracutaneous malignancies, including lymphomas. Cutaneous lymphomas in immunocompromised patients have some peculiar aspects that warrant discussion in a separate chapter. Although in organs other than the skin B-cell lymphomas clearly predominate also in immunocompromised patients, cutaneous T-cell lymphomas represent about one-third of the cutaneous lymphomas arising in the setting of immunosuppression [1].

The field of cutaneous (and extracutaneous) lymphomas in the setting of immune suppression is rapidly expanding – and confusing. Besides reports on "specific" entities, such as polymorphic or monomorphic post-transplant lymphoproliferative disorders, many different types of lymphoma resembling "conventional" Hodgkin and non-Hodgkin lymphomas may arise in immunosuppressed individuals, such as mycosis fungoides for example. In addition, even entities that are considered relatively specific for particular types of immune suppression, such as plasmablastic lymphoma of the oral cavity occurring in HIV-infected individuals, may occur in different settings and rarely in non-immunocompromised patients. In short, a precise classification of these entities is difficult and in many instances would duplicate the normal classification of cutaneous or extracutaneous lymphomas. In this context, a few considerations should be borne in mind.

• One of the main differences between lymphomas in immunocompetent and immunosuppressed individuals is represented by the more frequent association with infectious agents in immunosuppressed patients, particularly with Epstein–Barr virus (EBV), but also with many other viruses.

• The same infectious agent may be associated with different types of lymphoma. Thus, demonstration of a particular virus should be interpreted only in the setting of complete clinical, morphologic, phenotypic, and genetic information and cannot be considered specific for a particular type of lymphoma.

• Although some types of lymphoma are frequently associated with particular forms of immune suppression (e.g. plasmablastic lymphoma in HIV-infected patients), lymphomas with the same morphologic and phenotypic features may be observed in other types of immune suppression or even in immunocompetent individuals. In this context, a diagnosis of one of these particular lymphomas does not require demonstration of immune suppression if compelling evidence is present.

• There are many overlaps between entities included in the sections on different types of immune deficiency. In this context, it should be remembered that many lymphomas described in a specific section may be encountered also in patients with other types of impaired immune conditions.

• Finally, some lymphomas not included in this chapter may be associated with impairment of the immune system related to aging, such as EBV$^+$ diffuse large B-cell lymphoma of the elderly (see Chapter 13).

A last consideration concerns treatment: in many cases, reduction of the immune suppression combined with antiviral treatment results in remission of the lymphoma, and "conventional" therapeutic options are usually left for cases that are not responding to this approach.

CUTANEOUS POST-TRANSPLANT LYMPHOPROLIFERATIVE DISORDERS

Lymphoproliferative disorders are one of the most common malignancies in recipients of solid organ and bone marrow transplantation, developing in approximately 2% of patients (post-transplant lymphoproliferative disorders) [2]. They represent for the most part examples of EBV-associated lymphoproliferative disorders. Although cutaneous manifestations are rare, some patients may present with disease localized solely to the skin [3–9]. Most cases arise within the first year after organ or bone marrow transplantation, but the time interval between transplantation and the onset of a post-transplant lymphoproliferative disorder may be much longer (several years).

Skin Lymphoma: The Illustrated Guide. By L. Cerroni, K. Gatter and H. Kerl. Published 2009 Blackwell Publishing, ISBN: 978-1-4051-8554-7.

Post-transplant lymphoproliferative disorders occur more often in recipients of heart–lung allografts, and less commonly in those who receive renal allografts. Other risk factors include primary infection with EBV following transplantation, infection with cytomegalovirus, T-cell-specific immunosuppression, and younger age [10].

Post-transplant lymphoproliferative disorders are currently classified according to four major categories [2]:
1. early lesions (reactive plasmacytic hyperplasia, infectious mononucleosis-like lesions)
2. polymorphic post-transplant lymphoproliferative disorder
3. monomorphic post-transplant lymphoproliferative disorder, with clinicopathologic features corresponding to "conventional" entities of B- and NK/T-cell lymphomas
4. classic Hodgkin lymphoma type post-transplant lymphoproliferative disorder.

Most monomorphic lesions exhibit a B-cell phenotype, but in rare instances an NK/T-cell phenotype has been observed. The occurrence of NK/T-cell lymphomas seems to be more frequent in the skin than in other organs [1]. One case of mycosis fungoicles has been observed in a pediatric patient.

Clinical features

Patients are adults or children who have received allogenic solid organ or bone marrow transplantation and are under immunosuppressive treatment. Cutaneous lesions are variable, including erythematous plaques, nodules and tumors, sometimes ulcerated. They can be solitary, localized to a single anatomic region or generalized. Concomitant involvement of other organs can be observed and is usually associated with systemic symptoms, including elevated serum levels of lactic dehydrogenase. Precise staging investigations should always be performed, in order to evaluate the extent of involvement before planning the treatment.

Histopathology, immunophenotype and molecular genetics

Histopathologic features vary according to the subtype of post-transplant lymphoproliferative disorder. Early lesions show polyclonal (rarely monoclonal) proliferations of mature plasma cells with rare immunoblasts. Polymorphic post-transplant lymphoproliferative disorder is characterized by the presence of a monoclonal infiltrate of B lymphocytes, comprising the whole spectrum of maturation and including plasma cells, immunoblasts and intermediate-sized lymphoid cells (Fig. 15.1). In monomorphic post-transplant lymphoproliferative disorder, the histopathologic picture is that of a malignant lymphoma (diffuse large B-cell lymphoma, Burkitt lymphoma, plasma cell myeloma or extramedullary plasmacytoma). Cases involving the skin present mostly with the features of diffuse large B-cell lymphoma. In rare cases, a plasmablastic morphology can be observed, similar to plasmablastic lymphoma arising in HIV-infected individuals [11,12]. One case resembling lymphomatoid granulomatosis has been described as well [13].

In rare instances, the aspects may be those of a peripheral NK/T-cell lymphoma not otherwise specified. Expression of α/β or γ/δ T-cell receptors (TCRs), as well as of CD4, CD8, CD30 and CD56, is variable in these cases. Analysis of phenotypic and molecular features of a large group of cases confirmed the diversity of different cases of monomorphic post-transplant lymphoproliferative disorders [14].

In the skin, the occurrence of cases indistinguishable from mycosis fungoides or cutaneous CD30+ anaplastic large cell lymphoma has been reported [1,15–18]. However, the prognosis seems worse than that of conventional examples of these lymphomas and similar to that of other post-transplant lymphoproliferative disorders [1]. A case of subcutaneous "panniculitis-like" T-cell lymphoma has been observed in a cardiac allograft recipient [19]. Although cutaneous T-cell lymphomas in immunocompromised patients are usually not associated with EBV infection, EBV+ cases can be observed rarely [20].

Genetic analyses showed that gains of chromosomes 5p and 11p and deletions of chromosome 12p were common in the diffuse large B-cell lymphoma variant of post-transplant lymphoproliferative disorders, and that some overlapping features between diffuse large B-cell lymphomas in immunocompetent and immunosuppressed individuals could be observed [21]. High levels of hypermethylation of the tumor suppressor gene *p16* have been observed in one EBV-associated case, supporting the evidence for a carcinogenic role of EBV in positive cases [22].

Treatment and prognosis

Reduction of immunosuppression, often associated with antiviral therapy, is the main strategy for treatment of post-transplant lymphoproliferative disorders [23–25]. Regression of the lesions may take place over a period of a few weeks up to a few months. Lesions that do not respond to these measures may be treated by more conventional modalities, including radiotherapy, interferon-α, anti-CD20 antibody (rituximab) (only for cases with B-cell phenotype), and systemic chemotherapy.

Plasmacytic hyperplasia almost always responds completely to mild reduction of immunosuppression. The prognosis of polymorphic or monomorphic post-transplant lymphoproliferative disorders limited to the skin seems to be more favorable than that of extracutaneous post-transplant lymphoproliferative disorders. However, mycosis fungoides-like cases in immunosuppressed individuals do not share the same favorable prognosis of conventional mycosis fungoides in immunocompetent hosts [1].

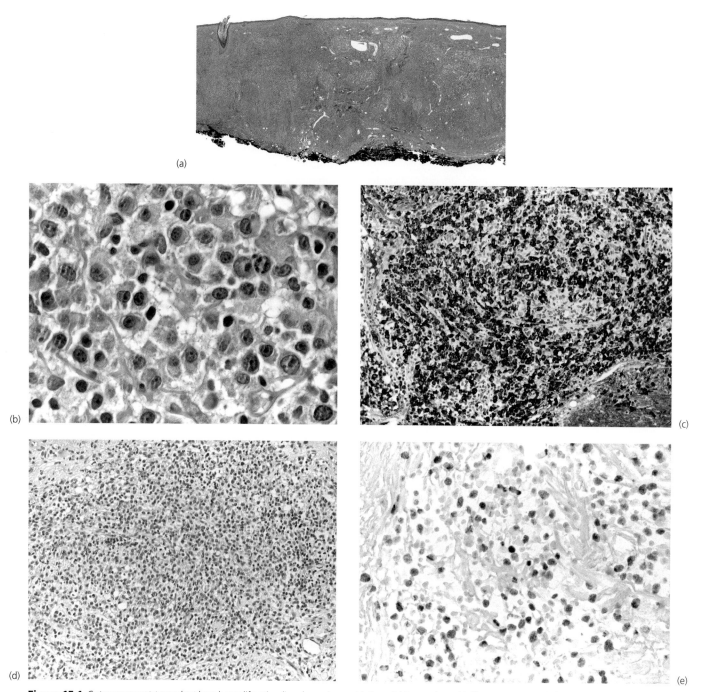

Figure 15.1 Cutaneous post-transplant lymphoproliferative disorder, polymorphic type. (a) Dense dermal infiltrates composed of (b) small, medium-sized and large cells admixed with plasma cells; (c) the cells are positive for κ, but not for (d) λ immunoglobulin light-chain; (e) note positive signal upon *in situ* hybridization for EBV (EBER-1).

Résumé

Cutaneous post-transplant lymphoproliferative disorders

Clinical	Children and adults. Onset of skin lesions usually within 1 year from organ transplantation. More frequent in recipients of heart–lung allografts. Four categories: reactive plasmacytic hyperplasia, polymorphic or monomorphic post-transplant lymphoproliferative disorder, classic Hodgkin lymphoma type post-transplant lymphoproliferative disorder. In the skin relatively high frequency of cases with T-cell phenotype, often indistinguishable from conventional mycosis fungoides or CD30$^+$ anaplastic large cell lymphoma.
Morphology	Mature plasma cells (plasmacytic hyperplasia); plasma cells, immunoblasts, intermediate cells (polymorphic type); clear-cut features of lymphoma (monomorphic type).
Immunology	CD20, 79a +(−) LMP-1 +(−) EBER-1 +(−) (cases with T-cell phenotype only rarely associated with EBV infection) CD3, 5 −(+) (in the skin about 1/3 of cases have a T-cell phenotype)
Genetics	Monoclonal rearrangement of the J$_H$ gene (polymorphic and monomorphic types). Gains of chromosomes 5p and 11p and deletions of chromosome 12p.
Treatment guidelines	Reduction of immunosuppression. Antiviral therapy. Cases that do not respond may be treated with rituximab (cases with B-cell phenotype), interferon-α, radiotherapy or systemic chemotherapy.

CUTANEOUS LYMPHOMAS IN HIV-INFECTED INDIVIDUALS

The onset of cutaneous or mucosal lymphomas caused by viral-induced immunosuppression has been observed in individuals with HIV-related acquired immunodeficiency syndrome (AIDS) [26–29]. It has been estimated that HIV-infected patients have a risk of developing a malignant lymphoma up to 200-fold higher than normal individuals. There are some overlapping features between the lymphomas arising in HIV$^+$ patients and those observed after solid organ or bone marrow transplantation. Besides cutaneous and mucosal lymphomas, HIV-infected individuals may develop many other extracutaneous lymphomas, particularly diffuse large B-cell lymphoma, Burkitt lymphoma and primary effusion lymphoma.

Cutaneous lesions may represent examples of "common" skin lymphomas such as mycosis fungoides, CD30$^+$ anaplastic large cell lymphoma or diffuse large B-cell lymphoma, leg type, similar to what can be observed in cutaneous lymphomas arising after solid organ transplantation [30–32]. In contrast to cutaneous lymphomas in non-infected individuals, however, mycosis fungoides represents a minority of the cases arising in HIV$^+$ patients, whereas B-cell lymphomas are more common.

The entity of plasmablastic lymphoma of the oral cavity has been reported mainly (but not exclusively) in HIV$^+$ individuals [33–38]. Cases have been observed less frequently in other types of immunosuppression or rarely in elderly immunocompetent individuals. Although earlier reports suggested an association of plasmablastic lymphoma with human herpesvirus 8 (HHV-8) infection [39], it has been demonstrated that true plasmablastic lymphomas are HHV-8$^-$ [40,41]. In rare patients, HHV-8-associated plasmablastic lymphoma has been observed concomitantly to Kaposi sarcoma and multicentric Castleman disease, suggesting that in this peculiar subgroup of patients HHV-8 may play a role in the development of the lymphoma [41,42]. It has been suggested that HHV-8$^+$ cases should be considered as solid variants of primary effusion lymphomas rather than as plasmablastic lymphoma [41,43].

Association with EBV has been documented in most cases of plasmablastic lymphoma and other cutaneous B-cell lymphoma associated with HIV infection, and rarely also in cases of HIV-related cutaneous CD30$^+$ anaplastic large cell lymphoma. Cases of HIV-related cutaneous CD30$^+$ anaplastic large cell lymphoma positive for HHV-8 have been documented as well [44]. Infection with human T-lymphotropic virus 2 (HTLV-II) has been detected in one HIV patient with a cutaneous T-cell lymphoma [45].

Clinical features

Patients are adults who are infected with HIV and have a very low CD4 count, but rarely children can be affected as well [26,46,47]. The onset of a cutaneous lymphoma may represent the first AIDS-defining illness in some of these patients. Cutaneous lesions are variable, depending on the type of lymphoma, and are not different from those observed in non-HIV-infected individuals. Rarely, a post-transplant lymphoproliferative disorder-like polymorphic infiltrate may be observed [48]. Accurate staging investigations should be performed in order to evaluate the extent (if any) of extra-cutaneous involvement.

In patients with HIV infection, mycosis fungoides should be distinguished from benign CD8$^+$ cutaneous infiltrates, which may reveal similar clinicopathologic features (see Chapter 22).

Plasmablastic lymphoma presents mostly with nodules and tumors arising in the oral mucosa (or at other mucosal sites), but rarely cutaneous cases have been reported [49].

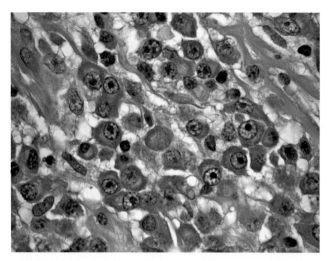

Figure 15.2 Cutaneous plasmablastic lymphoma in an HIV-infected individual. Note plasmablasts with eccentric nuclei, prominent nucleoli and abundant cytoplasm, admixed with plasma cells.

Histopathology, immunophenotype and molecular genetics

Histopathologic, immunophenotypical and molecular genetic features are similar to those observed in the corresponding lymphoma entities arising in non-HIV-infected individuals. However, in cases of diffuse large B-cell lymphoma, plasmablastic differentiation (Fig. 15.2) and association with EBV (positivity for LMP-1 and/or EBER-1) are more commonly seen.

Plasmablastic lymphoma shows a spectrum of morphologic presentations ranging from plasmablasts (large cells resembling immunoblasts) to more mature-looking plasma cells. The neoplastic cells are usually negative for CD20 but strongly positive for CD38, CD138 and multiple myeloma oncogene-1 (MUM-1), and express monoclonal immunoglobulins in the majority of cases. Two different phenotypic variants have been recently described, the first carrying a full plasmablastic phenotype, while the second shows a defective phenotype [50].

Treatment and prognosis

Mycosis fungoides in HIV⁺ patients should be managed according to standard protocols (see Chapter 2) [26,51]. Solitary or localized lesions of other lymphomas may be treated with local radiotherapy. Antiviral treatment should be accurately verified.

As these lymphomas arise in patients who are profoundly immunocompromised, death often ensues, resulting from complications of AIDS rather than from direct lymphoma spread. In this context, the use of conservative strategies for treatment of the cutaneous lymphomas has been advocated [26].

Plasmablastic lymphoma is extremely aggressive and survival is usually very short (<1 year). Better management of the underlying HIV infection may improve the prognosis in these

patients. In general, the combination of anti-cancer and antiviral treatments may improve the prognosis as well [52].

Résumé

HIV-associated cutaneous lymphomas

Clinical	Adults with HIV infection and very low CD4 cell count (children rarely affected). Clinical features may be those of "common" types of cutaneous lymphomas (e.g. mycosis fungoides, CD30⁺ anaplastic large cell lymphoma, diffuse large B-cell lymphoma, leg type). Plasmablastic lymphoma is encountered mainly in the oral mucosa in HIV⁺ individuals.
Morphology	Similar to the non-HIV-related counterparts; in plasmablastic lymphomas, spectrum of morphologic variability from immunoblast-like cells to more mature-looking plasma cells.
Immunology	CD20, 79a + (B-cell types) CD3, 5 + (T-cell types) CD30 + (CD30⁺ anaplastic large cell lymphoma) LMP-1, EBER-1 + (especially B-cell lymphomas) MUM-1, CD38, CD138 + (plasmablastic lymphoma)
Genetics	Monoclonal rearrangement of the TCR or J_H genes depending on the type.
Treatment guidelines	Radiotherapy (solitary or localized lesions); mycosis fungoides should be managed according to standard treatment regimens; antiviral therapy should be verified.

OTHER CUTANEOUS LYMPHOMAS ASSOCIATED WITH IMMUNE DYSREGULATION

These include congenital immune deficiencies, cutaneous lymphomas arising under treatment with methotrexate, and immunomodulatory treatment-related lymphoid proliferations.

Cutaneous (or extracutaneous) lymphomas in patients under methotrexate therapy are well known. In recent years, onset of cutaneous or extracutaneous lymphomas has been described also in patients undergoing treatment with immunosuppressive [53,54] or immunomodulatory drugs ("biologics") such as infliximab or etanercept, among many others. In some cases of mycosis fungoides a wrong diagnosis of atopic dermatitis or psoriasis had been made, and treatment with one of the many immunologic agents had been started, resulting in rapid progression of the disease (see also Chapter 2) [55–57]. These particular cases have been termed "monoclonal antibody immunomodulator-related lymphoid proliferations"

[58]. The lymphomas occurring in these settings have clinico-pathologic features similar to corresponding entities observed in patients who do not take the drugs, the main difference being represented by a higher rate of association with EBV infection detected in methotrexate-associated lymphomas. These lymphomas are included in two chapters in the new World Health Organization (WHO) classification of tumors of hematopoietic and lymphoid tissues [59,60]. In some cases rapid histopathologic progression from early changes to fully developed lesions has been documented [61]. In over half of the cases associated with methotrexate treatment, the lesions regress upon withdrawal of methotrexate.

Besides iatrogenic-induced or infection-related immuno-suppression, cutaneous lymphomas may arise in the setting of congenital immunodeficiency disorders such as Wiskott–Aldrich syndrome or ataxia-telangiectasia, among many others [20,59]. The most frequent lymphoma type observed in this group of patients is diffuse large B-cell lymphoma and clini-copathologic features are the same as for lesions arising in immunocompetent hosts. Lymphomatoid granulomatosis is also found at a higher frequency, but many other Hodgkin and non-Hodgkin lymphomas can be observed in this group of patients. The frequency of different types of lymphomas is different in the various types of congenital immunodeficiency disorders. The treatment is directed at both the underlying immune deficiency and the cutaneous lymphomas, depend-ing also on the lymphoma type.

References

1. Lok C, Viseux V, Denoeux JP, Bagot M. Post-transplant cutaneous T-cell lymphomas. *Crit Rev Oncol Hematol* 2005;**56**:137–145.
2. Swerdlow SH, Webber SA, Chadburn A, Ferry JA. Post-transplant lymphoproliferative disorders. In: Swerdlow SH, Campo E, Harris NL *et al.*, eds. *WHO Classification of Tumours of Haematopoietic and Lymphoid Tissues*. Lyon: IARC Press, 2008: 343–349.
3. Pacheco TR, Hinthner L, Fitzpatrick J. Extramedullary plasma-cytoma in cardiac transplant recipients. *J Am Acad Dermatol* 2003; **49**:S255–258.
4. Seckin D, Demirhan B, Gülec TO, Arikan U, Haberal M. Post-transplantation primary cutaneous CD30 (Ki1)-positive large-cell lymphoma. *J Am Acad Dermatol* 2001;**45**:S197–199.
5. Ward HA, Russo GG, McBurney E, Millikan LE, Boh EE. Post-transplant primary cutaneous T-cell lymphoma. *J Am Acad Dermatol* 2001;**44**:675–680.
6. Schumann KW, Oriba HA, Bergfeld WF, Hsi ED, Hollandsworth K. Cutaneous presentation of post-transplant lymphoproliferative disorder. *J Am Acad Dermatol* 2000;**42**:923–926.
7. Chai C, White WL, Shea CR, Prieto VG. Epstein–Barr virus asso-ciated lymphoproliferative-disorders primarily involving the skin. *J Cutan Pathol* 1999;**26**:242–247.
8. Gonthier DM, Hartman G, Holley JL. Post-transplant lympho-proliferative disorder presenting as an isolated skin lesion. *Am J Kidney Dis* 1992;**19**:600–603.
9. McGregor JM, Yu CCW, Lu QL *et al.* Post-transplant cutaneous lymphoma. *J Am Acad Dermatol* 1993;**29**:549–554.
10. Harris NL, Swerdlow SH. Post-transplant lymphoproliferative disorders: summary of Society for Hematopathology Workshop. *Semin Diagn Pathol* 1997;**14**:8–14.
11. Nicol I, Boye T, Carsuzaa F *et al.* Post-transplant plasmablastic lymphoma of the skin. *Br J Dermatol* 2003;**149**:889–891.
12. Samolitis NJ, Bharadwaj JS, Weis JR, Harris RM. Post-transplant lymphoproliferative disorder limited to the skin. *J Cutan Pathol* 2004;**31**:453–457.
13. Kwon EJ, Katz KA, Draft KS *et al.* Posttransplantation lymphoproliferative disease with features of lymphomatoid granulomatosis in a lung transplant patient. *J Am Acad Dermatol* 2006;**54**:657–663.
14. Capello D, Cerri M, Muti G *et al.* Molecular histogenesis of post-transplantation lymphoproliferative disorders. *Blood* 2003;**102**: 3775–3785.
15. Ravat FE, Spittle MF, Russel-Jones R. Primary cutaneous T-cell lymphoma occurring after organ transplantation. *J Am Acad Dermatol* 2006;**54**:668–675.
16. Magro CM, Weinerman DJ, Porcu PL, Morrison CD. Post-transplant EBV-negative anaplastic large-cell lymphoma with dual rearrangement: a propos of two cases and review of the literature. *J Cutan Pathol* 2007;**34**(suppl 1):1–8.
17. Coyne JD, Banerjee SS, Bromley M, Mills S, Diss TC, Harris M. Post-transplant T-cell lymphoproliferative disorder/T-cell lym-phoma: a report of three cases of T-anaplastic large-cell lymphoma with cutaneous presentation and a review of the literature. *Histopathology* 2004;**44**:387–393.
18. Belloni Fortina A, Montesco MC, Piaserico S, *et al.* Primary Cutaneous CD30+ Anaplastic Large Cell Lymphoma in a Heart Transplant Patient: Case Report and Literature Review. *Acta Derm Venereol (Stockh)* 2009;**89**:74–77.
19. Bragman SG, Yeaney GA, Greig BW, Vnencak-Jones CL, Hamilton KS. Subcutaneous panniculitic T-cell lymphoma in a cardiac allograft recipient. *J Cut Pathol* 2005;**32**:366–370.
20. Wallet-Faber N, Bodemer C, Blanche S *et al.* Primary cutaneous Epstein–Barr virus-related lymphoproliferative disorders in 4 immunosuppressed children. *J Am Acad Dermatol* 2008;**58**:74–80.
21. Rinaldi A, Kwee I, Poretti G *et al.* Comparative genome-wide profiling of post-transplant lymphoproliferative disorders and diffuse large B-cell lymphomas. *Br J Haematol* 2006;**134**:27–36.
22. Arbiser JL, Mann KP, Losken EM *et al.* Presence of p16 hyperme-thylation and Epstein-Barr virus infection in transplant-associated hematolymphoid neoplasms of the skin. *J Am Acad Dermatol* 2006;**55**:794–798.
23. Starzl TE, Nalesnik MA, Porter KA *et al.* Reversibility of lymphomas and lymphoproliferative lesions developing under cyclosporin-steroid therapy. *Lancet* 1984;**8377**: 583–587.
24. Green M. Management of Epstein–Barr virus-induced post-transplant lymphoproliferative disease in recipients of solid organ transplantation. *Am J Transplant* 2001;**1**:103–108.
25. Blokx WAM, Andriessen MPM, van Hamersvelt HW, van Krieken JHJM. Initial spontaneous remission of post-transplantation Epstein–Barr virus-related B-cell lymphoproliferative disorder of the skin in a renal transplant recipient: case report and review of the literature on cutaneous B-cell post-transplantation lym-phoproliferative disease. *Am J Dermatopathol* 2002;**24**:414–422.
26. Beylot-Barry M, Vergier B, Masquelier B *et al.* The spectrum of cutaneous lymphomas in HIV infection: a study of 21 cases. *Am J Surg Pathol* 1999;**23**:1208–1216.

27. Kerschmann RL, Berger TG, Weiss LM *et al.* Cutaneous presentations of lymphoma in human immunodeficiency virus disease: predominance of T-cell lineage. *Arch Dermatol* 1995;**131**:1281–1288.

28. Raphael M, Said J, Borisch B, Cesarman E, Harris NL. Lymphomas associated with HIV infection. In: Swerdlow SH, Campo E, Harris NL *et al.*, eds. *WHO Classification of Tumours of Haematopoietic and Lymphoid Tissues*. Lyon: IARC Press, 2008: 340–342.

29. Ribera JM, Navarro JT. Human immunodeficiency virus-related non-Hodgkin's lymphoma. *Haematologica* 2008;**93**:1129–1132.

30. Chadburn A, Cesarman E, Jagirdar J, Subar M, Mir RN, Knowles DM. CD30 (Ki-1) positive anaplastic large cell lymphomas in individuals infected with the human immunodeficiency virus. *Cancer* 1993;**72**:3078–3090.

31. Jhala DN, Medeiros LJ, Lopez-Terrada D, Jhala NC, Krishnan B, Shahab I. Neutrophil-rich anaplastic large cell lymphoma of T-cell lineage. A report of two cases arising in HIV-positive patients. *Am J Clin Pathol* 2000;**114**:478–482.

32. Katano H, Suda T, Morishita Y, *et al.* Human herpesvirus 8-associated solid lymphomas that occur in AIDS patients take anaplastic large cell morphology. *Mod Pathol* 2000;**13**:77–85.

33. Delecluse HJ, Anagnostopoulos I, Dallenbach F *et al.* Plasmablastic lymphomas of the oral cavity: a new entity associated with the human immunodeficiency virus infection. *Blood* 1997;**89**:1413–1420.

34. Carbone A, Gloghini A, Gaidano G. Is plasmablastic lymphoma of the oral cavity an HHV8 associated disease? *Am J Surg Pathol* 2004;**28**:1251–1252.

35. Verma S, Nuovo GJ, Porcu P, Baiocchi RA, Crowson AN, Magro CM. Epstein–Barr virus- and human herpesvirus 8-associated primary cutaneous plasmablastic lymphoma in the setting of renal transplantation. *J Cutan Pathol* 2005;**32**:35–39.

36. Colomo L, Loong F, Rives S *et al.* Diffuse large B-cell lymphomas with plasmablastic differentiation represent a heterogeneous group of disease entities. *Am J Surg Pathol* 2004;**28**:736–747.

37. Stein H, Harris NL, Campo E. Plasmablastic lymphoma. In: Swerdlow SH, Campo E, Harris NL *et al.*, eds. *WHO Classification of Tumours of Haematopoietic and Lymphoid Tissues*. Lyon: IARC Press, 2008: 256–257.

38. Castillo J, Pantanowitz L, Dezube BJ. HIV-associated plasmablastic lymphoma: lessons learned from 112 published cases. *Am J Hematol* 2008;**83**:804–809.

39. Cioc AM, Allen C, Kalmar JR *et al.* Oral plasmablastic lymphomas in AIDS patients are associated with human herpesvirus 8. *Am J Surg Pathol* 2004;**28**:41–46.

40. Goedhals J, Beukes CA, Hardie D. HHV8 in plasmablastic lymphoma. *Am J Surg Pathol* 2008;**32**:172.

41. Carbone A, Gloghini A, Gaidano G. KSHV/HHV8 doesn't play a significant role in the development of plasmablastic lymphoma of the oral cavity. *Am J Surg Pathol* 2008;**32**:172–174.

42. Liu W, Lacouture ME, Jiang J *et al.* KSHV/HHV8-associated primary cutaneous plasmablastic lymphoma in a patient with Castleman's disease and Kaposi's sarcoma. *J Cutan Pathol* 2006;**33** (suppl. 2): 46–51.

43. Said J, Cesarman E. Primary effusion lymphoma. In: Swerdlow SH, Campo E, Harris NL *et al.*, eds. *WHO Classification of Tumours of Haematopoietic and Lymphoid Tissues*. Lyon: IARC Press, 2008: 260–261.

44. Fardet L, Blanche S, Brousse N, Bodemer C, Fraitag S. Cutaneous EBV-related lymphoproliferative disorder in a 15-year-old boy with AIDS: an unusual clinical presentation. *J Pediatr Hematol Oncol* 2002;**24**:666–669.

45. Gandemer V, Verkarre V, Quartier P, Brousse N, Blanche S. Lymphomes chez l'enfant infecte par le HIV-1. *Arch Pediatr* 2000; **7**:738–744.

46. Nador RG, Chadburn A, Gundappa G *et al.* Human immunodeficiency virus (HIV)-associated polymorphic lymphoproliferative disorders. *Am J Surg Pathol* 2003;**27**:293–302.

47. Jordan LB, Lessells AM, Goodlad JR. Plasmablastic lymphoma arising at a cutaneous site. *Histopathology* 2005;**46**:113–115.

48. Montes-Moreno S, Gonzalez-Medina AR, Rodriguez-Pinilla SM, Maestre L, Sanchez-Verde L, Piris MA. Is there an immunophenotype for plasmablastic lymphoma? Immunohistochemical evaluation of the phenotype with new specific markers against XBP1, Blimp1, GCET1 and KLHL6. *J Haematopathol* 2008;**1**:208–209.

49. Nakamura K, Katano H, Hoshino Y *et al.* Human herpesvirus type 8 and Epstein-Barr virus-associated cutaneous lymphoma taking anaplastic large cell morphology in a man with HIV infection. *Br J Dermatol* 1999;**141**:141–145.

50. Poiesz B, Dube D, Dube S *et al.* HTLV-II-associated cutaneous T-cell lymphoma in a patient with HIV-1 infection. *N Engl J Med* 2000;**342**:930–936.

51. Paech V, Lorenzen T, Stoehr A *et al.* Remission of cutaneous mycosis fungoides in a patient with advanced HIV-infection. *Eur J Med Res* 2002;**7**:477–479.

52. Carbone A, Cesarman E, Spina M, Gloghini A, Schulz TF. HIV-associated lymphomas and gamma-herpesviruses. *Blood* 2009; **113**:1213–1224.

53. Corazza M, Zampino MR, Montanari A, Altieri E, Virgili A. Primary cutaneous CD30+ large T-cell lymphoma in a patient with psoriasis treated with cyclosporine. *Dermatology* 2003;**206**:330–333.

54. Kirby B, Owen CM, Blewitt RW, Yates VM. Cutaneous T-cell lymphoma developing in a patient on cyclosporin therapy. *J Am Acad Dermatol* 2002;**47**:s165–s167.

55. Hernandez C, Worobec SM, Gaitonde S, Kiripolski ML, Aquino K. Progression of undiagnosed cutaneous T-cell lymphoma during efalizumab therapy. *Arch Dermatol* 2009;**145**:92–94.

56. Lafaille P, Bouffard D, Provost N. Exacerbation of undiagnosed mycosis fungoides during treatment with etanercept. *Arch Dermatol* 2009;**145**:94–95.

57. Chuang GS, Wasserman DI, Byers HR, Demierre MF. Hypopigmented T-cell dyscrasia evolving to hypopigmented mycosis fungoides during etanercept therapy. *J Am Acad Dermatol* 2008;**59**:s121–s122.

58. O'Malley DP, Chen S, Perkins SL *et al.* Monoclonal antibody immunomodulator-related lymphoid proliferations. *J Haematopathol* 2008;**1**:228–229.

59. Van Krieken JH, Onciu M, Elenitoba-Johnson KSJ, Jaffe ES. Lymphoproliferative diseases associated with primary immune disorders. In: Swerdlow SH, Campo E, Harris NL *et al.*, eds. *WHO Classification of Tumours of Haematopoietic and Lymphoid Tissues*. Lyon: IARC Press, 2008: 336–339.

60. Gaulard P, Swerdlow SH, Harris NL, Jaffe ES, Sundström C. Other iatrogenic immunodeficiency-associated lymphoproliferative disorders. In: Swerdlow SH, Campo E, Harris NL *et al.*, eds. *WHO Classification of Tumours of Haematopoietic and Lymphoid Tissues*. Lyon: IARC Press, 2008: 350–351.

61. Clarke LE, Junkins-Hopkins JM, Seykora JT, Adler DJ, Elenitsas R. Methotrexate-associated lymphoproliferative disorder in a patient with rheumatoid arthritis presenting in the skin. *J Am Acad Dermatol* 2007;**56**:686–690.

Section 4: Cutaneous manifestations of precursor hematologic neoplasms

Blastic plasmacytoid dendritic cell neoplasm (CD4$^+$/CD56$^+$ hematodermic neoplasm)

Blastic plasmacytoid dendritic cell neoplasm has been the source of considerable research and progress in recent years. One of the consequences is that this neoplasm has changed names several times: in the last edition of this book it was still mentioned according to the old World Health Organization (WHO) terminology of "blastic NK cell lymphoma;" the WHO-European Organization for Research and Treatment of Cancer (EORTC) classification of primary cutaneous lymphomas published in 2005 listed it as "CD4$^+$/CD56$^+$ hematodermic neoplasm" [1], and the term "blastic plasmacytoid dendritic cell neoplasm" has been adopted by the new WHO classification of tumors of hematopoietic and lymphoid tissues published in 2008 [2]. The new terminology derives from evidence that neoplastic cells differentiate toward a common myeloid and lymphoid cell precursor, identified recently as the plasmacytoid type 2 dendritic cell ("plasmacytoid monocyte") [3–6]. Several other names have been used in the past for this hematologic neoplasm, including "early plasmacytoid dendritic cell leukemia–lymphoma" [7,8] and "agranular CD4 CD56 hematodermic neoplasms" [4,6,9–11] among others. In fact, among all hematological neoplasms this is probably the entity that has been reported in the literature under more names in the last few years. Malignant transformation of neoplastic cells occurs at a very early stage of differentiation, so the blastic plasmacytoid dendritic cell neoplasm belongs to the precursor hematologic neoplasms.

A relationship between the blastic plasmacytoid dendritic cell neoplasm and myelogenous leukemia has been postulated [12–17], with evolution into myelogenous leukemia or association with previous myelodysplastic syndrome being documented in a few patients [13,18]. However, typical cases of acute myeloid leukemia involving the skin usually have a different phenotype, and positivity for CD56 is rare (see Chapter 19) [19]. A complete phenotypic analysis is necessary for differentiation of blastic plasmacytoid dendritic cell neoplasm from myelogenous leukemia (see below). In this context, it is interesting to note that overlapping myeloid and lymphoid features are known also in other neoplasms such as chronic myelogenous leukemia, in which blast crisis in 10% of the cases reveals a B- or, more rarely, a T-cell phenotype. Recently, studies by comparative genomic hybridization have revealed different profiles of blastic plasmacytoid dendritic cell neoplasm and cutaneous lesions of myelogenous leukemia [20].

In most cases, at presentation blastic plasmacytoid dendritic cell neoplasm is confined to the skin or skin lesions are the first manifestation of the disease [21–26]. Leukemic spread after variable (usually short) periods of time is the rule [22], indicating that primary cutaneous cases most likely represent examples of so-called "aleukemic leukemia cutis" [27]. The recent identification of non-neoplastic plasmacytoid monocytes within the skin provides a theoretical background to the frequent occurrence of these lymphomas with lesions confined to the skin [28].

Clinical features

Patients are mostly elderly adults, although cases in younger individuals, including small children, have been reported [9,22–25,29–32]. There is a predominance of males. Clinically, they present with solitary (rarely), localized or, more commonly, generalized plaques and tumors with a characteristic "bruise-like" violaceous aspect (Figs 16.1, 16.2) due to intratumoral hemorrhage. Ulceration is uncommon. Mucosal regions may be involved (Fig. 16.3). The morphology of

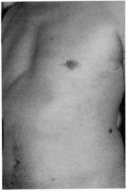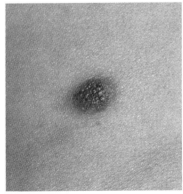

Figure 16.1 Blastic plasmacytoid dendritic cell neoplasm. Small solitary tumor on the flank. Note deep red ("bruise-like") color.

Skin Lymphoma: The Illustrated Guide. By L. Cerroni, K. Gatter and H. Kerl. Published 2009 Blackwell Publishing, ISBN: 978-1-4051-8554-7.

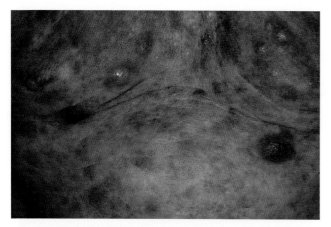

Figure 16.2 Blastic plasmacytoid dendritic cell neoplasm . Multiple plaques and tumors on the chest. Note "bruise-like" violaceous aspect.

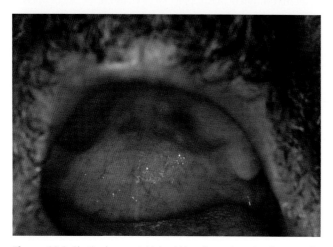

Figure 16.3 Blastic plasmacytoid dendritic cell neoplasm. Involvement of the oral mucosa.

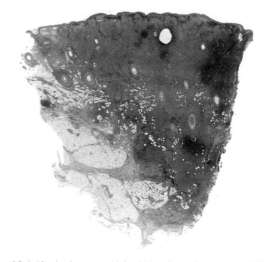

Figure 16.4 Blastic plasmacytoid dendritic cell neoplasm. Dense diffuse infiltrate involving the entire dermis and the superficial part of the subcutaneous fat.

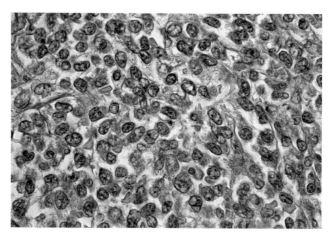

Figure 16.5 Blastic plasmacytoid dendritic cell neoplasm. Monomorphic proliferation of medium-sized cells.

cutaneous lesions is similar to that of the skin manifestations of myelogenous leukemia. In a distinct proportion of patients (approximately 30–40%), skin lesions are accompanied by general symptoms and extracutaneous manifestations in the blood, bone marrow and/or other organs. Lymph nodes are involved in approximately half of the cases at presentation. Thrombocytopenia, anemia and neutropenia are commonly found [4].

Skin lesions are the first manifestation of the disease in over 90% of patients. In patients with primary cutaneous disease, the time interval between the onset of skin lesions and leukemic spread is variable, usually between a few weeks and several months.

Histopathology, immunophenotype and molecular genetics

Histopathology
Histologically, blastic plasmacytoid dendritic cell neoplasm is characterized by a diffuse monomorphous infiltrate of medium-sized neoplastic cells with a blastoid morphology (Figs 16.4, 16.5). The epidermis is not involved as a rule, whereas involvement of the subcutaneous tissues is common. Angio-centricity and/or angiodestruction, necrosis and granulomatous reactions are uncommon (Fig. 16.6). The morphologic features are similar to those of skin involvement in myelogenous leukemia or myeloid sarcoma.

In early lesions there are perivascular infiltrates of blastoid cells, sometimes admixed with reactive lymphocytes (Fig. 16.7). In some cases we have observed peculiar morphologic features characterized by a certain degree of pleomorphism of the cells with elongated and twisted nuclei resembling large centrocytes of follicle center lymphoma, diffuse type (Fig. 16.8). As Bcl-6 and multiple myeloma oncogene 1 (MUM-1) may be positive in a proportion of cells in blastic plasmacytoid dendritic cell neoplasm, these morphologic features may be the source of a diagnostic pitfall.

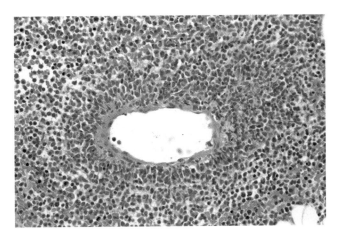

Figure 16.6 Blastic plasmacytoid dendritic cell neoplasm. Angiocentric infiltrate of blastoid cells.

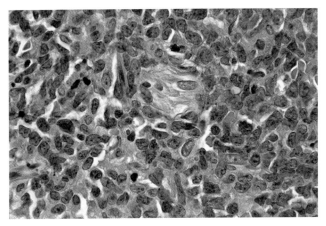

Figure 16.8 Blastic plasmacytoid dendritic cell neoplasm. The neoplastic cells reveal partly a conventional blastoid morphology, partly elongated, twisted, pleomorphic nuclei resembling large centrocytes (see text).

Immunophenotype

Phenotypically, the neoplastic cells are positive for CD4 and CD56 (Fig. 16.9) [6,22,23,33]. TdT is positive in the majority of the cases in a variable proportion of the cells (Fig. 16.10a), whereas myeloid antigens, NK cell markers and cytotoxic proteins are negative (Fig. 16.10b, d). Cases positive for CD68 have been reported (Fig. 16.11), but in our experience CD68 is usually negative (Fig 16.10c) [6,11,23,34,35]. Petrella *et al* described positivity for CD123 in all their cases in one series, a finding confirmed in subsequent studies (Fig. 16.12) [6,36]. The positivity for CD123 underlines the relationship with plasmacytoid dendritic cells 2, while the positivity for TdT

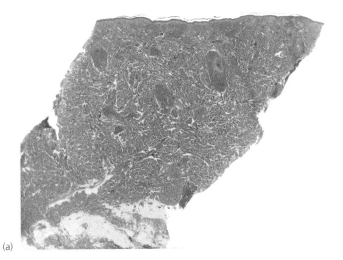

(a)

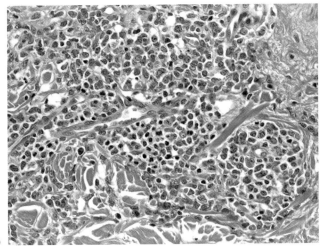

(b)

Figure 16.7 Blastic plasmacytoid dendritic cell neoplasm. Early lesion showing (a) perivascular infiltrates of (b) medium-sized blastoid cells.

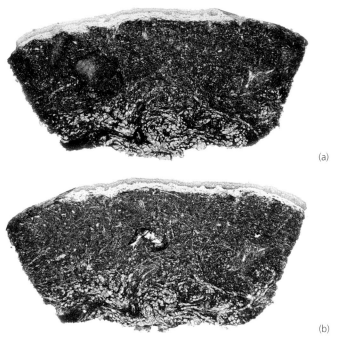

(a)

(b)

Figure 16.9 Blastic plasmacytoid dendritic cell neoplasm. Positive reaction for (a) CD56 and (b) CD4.

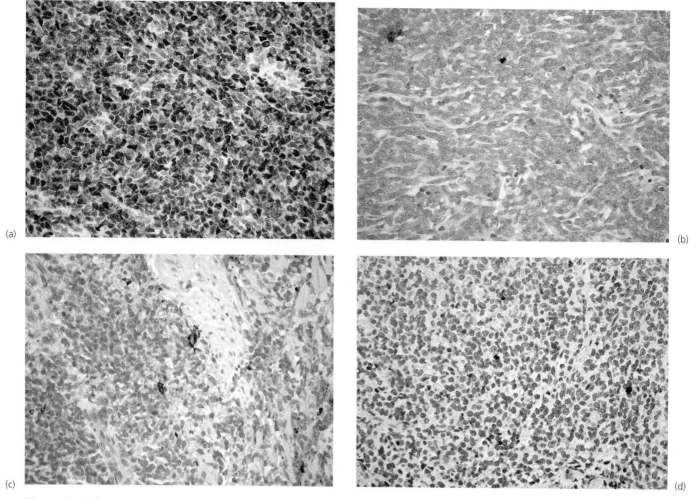

Figure 16.10 Blastic plasmacytoid dendritic cell neoplasm. Positivity for (a) TdT and negativity for (b) myeloperoxidase, (c) CD68 and (d) TIA-1.

confirms the origin from a precursor cell. Neoplastic cells in a proportion of cases may be positive for CD2, CD7, and CD45Ra. Other markers positive in blastic plasmacytoid dendritic cell neoplasms are Bcl-2, CD43, CD101, HLA-DR, and BDCA-2 (Fig. 16.13a) [37–39]. In some cases we have also observed focal positivity for Bcl-6 and MUM-1 (Fig. 16.13b, c). Finally, several new markers have been investigated in blastic plasmacytoid dendritic cell neoplasm, particularly concerning its differentiation from myelogenous leukemia. The most useful monoclonal antibodies in this respect seem to be BCL11A, CD2AP, and ICSBP/IRF8, which are positive in blastic plasmacytoid dendritic cell neoplasm but usually negative in myelogenous leukemia (Fig. 16.13d). The pattern of expression of nucleophosmin, an estrogen-regulated nucleolar protein that is expressed in a mutated form in the cytoplasm in one-third of the cases of adult de novo acute myeloid leukemia, differs between blastic plasmacytoid dendritic cell neoplasms (nuclear pattern) and myelogenous leukemia (cytoplasmic pattern) [40]. These observations lend support to the distinction of blastic plasmacytoid dendritic cell neoplasm from myelogenous

leukemia. The usefulness of all these new markers, however, should be confirmed in larger studies.

Although the previous term adopted for this entity was "CD4+/CD56+ hematodermic neoplasm," cases negative for CD4 have been recorded [41,42], and CD56 can be negative as well [43,44]. As CD123, too, may be negative in some cases, the three markers most widely used for diagnosis of this rare entity should always be used together and in conjunction with a broad panel of antibodies directed toward lymphoid and myeloid lineages, keeping in mind that only integration of all stainings can allow a precise diagnosis.

Expression of the lymphoid proto-oncogene *TCL1* was demonstrated in the majority of blastic plasmacytoid dendritic cell neoplasms in one series, as well as in nodal plasmacytoid dendritic cells, again emphasizing the likely derivation of this unusual neoplasm from these cells [36,45,46].

Molecular genetics

There is no association with Epstein–Barr virus (EBV) infection. Molecular genetic studies reveal that the T-cell receptor

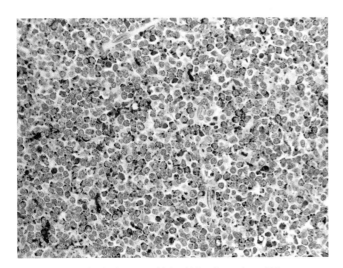

Figure 16.11 Blastic plasmacytoid dendritic cell neoplasm. This case reveals positivity of the majority of neoplastic cells for CD68. In our experience, this pattern is the exception rather than the rule.

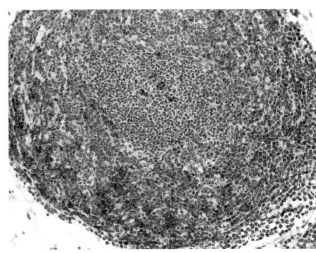

Figure 16.12 Blastic plasmacytoid dendritic cell neoplasm. Positivity of neoplastic cells (periphery of nodule) for CD123. Negative cells in the center of the nodule represent small reactive lymphocytes.

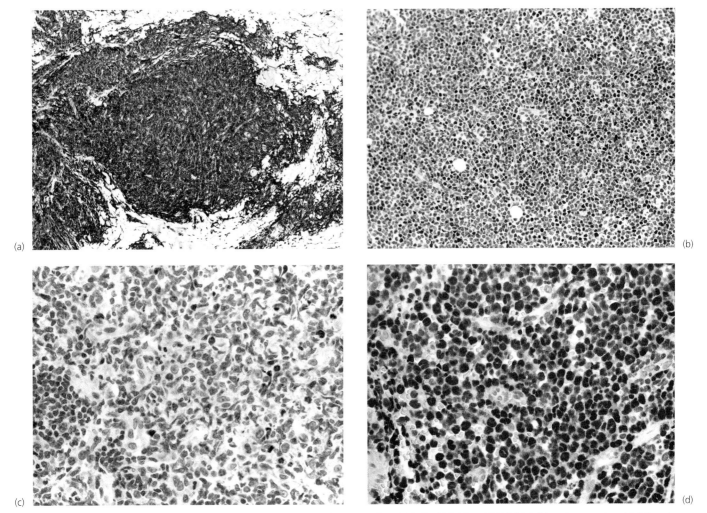

(a)

(b)

(c)

(d)

Figure 16.13 Blastic plasmacytoid dendritic cell neoplasm. Phenotypic features with positivity for (a) Bcl-2 and (b) MUM-1, (c) weak expression of Bcl-6, and (d) nuclear positivity for IRF8.

(TCR) and immunoglobulin heavy chain (J_H) genes are in germline configuration, but exceptional cases with TCR gene rearrangement have been observed [47,48]. Thus, although for practical purposes a monoclonal rearrangement of the TCR and/or J_H genes rules out the diagnosis of blastic plasmacytoid dendritic cell neoplasm, care should be taken in the interpretation of molecular results. One potential pitfall may be represented by the presence of small oligoclonal populations of reactive T- and B-lymphocytes within the infiltrate.

Complex karyotypes and chromosomal abnormalities involving chromosomes 5q, 6q, 12p, 13q, 15q and 9 have been observed in blastic plasmacytoid dendritic cell neoplasm [3]. Gain of chromosome 7q and 22 and loss of chromosomes 3p and 13q was demonstrated by comparative genome hybridization in one study [49], while recurrent deletion of regions on chromosome 4 (4q34), chromosome 9 (9p13–p11 and 9q12–q34), and chromosome 13 (13q12–q31) was found in another study [20], and losses of 9/9p and 13q and gain of 7 in a third [50]. The least common denominator of these studies seems to be the presence of abnormalities involving chromosomes 9 and 13, which reflects our experience as well. Different results may be due to the differences existing between lesions in early or advanced stages of the disease, as well as the site of involvement of the lesions studied.

Treatment

Treatment of patients with blastic plasmacytoid dendritic cell neoplasm should be carried out in a hematologic setting. The neoplasm should be considered as a form of precursor aleukemic leukemia cutis and treated accordingly.

The chemotherapy schemes used are those applied for acute leukemias. Although systemic chemotherapy is usually followed by rapid, complete primary responses, remissions are short and recurrences are the rule [51]. The few patients with prolonged survival (and possibly cure) reported in the literature received allogenic stem cell transplantation [4,7, 18,52]. Solitary lesions may be treated with radiotherapy, but systemic chemotherapy should be administered as well. Remission has been documented in a patient treated with pralatrexate [53], and maintenance treatment with etoposide after systemic chemotherapy was successful in another [54].

Prognosis

Blastic plasmacytoid dendritic cell neoplasm is a very aggressive disorder, and the prognosis is very poor. The estimated 5-year survival is 0% [55]. Patients usually succumb within 1 year and only in exceptional cases have longer survivals been reported [4,7,9,32]. Although presentation with solitary or localized skin lesions may be associated with a longer survival, at present there is no evidence that long-term survival can be achieved with conventional treatments, even for these patients. As already mentioned, allogenic bone marrow transplantation may yield better results, and should be offered as the first therapeutic option whenever possible [4,7,18,52].

Young age (<40 years) and TdT expression in >50% of the neoplastic cells were independent prognostic variables associated with a better prognosis in one study [37]. Skin involvement represented an unfavorable prognostic sign in another study; however, as already mentioned, cutaneous manifestations are found in the vast majority of patients [56].

Résumé

Clinical	Adults, elderly (rarely children). Localized or generalized "bruise-like" violaceous plaques and tumors. Ulceration uncommon. No preferential location reported.
Morphology	Monomorphous infiltrate of medium-sized cells within the entire dermis and subcutis. The epidermis is spared. Cytomorphology: blastoid cells.
Immunology	CD4, 56, 123 + TIA-1 – CD3, 5, 20 – TdT +/– TCL-1 + CD68 –(+) Myeloperoxidase –
Genetics	Germline configuration of the TCR and J_H genes. No evidence of EBV infection.
Treatment guidelines	Systemic chemotherapy, allogenic bone marrow transplantation.

References

1. Willemze R, Jaffe ES, Burg G et al. WHO-EORTC classification for cutaneous lymphomas. *Blood* 2005;**105**:3768–3785.
2. Facchetti F, Jones DM, Petrella T. Blastic plasmacytoid dendritic cell neoplasm. In: Swerdlow SH, Campo E, Harris NL et al., eds. *WHO Classification of Tumours of Haematopoietic and Lymphoid Tissues*. Lyon: IARC Press, 2008: 145–147.
3. Chaperot L, Bendriss N, Manches O et al. Identification of a leukemic counterpart of the plasmacytoid dendritic cells. *Blood* 2001;**97**:3210–3217.
4. Feuillard J, Jacob MC, Valensi F et al. Clinical and biologic features of CD4 CD56 malignancies. *Blood* 2002;**99**:1556–1563.
5. Leroux D, Mugneret F, Callanan M et al. CD4, CD56 DC2 acute leukemia is characterized by recurrent clonal chromosomal changes affecting 6 major targets: a study of 21 cases by the Groupe Français de Cytogenetique Hematologique. *Blood* 2002;**99**:4154–4159.

6. Petrella T, Comeau MR, Maynadié M *et al.* Agranular CD4 CD56 hematodermic neoplasm (blastic NK-cell lymphoma) originates from a population of CD56[7] precursor cells related to plasmacytoid monocytes. *Am J Surg Pathol* 2002;**26**:852–862.

7. Jacob MC, Chaperot L, Mossuz P *et al.* CD4 CD56 lineage negative malignancies: a new entity developed from malignant early plasmacytoid dendritic cells. *Haematologica* 2003;**88**:941–955.

8. Garnache-Ottou F, Feuillard J, Saas P. Plasmacytoid dendritic cell leukaemia/lymphoma: towards a well defined entity? *Br J Haematol* 2007;**136**;539–548.

9. Dummer R, Potoczna N, Haffner AC *et al.* A primary cutaneous non-T, non-B CD4, CD56 lymphoma. *Arch Dermatol* 1996;**132**: 550–553.

10. Kato N, Yasukawa K, Kimura K *et al.* CD2 CD4 CD56 hematodermic/hematolymphoid malignancy. *J Am Acad Dermatol* 2001;**44**: 231–238.

11. Petrella T, Dalac S, Maynadie M *et al.* CD4 CD56 cutaneous neoplasms: a distinct hematological entity? Groupe Français d'Etude des Lymphomes Cutanés (GFELC). *Am J Surg Pathol* 1999;**23**: 137–146.

12. Bagot M, Bouloc A, Charue D *et al.* Do primary cutaneous non-T non-B CD4 CD56 lymphomas belong to the myelo-monocytic lineage? *J Invest Dermatol* 1998;**111**:1242–1244.

13. Khoury JD, Medeiros LJ, Manning JT *et al.* CD56 TdT blastic natural killer cell tumor of the skin: primitive systemic malignancy related to myelomonocytic leukemia. *Cancer* 2002;**94**:2401–2408.

14. Scott AA, Head DR, Kopecky KJ *et al.* HLA-DR, CD33, CD56, CD16 myeloid natural killer cell acute leukemia: a previously unrecognized form of acute leukemia potentially misdiagnosed as French-American-British acute myeloid leukemia-M3. *Blood* 1994;**84**:244–255.

15. Suzuki R, Nakamura S. Malignancies of natural killer (NK) cell precursor: myeloid/NK cell precursor acute leukemia and blastic plasmacytoid dendritic cell neoplasm /leukemia. *Leuk Res* 1999; **23**:615–624.

16. Kazakov DV, Mentzel T, Burg G, Dummer R, Kempf W. Blastic natural killer-cell lymphoma of the skin associated with myelodysplastic syndrome of myelogenous leukaemia: a coincidence or more? *Br J Dermatol* 2003;**149**:869–876.

17. Bekkenk MW, Jansen PM, Meijer CJLM, Willemze R. CD56+ hematological neoplasms presenting in the skin – a retrospective analysis of 23 new cases and 130 cases from the literature. *Ann Oncol* 2004;**15**:1097–1108.

18. Assaf C, Gellrich S, Whittaker S *et al.* CD56-positive haematological neoplasms of the skin: a multicentre study of the Cutaneous Lymphoma Project Group of the European Organisation for Research and Treatment of Cancer. *J Clin Pathol* 2007;**60**:981–989.

19. Kaddu S, Zenahlik P, Beham-Schmid C, Kerl H, Cerroni L. Specific cutaneous infiltrates in patients with myelogenous leukemia: a clinicopathologic study of 26 patients with assessment of diagnostic criteria. *J Am Acad Dermatol* 1999;**40**:966–978.

20. Dijkman R, van Doorn R, Szuhai K, Willemze R, Vermeer MH, Tensen CP. Gene-expression profiling and array-based CGH classify CD4CD56 hematodermic neoplasm and cutaneous myelomonocytic leukemia as distinct disease entities. *Blood* 2007;**109**:1720–1727.

21. Bower CP, Standen GR, Pawade J, Knechtli CJ, Kennedy CTC. Cutaneous presentation of steroid responsive blastoid natural killer cell lymphoma. *Br J Dermatol* 2000;**142**:1017–1020.

22. Chan JKC, Jaffe ES, Ralfkiaer E. Blastic NK-cell lymphoma. In: Jaffe ES, Harris NL, Stein H *et al.*, eds. *World Health Organization Classification of Tumours: Tumours of Haematopoietic and Lymphoid Tissues.* Lyon: IARC Press, 2001: 214–215.

23. Massone C, Chott A, Metze D *et al.* Subcutaneous, blastic natural killer (NK) NK/T-cell and other cytotoxic lymphomas of the skin: a morphologic, immunophenotypic and molecular study of 50 patients. *Am J Surg Pathol* 2004;**28**:719–735.

24. Nagatani T, Okazawa H, Kambara T *et al.* Cutaneous monomorphous CD4- and CD56-positive large-cell lymphoma. *Dermatology* 2000;**200**:202–208.

25. Radonich MA, Lazova R, Bolognia J. Cutaneous natural killer/T-cell lymphoma. *J Am Acad Dermatol* 2002;**46**:451–456.

26. Child FJ, Mitschell TJ, Whittaker SJ *et al.* Blastic natural killer cell and extranodal natural killer cell-like T-cell lymphoma presenting in the skin: report of six cases from the UK. *Br J Dermatol* 2003;**148**:507–515.

27. Husak R, Blume-Peytaki U, Orfanos CE. Aleukemic leukemia cutis in an adolescent boy. *N Engl J Med* 1999;**340**:893–894.

28. Wollenberg A, Wagner M, Gunther S *et al.* Plasmacytoid dendritic cells: a new cutaneous dendritic cell subset with distinct role in inflammatory skin diseases. *J Invest Dermatol* 2002;**119**:1096–1102.

29. Chang SE, Choi HJ, Huh J *et al.* A case of primary cutaneous CD56, TdT, CD4, blastic NK-cell lymphoma in a 19-year-old woman. *Am J Dermatopathol* 2002;**24**:72–75.

30. Fass J, Tichy EH, Kraus EW *et al.* Cutaneous tumors as the initial presentation of non-T, non-B, nonmyeloid CD4+ CD56+ hematolymphoid malignancy in an adolescent boy. *Ped Dermatol* 2005;**22**:19–22.

31. Hu SCS, Tsai KB, Chen GS, Chen PH. Infantile CD4+/CD56+ dematodermic neoplasm. *Haematologica* 2007;**92**,91–93.

32. Brody J, Allen S, Schulman P *et al.* Acute agranular CD4-positive natural killer cell leukemia: comprehensive clinicopathologic studies including virologic and *in vitro* culture with inducing agents. *Cancer* 1995;**75**:2474–2483.

33. Santucci M, Pimpinelli N, Massi D *et al.* Cytotoxic natural killer cell cutaneous lymphomas: report of the EORTC cutaneous lymphoma task force workshop. *Cancer* 2003;**97**:610–627.

34. Ko YH, Kim SH, Ree HJ. Blastic NK-cell lymphoma expressing terminal deoxynucleotidyl transferase with Homer-Wright type pseudorosettes formation. *Histopathology* 1998;**33**:547–553.

35. Nakamura S, Koshikawa T, Yatabe Y, Suchi T. Lymphoblastic lymphoma expressing CD56 and TdT. *Am J Surg Pathol* 1998;**22**: 135–137.

36. Herling M, Teitell MA, Shen RR, Medeiros LJ, Jones D. TCL1 expression in plasmacytoid dendritic cells (DC2s) and the related CD4 CD56 blastic tumors of skin. *Blood* 2003;**101**:5007–5009.

37. Meyer N, Petrella T, Poszepczynska-Guigne E *et al.* CD4+ CD56+ blastic tumor cells express CD101 molecules. *J Invest Dermatol* 2005;**124**:668–669.

38. Jaye DL, Geigerman CM, Herling M, Eastburn K, Waller EK, Jones D. Expression of the plasmacytoid dendritic cell marker BDCA-2 supports a spectrum of maturation among CD4+ CD56+ hematodermic neoplasms. *Mod Pathol* 2006;**19**:1555–1562.

39. Pilichowska ME, Fleming MD, Pinkus JL, Pinkus GS. CD4+/ CD56+ hematodermic neoplasm ("blastic natural killer cell lymphoma"). Neoplastic cells express the immature dendritic cell marker BDCA-2 and produce interferon. *Am J Clin Pathol* 2007;**128**:445–453.

40. Facchetti F, Pileri SA, Agostinelli C, et al. Cytoplasmic nucleophosmin is not detected in blastic plasmacytoid dendritic cell neoplasm. *Haematologica* 2009;**94**:285–288.

41. Argyrakos T, Rontogianni D, Karmiris T *et al.* Blastic natural killer (NK)-cell lymphoma: report of an unusual CD4 negative case and review of the CD4 negative neoplasms with blastic features in the literature. *Leukem Lymph* 2004;**45**:2127–2133.

42. Ascani S, Massone C, Ferrara G *et al.* CD4-negative variant of CD4+/CD56+ hematodermic neoplasm: description of three cases. *J Cutan Pathol* 2008;**35**:911–915.

43. Petrella T, Teitell MA, Spiekermann C *et al.* A CD56-negative case of blastic natural killer-cell lymphoma (agranular CD4/CD56 haematodermic neoplasm). *Br J Dermatol* 2004;**150**:174–176.

44. Marafioti T, Paterson JC, Ballabio E *et al.* Novel markers of normal and neoplastic human plasmacytoid dendritic cells. *Blood* 2008;**111**:3778–3792.

45. Herling MH, Teitell MA, Shen RR, Medeiros LJ, Jones D. TCL1 expression in plasmacytoid dendritic cells (DC2s) and the related CD4 CD56 blastic tumors of skin. *Blood* 2003;**101**:5007–5009.

46. Petrella T, Meijer CJLM, Dalac S *et al.* TCL1 and CLA expression in agranular CD4/CD56 hematodermic neoplasms (blastic NK-cell lymphomas) and leukemia cutis. *Am J Clin Pathol* 2004; **122**:307–313.

47. Stetsenko GY, McFarlane R, Kalus A *et al.* CD4+/CD56+ hematodermic neoplasm: report of a rare variant with a T-cell receptor gene rearrangement. *J Cutan Pathol* 2008;**35**:579–584.

48. Liu XY, Atkins RC, Feusner JH, Rowland JM. Blastic NK-cell-like lymphoma with T-cell receptor gene rearrangement. *Am J Hematol* 2004;**75**:251–253.

49. Hallermann C, Middel P, Griesinger F, Gunawan B, Bertsch HP, Neumann C. CD4+ CD56+ blastic tumor of the skin: cytogenetic observations and further evidence of an origin from plasmacytoid dendritic cells. *Eur J Dermatol* 2004;**14**:317–322.

50. Mao X, Onadim Z, Price EA *et al.* Genomic alterations in blastic natural killer/extranodal natural killer-like T cell lymphoma with cutaneous involvement. *J Invest Dermatol* 2003;**121**:618–627.

51. DiGiuseppe JA, Louie DC, Williams JE *et al.* Blastic natural killer cell leukemia-lymphoma: a clinicopathologic study. *Am J Surg Pathol* 1997;**21**:1223–1230.

52. Hyakuna N, Toguchi S, Higa T *et al.* Childhood blastic NK cell leukemia successfully treated with L-asparaginase and allogeneic bone marrow transplantation. *Pediatr Blood Cancer* 2004;**42**:631–634.

53. Leitenberger JJ, Berthelot CN, Polder KD *et al.* CD4+ CD56+ hematodermic/plasmacytoid dendritic cell tumor with response to pralatrexate. *J Am Acad Dermatol* 2008;**58**:480–484.

54. Hatano Y, Ogata M, Ohishi M *et al.* Maintenance of long-term remission using oral administration of low-dose etoposide in a patient demonstrating a relapse of blastic natural killer-cell lymphoma. *Clin Exp Dermatol* 2006;**32**:96–97.

55. Fink-Puches R, Zenahlik P, Bäck B *et al.* Primary cutaneous lymphomas: applicability of current classification schemes (European Organization for Research and Treatment of Cancer, World Health Organization) based on clinicopathologic features observed in a large group of patients. *Blood* 2002;**99**:800–805.

56. Suzuki R, Nakamura S, Suzumiya J *et al.* Blastic natural killer cell lymphoma/leukemia (CD56-positive) blastic tumor. Prognostication and categorization according to anatomic sites of involvement. *Cancer* 2005;**104**:1022–1031.

17 Cutaneous lymphoblastic lymphomas

Lymphoblastic lymphomas are precursor hematologic neoplasms with aggressive behavior and relatively frequent skin involvement [1]. In spite of extensive staging investigations, the skin may appear as the only involved site in some patients, particularly in the B-cell variant of the disease. In our opinion, however, it is difficult to conceive of a truly "primary" cutaneous lymphoblastic lymphoma, and cases with skin manifestations and negative staging should be managed as a systemic disease from the outset. These cases may resemble conceptually the so-called "aleukemic" leukemia cutis or the blastic plasmacytoid dendritic cell neoplasm, where apparent exclusive cutaneous involvement is invariably followed by overt leukemic manifestations, usually in a matter of a few months.

The distinction between leukemic and lymphomatous forms depends on the involvement of the peripheral blood and bone marrow, and is sometimes arbitrary. Although lymphoblastic lymphomas are divided into B and T types, rarely neoplastic cells do not express B- or T-cell markers, thus having a so-called "null" phenotype. Distinction of these cases from other precursor neoplasms (e.g. natural killer (NK), myeloid) is extremely difficult, as some degree of overlapping phenotypic features may be observed.

CUTANEOUS B-LYMPHOBLASTIC LYMPHOMA

B-lymphoblastic lymphoma is a malignant proliferation of precursor B lymphocytes [2]. Cutaneous involvement is not rare but exact data are not available. Although patients usually have secondary skin manifestations of acute lymphoblastic leukemia with bone marrow and peripheral blood involvement, primary skin involvement has been observed occasionally [3–11].

It must be stressed that histologic features alone do not allow one to differentiate lymphoblastic lymphomas of B phenotype from those of T cell lineage (see next section).

Clinical features

Children and young adults are usually affected, but cases in neonates have been also observed [3–15]. Clinically patients present with large erythematous tumors, usually solitary, commonly located on the head and neck (Fig. 17.1). In patients with precursor B-lymphoblastic leukemia, cutaneous involvement may be the first sign of recurrence after successful first-line treatment. In these cases skin manifestations may be characterized by solitary or localized papules and tumors that may be difficult to recognize (Fig. 17.2).

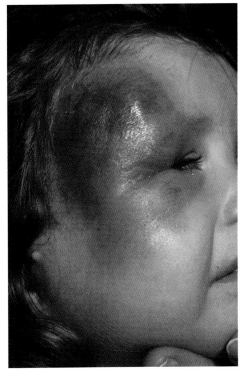

Figure 17.1 Cutaneous B-lymphoblastic lymphoma. Large tumor on the face of an 18-month-old child.

Skin Lymphoma: The Illustrated Guide. By L. Cerroni, K. Gatter and H. Kerl. Published 2009 Blackwell Publishing, ISBN: 978-1-4051-8554-7.

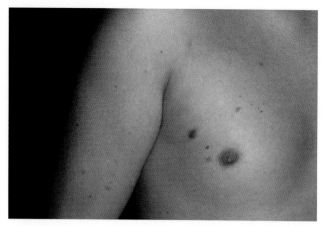

Figure 17.2 Cutaneous B-lymphoblastic lymphoma. Small erythematous papule on the chest as first sign of recurrence of acute lymphoblastic leukemia in a 28-year-old man (histopathologic and immunophenotypical features are depicted in Fig. 17.6).

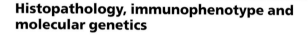

Histopathology, immunophenotype and molecular genetics

Histopathology

Dense, diffuse monomorphous infiltrates are found within the dermis and the subcutaneous fat. Cytomorphologically the lymphoblasts are medium-sized cells with round, oval or convoluted nuclei, fine chromatin, inconspicuous nucleoli, and scant cytoplasm (Fig. 17.3). Mitoses and necrotic ("apoptotic") cells are frequent, and "starry sky" or "mosaic stone"-like patterns may be seen (Figs 17.4, 17.5). In secondary skin involvement from B-lymphoblastic leukemia, the pattern at low power may mimic that of an inflammatory skin condition, emphasizing the need for careful histologic and immuno-histochemical examination to make a confident diagnosis (Fig. 17.6a, b).

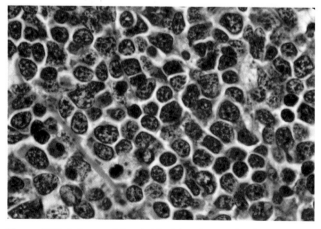

Figure 17.3 Cutaneous B-lymphoblastic lymphoma. B lymphoblasts with round nuclei and finely dispersed chromatin.

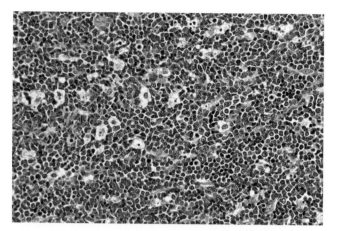

Figure 17.4 Cutaneous B-lymphoblastic lymphoma. Monomorphous proliferation of medium-sized cells. Note "starry sky" pattern.

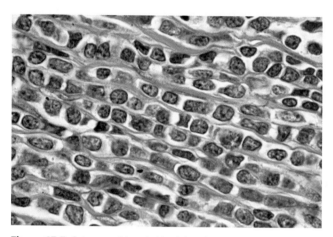

Figure 17.5 Cutaneous B-lymphoblastic lymphoma. Note "mosaic stone"-like arrangement of neoplastic cells.

Immunophenotype

Cutaneous B-lymphoblastic lymphoma expresses usually CD79a, TdT, CD10 (common acute lymphoblastic leukemia/ lymphoma antigen – CALLA), paired box gene (PAX)-5 and cytoplasmic μ heavy chains without surface immunoglobulins (Figs 17.6c, d, 17.7). CD20 is positive in the majority of cases. A proportion of cases are also positive for CD99 and CD34. Expression of the various markers is related to the stage of differentiation of the cells, and B-cell markers may be negative in some cases.

Molecular genetics

Molecular genetics shows a monoclonal rearrangement of the immunoglobulin heavy chain (J_H) genes in virtually all cases. Although a polyclonal pattern of the T-cell receptor (TCR) genes is more commonly found, in a variable proportion of cases a concomitant monoclonal rearrangement of TCR and J_H genes can be observed, giving rise to potential pitfalls in the molecular diagnosis of the tumor.

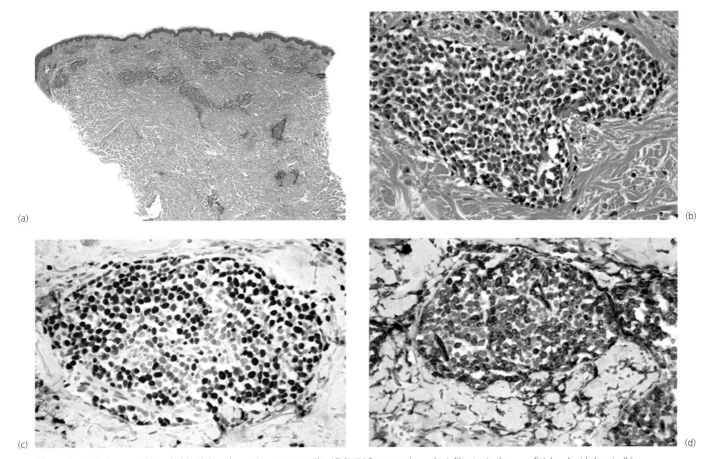

(a)

(b)

(c)

(d)

Figure 17.6 Cutaneous B-lymphoblastic lymphoma (same case as Fig. 17.2). (a) Dense perivascular infiltrates in the superficial and mid-dermis. (b) Monomorphous medium-sized cells predominate. Most neoplastic cells show nuclear positivity for (c) TdT and (d) CD34.

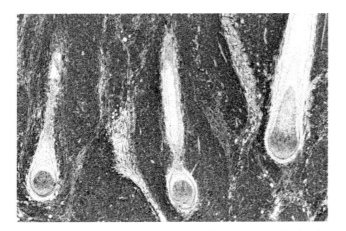

Figure 17.7 Cutaneous B-lymphoblastic lymphoma. Most neoplastic cells show positivity for CD10.

Table 17.1 Classification of precursor lymphoid neoplasms according to the WHO [1]

B-lymphoblastic leukemia/lymphoma, NOS
B-lymphoblastic leukemia/lymphoma with recurrent genetic
  abnormalities
  B-lymphoblastic leukemia/lymphoma with t(9;22)(q34;q11.2);
    BCR-ABL1
  B-lymphoblastic leukemia/lymphoma with t(v;11q23); *MLL* rearranged
  B-lymphoblastic leukemia/lymphoma with t(12;21)(p13;q22);
    TEL-AML1 (ETV6-RUNX1)
  B-lymphoblastic leukemia/lymphoma with hyperdiploidy
  B-lymphoblastic leukemia/lymphoma with hypodiploidy (hypodiploid
    ALL)
  B-lymphoblastic leukemia/lymphoma with t(5;14)(q31;q32); *IL3-IGH*
  B-lymphoblastic leukemia/lymphoma with t(1;19)(q23;p13.3);
    E2A-PBX1 (TCF3-PBX1)
T-lymphoblastic leukemia/lymphoma

Several genetic aberrations have been described in B-lymphoblastic lymphoma, resulting in the identification of specific groups listed in the new World Health Organization (WHO) classification of tumors of hematopoietic and lymphoid tissues [1]. Table 17.1 summarizes the new classification of lymphoblastic lymphomas according to the WHO. Two cases of primary cutaneous B-lymphoblastic lymphoma with specific genetic changes have been recently reported in adult patients, underlining that all subtypes of lymphoblastic leukemia/lymphoma may involve the skin [16].

Differential diagnosis

The differential diagnosis of cutaneous B-lymphoblastic lymphoma includes several entities that may show similar morphologic features. Mantle cell lymphoma contains cells with more cleaved or irregularly shaped nuclei and with a characteristic immunophenotype (CD5+, cyclin-D1+, CD10−, TdT−) (see Chapter 13). Myelomonocytic leukemia shows a proliferation of immature myeloid cells with figurate or "Indian-line" patterns that stain positive for myeloid markers (e.g. naphtol-ASD-chloracetate-esterase and myeloperoxidase among others) and do not reveal a monoclonal rearrangement of the J_H gene (see Chapter 19). Blastic plasmacytoid dendritic cell neoplasm is characterized by a strong positivity for CD4 and CD56 in addition to a variable positivity for TdT, as well as by lack of rearrangement of the J_H gene (see Chapter 16). The differential diagnosis may also include cutaneous Merkel cell tumors and metastatic neuroendocrine carcinomas, which are characterized by the co-expression of cytokeratin filaments, neurofilament proteins, and various other neuroendocrine markers (e.g. chromogranin-A), in addition to the lack of expression of lymphoid markers and absence of J_H gene rearrangement.

Treatment and prognosis

These patients should be managed in a hematologic setting. The treatment of choice is systemic chemotherapy, often with bone marrow transplantation. Patients with localized skin disease appear to have a relatively good prognosis but treatment strategies should be the same as those for systemic variants of the disease.

CUTANEOUS T-LYMPHOBLASTIC LYMPHOMA

T-lymphoblastic lymphoma is a malignant proliferation of precursor T lymphocytes [17]. The exact incidence of specific skin involvement in these patients is not known. As already mentioned for the B-cell variant of lymphoblastic lymphoma, it should be stressed that histologic features alone do not allow one to differentiate lymphoblastic lymphomas of T phenotype from those of B-cell lineage [3]. In the skin, T-lymphoblastic lymphoma almost always represents a secondary manifestation of a primary extracutaneous disease [3,18].

Clinical features

Although T-lymphoblastic lymphoma is observed mainly in children and adolescents, reports of cutaneous involvement are mainly in adult patients [3,4]. Clinically patients present with localized or generalized large cutaneous-subcutaneous tumors (Fig. 17.8) [3,4]. Involvement of the mediastinum (thymus) is common, and the central nervous system may be involved as well.

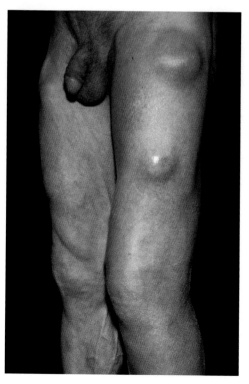

Figure 17.8 Cutaneous T-lymphoblastic lymphoma. Subcutaneous tumors on the leg.

Résumé		
Cutaneous B-lymphoblastic lymphoma		
Clinical	Children, young adults. Solitary tumors. Preferential location: head and neck.	
Morphology	Nodular or diffuse infiltrates characterized by monomorphous proliferations of lymphoblasts.	
Immunology	CD79a	+
	CD20	+(−)
	CD10	+
	PAX5	+
	CD34	+/−
	TdT	+
Genetics	Monoclonal rearrangement of the J_H gene detected in the majority of cases. TCR genes may be clonally rearranged as well.	
Treatment guidelines	Systemic chemotherapy; bone marrow transplantation.	

Histopathology, immunophenotype and molecular genetics

Histology reveals a monomorphous proliferation of medium-sized cells characterized by round or convoluted nuclei with finely dispersed chromatin and scanty cytoplasm (Fig. 17.9). A "starry sky" pattern is often observed at low magnification due to the presence of macrophages with inclusion bodies. There are abundant mitoses and necrotic (apoptotic) cells.

The immunophenotype of neoplastic cells is variable, depending also upon their degree of differentiation. TdT is positive in all cases (Fig. 17.10), and most cases express cytoplasmic CD3 and CD7 as well. Both CD4 and CD8 can be positive or negative. CD1a, CD2, CD5, CD99 and CD34 are other useful markers, but are not constantly positive. Expression of B-cell (CD79a) or myeloid cell markers (CD13, CD33) is present in a minority of cases and may be the source of diagnostic pitfalls.

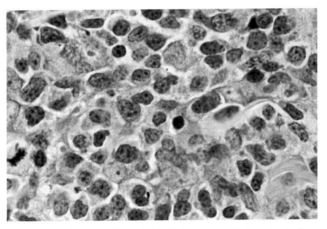

Figure 17.9 Cutaneous T-lymphoblastic lymphoma. Medium-sized cells, some with convoluted nuclei, with finely dispersed chromatin.

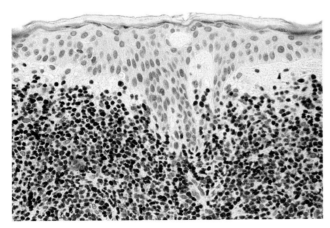

Figure 17.10 Cutaneous T-lymphoblastic lymphoma. Positive nuclear staining for TdT.

Molecular genetics usually shows monoclonally rearranged TCR and germline J_H genes, but clonal rearrangements of both TCR and J_H genes can be observed in a minority of cases. Several genetic abnormalities have been detected in T-lymphoblastic leukemia/lymphoma, particularly involving the *TCR* loci at 14q11.2 (TCR α and δ), 7q35 (TCR β), and 7p14-15 (TCR γ) [17].

Treatment and prognosis

The treatment of choice is systemic chemotherapy, possibly followed by bone marrow transplantation. Patients are treated with schemes similar to those for other types of acute lymphoblastic leukemia/lymphoma.

Résumé

Cutaneous T-lymphoblastic lymphoma

Clinical	Skin involvement mainly in adults. Localized or generalized large cutaneous or subcutaneous tumors.
Morphology	Monomorphous proliferation of medium-sized cells with round or convoluted nuclei with finely dispersed chromatin and scanty cytoplasm.
Immunology	TdT + Cytoplasmic CD3 + CD1a, 2, 7 + CD34 + (−) CD99 +/−
Genetics	Monoclonal rearrangement of the TCR genes. In a minority of cases clonal rearrangement of both TCR and J_H genes.
Treatment guidelines	Systemic chemotherapy, bone marrow transplantation.

References

1. Swerdlow SH, Campo E, Harris NL *et al*, eds. *WHO Classification of Tumours of Haematopoietic and Lymphoid Tissues*. Lyon: IARC Press, 2008: 167–178.
2. Borowitz MJ, Chan JKC. B lymphoblastic leukaemia/lymphoma, not otherwise specified. In: Swerdlow SH, Campo E, Harris NL *et al.*, eds. *WHO Classification of Tumours of Haematopoietic and Lymphoid Tissues*. Lyon: IARC Press, 2008: 168–170.
3. Chimenti S, Fink-Puches R, Peris K *et al.* Cutaneous involvement in lymphoblastic lymphoma. *J Cut Pathol* 1999;**26**:379–385.
4. Sander CA, Medeiros LJ, Abruzzo LV, Horak ID, Jaffe ES. Lymphoblastic lymphoma presenting in cutaneous sites: A clinico-pathologic analysis of six cases. *J Am Acad Dermatol* 1991;**25**: 1023–1031.

5. Schmitt IM, Manente L, Di Matteo A, Felici F, Giangiacomi M, Chimenti S. Lymphoblastic lymphoma of the pre-B phenotype with cutaneous presentation. *Dermatology* 1997;**195**:289–292.

6. Trupiano JK, Bringelsen K, Hsi E. Primary cutaneous lymphoblastic lymphoma presenting in an 8-week old infant. *J Cutan Pathol* 2002;**29**:107–112.

7. Grümayer ER, Ladenstein RL, Slavc I *et al.* B-cell differentiation pattern of cutaneous lymphomas in infancy and childhood. *Cancer* 1988;**61**:303–308.

8. Kamps WA, Poppema S. Pre-B-cell non-Hodgkin's lymphoma in childhood. *Am J Clin Pathol* 1988;**90**:103–107.

9. Cerroni L, Kerl H. Cutaneous B-lymphoblastic lymphoma. In: Burg G, LeBoit PE, Kempf W, Müller B, eds. *Cutaneous Lymphomas. Unusual Cases.* Darmstadt: Steinkopff Verlag, 2001: 68–69.

10. Kim JY, Kim YC, Lee ES. Precursor B-cell lymphoblastic lymphoma involving the skin. *J Cutan Pathol* 2006;**33**:649–653.

11. Choi JE, Ahn H, Kye YC, Kim SN. Precursor B-cell lymphoblastic lymphoma presenting as solitary infiltrative plaque in a child. *Acta Derm Venereol (Stockh)* 2008;**88**:282–284.

12. Kahwash SB, Qualman SJ. Cutaneous lymphoblastic lymphoma in children: report of six cases with precursor B-cell lineage. *Pediatr Dev Pathol* 2002;**5**:45–53.

13. Maitra A, McKenna RW, Weinberg AG, Schneider NR, Kroft SH. Precursor B-cell lymphoblastic lymphoma. A study of nine cases lacking blood and bone marrow involvement and review of the literature. *Am J Clin Pathol* 2001;**115**:868–875.

14. Lin P, Jones D, Dorfman DM, Medeiros LJ. Precursor B-cell lymphoblastic lymphoma: a predominantly extranodal tumor with low propensity for leukemic involvement. *Am J Surg Pathol* 2000;**24**:1480–1490.

15. Yen A, Sanchez R, Oblender M, Raimer S. Leukemia cutis: Darier's sign in a neonate with acute lymphoblastic leukemia. *J Am Acad Dermatol* 1996;**34**:375–378.

16. Shafer D, Wu H, Al-Saleem T *et al.* Cutaneous precursor B-cell lymphoblastic lymphoma in 2 adult patients. Clinicopathologic and molecular cytogenetic studies with a review of the literature. *Arch Dermatol* 2008;**144**:1155–1162.

17. Borowitz MJ, Chan JKC. T lymphoblastic leukaemia/lymphoma. In: Swerdlow SH, Campo E, Harris NL *et al.*, eds. *WHO Classification of Tumours of Haematopoietic and Lymphoid Tissues.* Lyon: IARC Press, 2008: 176–178.

18. van Zuuren EJ, Wintzen M, Jansen PM, Willemze R. Aleukaemic leukaemia cutis in a patient with acute T-cell lymphoblastic leukaemia. *Clin Exp Dermatol* 2003;**28**:330–332.

Section 5: Specific cutaneous manifestations of leukemias

18 Cutaneous manifestations of B-cell chronic lymphocytic leukemia

B-cell chronic lymphocytic leukemia (B-CLL) represents the most frequent type of chronic lymphocytic leukemia [1]. Cutaneous lesions in patients affected by B-CLL are common. In most instances they represent non-specific manifestations related to the impaired immune competence of these patients or to the ingestion of drugs; in some cases, however, neoplastic B lymphocytes are found within the skin [2]. Such lesions are referred to as specific cutaneous manifestations of the disease or "leukemia cutis." It must be remembered that under the same term of "leukemia cutis" specific manifestations of other types of leukemia, particularly myelogenous leukemia, have also been described.

Specific infiltrates of B-CLL have been frequently observed at the site of cutaneous inflammation (see next paragraph), showing that neoplastic cells retain at least in part the capability to answer chemotactic stimuli and to migrate to tissues where inflammation is present. In this context, neoplastic cells of the B-CLL have been observed in inflammatory lesions triggered by infectious organisms as well as in the inflammatory response elicited by cutaneous tumors.

Clinical features

Clinically patients present with localized or generalized erythematous papules, plaques or tumors [2–5]. Ulceration is uncommon. Peculiar clinical presentations include the so-called "facies leonina" and the onset of specific skin lesions at sites of previous herpes simplex or herpes zoster eruptions (Figs 18.1, 18.2) [6]. These latter were often classified in the past as pseudolymphoma [7,8], but are in fact specific cutaneous manifestations of the disease [6,9]. It has been demonstrated that lesions arising at typical sites of *Borrelia burgdorferi* infection (nipple, scrotum, earlobe) also represent specific manifestations of B-CLL triggered by infection with *B. burgdorferi* (Fig. 18.3) [10]. Lesions arising on the nipple were well known in the past and were termed "leukemia lymphatica mammillae" in old textbooks.

Skin Lymphoma: The Illustrated Guide. By L. Cerroni, K. Gatter and H. Kerl. Published 2009 Blackwell Publishing. ISBN: 978-1-4051-8554-7.

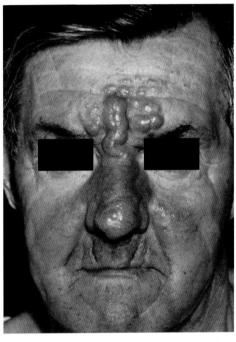

Figure 18.1 Cutaneous B-cell chronic lymphocytic leukemia (B-CLL). Nodules on the face conferring the aspect of the so-called "facies leonina."

Histopathology, immunophenotype and molecular genetics

Histopathology

Histology may show either a patchy perivascular and periadnexal pattern or the presence of dense, monomorphous, diffuse or nodular infiltrates of lymphocytes (Fig. 18.4) [6]. The subcutaneous fat is involved as a rule. The tumor is composed predominantly of small hyperchromatic lymphocytes without prominent atypical features (Fig. 18.5). Small nodular areas with larger cells showing features of prolymphocytes or paraimmunoblasts (so-called "proliferation centers") can be observed occasionally [6]. In some cases other cells such as eosinophils and epithelioid histiocytes can be found.

In patients with B-CLL, infiltrates of neoplastic lymphocytes may be observed in biopsy specimens of different cutaneous conditions, representing specific manifestations of the disease

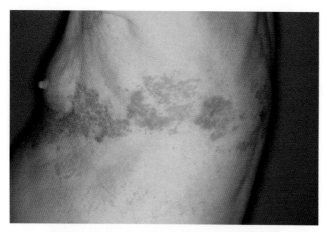

Figure 18.2 Cutaneous B-CLL. Specific skin manifestations at the site of a previous herpes zoster eruption.

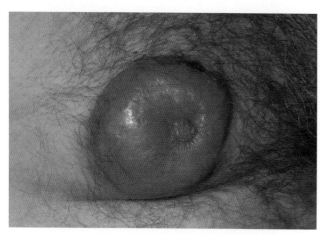

Figure 18.3 Cutaneous B-CLL. Specific skin manifestation at the site of a *Borrelia burgdorferi* infection (so-called "leukemia lymphatica mammillae").

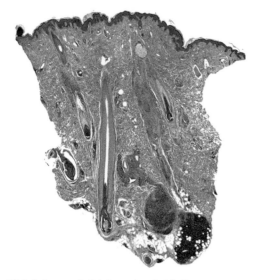

Figure 18.4 Cutaneous B-CLL. Dense lymphoid infiltrates within the dermis and subcutaneous fat.

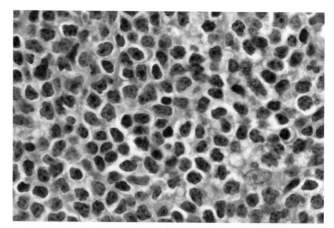

Figure 18.5 Cutaneous B-CLL. Monomorphous infiltrate of small lymphocytes.

at sites of skin inflammation caused by different etiologic factors [6,10,11]. A case of cutaneous "composite" lymphoma with features of both mycosis fungoides and B-CLL has been observed [12], probably representing a further example of the phenomenon just described. We have also observed a case of cutaneous intravascular large T-cell lymphoma arising in a patient with B-CLL, characterized by dermal vessels filled with cells of the intravascular lymphoma and surrounded by a perivascular infiltrate of CD20$^+$/CD5$^+$ small lymphocytes of the B-CLL. In the lymph nodes, composite lymphomas can be due to the association of two non-Hodgkin lymphoma (NHL) types, or of Hodgkin lymphoma and NHL. In the skin, composite lymphomas are very rare, and precise data on lymphoma types are not available.

Immunophenotype and molecular genetics

Immunohistology reveals the presence of B lymphocytes characterized by an aberrant immunophenotype (CD20$^+$, CD5$^+$, CD43$^+$) and by monoclonal expression of immunoglobulin

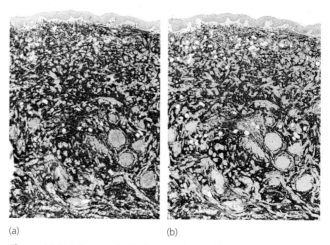

(a)   (b)

Figure 18.6 Cutaneous B-CLL. The neoplastic cells are positive for both (a) CD20 and (b) CD5.

light chains (Fig. 18.6) [6]. CD23 is usually positive, and CD5 may be negative in some cases. A variable population of reactive T lymphocytes is usually present.

Molecular genetics shows in most cases a monoclonal rearrangement of the immunoglobulin heavy chain (J_H) genes. There is evidence that two relevant prognostic subgroups of B-CLL can be defined according to the presence or absence of somatic hypermutations in the neoplastic cells [1]. Reports of cutaneous involvement in patients with B-CLL did not mention the mutation status of the original leukemia, so data on frequency of specific skin manifestations in the two subtypes are lacking.

Treatment and prognosis

Prognosis seems not to be affected by skin involvement [6]. The treatment must be planned according to the hematologic findings. Small solitary or clustered skin lesions may be removed surgically or by CO_2 laser vaporization. Larger lesions may be treated by radiotherapy. Positive responses to UV-B therapy and cladribine have been reported [13,14]. Alemtuzumab has been used in a patient with fludarabine-refractory B-CLL [15]. Rarely skin manifestations may regress slowly without any specific treatment [16].

Patients with somatic hypermutations (mutated B-CLL) have a better prognosis than those without mutations (unmutated B-CLL), especially in earlier stages of the disease.

Progression to diffuse large B-cell lymphoma (Richter's syndrome)

Large cell transformation of B-CLL (Richter's syndrome) has been reported occasionally in the skin [6,17–19]. Patients present clinically with solitary, large cutaneous tumors. Histology reveals features of a diffuse large B-cell lymphoma with many centroblasts and immunoblasts. Immunohistology shows positivity for B cell markers often with an aberrant profile similar to that described above (CD20[+], CD5[+], CD43[+]) and with monoclonal expression of immunoglobulin light chains.

Molecular genetics reveals the presence of a monoclonal rearrangement of the J_H genes. The clone may or may not be the same as that observed in the lymphocytes of the preceding B-CLL, meaning that in some cases Richter's syndrome represents the occurrence of a high-grade lymphoma unrelated to the previous B-CLL (a so-called "second lymphoma") [14]. It seems that Richter's syndrome in unmutated B-CLL is usually clonally related to the original neoplasm, whereas in unmutated B-CLL it represents more often a second lymphoma. The prognosis of patients with cutaneous Richter's syndrome (and with Richter's syndrome in general) is very poor and treatment is usually ineffective [2,19].

True skin lesions of Richter's syndrome should be distinguished from the rare onset of primary cutaneous B-cell lymphoma in patients with B-CLL, as prognosis and management are different [18].

Résumé

Clinical	Elderly. Solitary, grouped or generalized cutaneous papules, plaques and tumors. Possible onset at sites of previous inflammation (e.g. herpes simplex or herpes zoster infection, infection by *Borrelia burgdorferi*) or at sites of cutaneous tumors.
Morphology	Patchy or nodular infiltrates characterized by predominance of small lymphocytes. Predominance of large cells in Richter's syndrome.
Immunology	CD20 + CD5 +(−) CD43 + CD23 + sIg + (monoclonal)
Genetics	Monoclonal rearrangement of the J_H gene detected in the majority of cases. Somatic hypermutations detected in 50–60% of cases. Richter's syndrome may occur in the skin, and may be clonally related to the B-CLL (usually in unmutated cases) or not.
Treatment guidelines	Radiotherapy; excision of solitary lesions. Richter's syndrome should be managed aggressively in a hematologic setting.

TEACHING CASE

This 67-year-old man with a clinical history of B-CLL had herpes zoster on the right shoulder. Shortly after the herpes zoster resolved he developed several confluent papules, plaques and flat tumors at the site of the previous viral infection (Fig. 18.7a). The lesions did not respond to topical treatments. A biopsy revealed a specific infiltrate of the B-CLL with large cell transformation (Richter's syndrome) (Fig. 18.7b, c). Immunohistology showed an aberrant CD20$^+$/CD5$^+$ phenotype of neoplastic cells (Fig. 18.7d). Within a few weeks the patient experienced rapid progression of the B-CLL and he died 7 months after onset of specific skin manifestations.

Comment: In this patient specific skin manifestations of the B-CLL at the site of a previous herpes zoster eruption were the first sign of Richter's syndrome (large cell transformation), and preceded the final stage of the disease. Specific manifestations at sites of cutaneous inflammation are found more frequently in B-CLL patients without Richter's syndrome, but this case shows that exceptions can be observed. Although prognosis of B-CLL affecting the skin at sites of cutaneous inflammation is usually favorable, evidence of Richter's syndrome is always associated with poor prognosis and short survival.

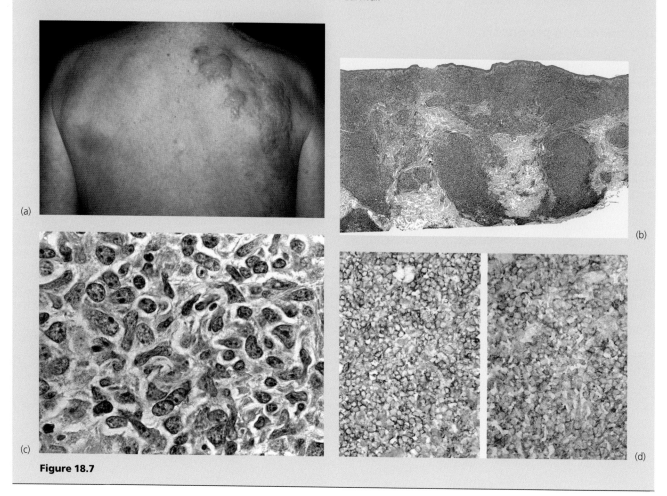

Figure 18.7

References

1. Müller-Hermelink HK, Monsterrat E, Catovsky D, Campo E, Harris NL, Stein H. Chronic lymphocytic leukaemia/small lymphocytic lymphoma. In: Swerdlow SH, Campo E, Harris NL *et al.*, eds. *WHO Classification of Tumours of Haematopoietic and Lymphoid Tissues.* Lyon: IARC Press, 2008: 180–182.

2. Cerroni L, Zenahlik P, Höfler G, Kaddu S, Smolle J, Kerl H. Specific cutaneous infiltrates of B-cell chronic lymphocytic leukemia. A clinicopathologic and prognostic study of 42 patients. *Am J Surg Pathol* 1996;**20**:1000–1010.

3. Paydas S, Zorludemir S. Leukaemia cutis and leukaemic vasculitis. *Br J Dermatol* 2000;**143**:773–779.

4. Schmid-Wendtner MH, Sander C, Volkenandt M, Wendtner CM. Chronic lymphocytic leukemia presenting with cutaneous lesions. *J Clin Oncol* 1999;**17**:1083–1085.

5. Agnew KL, Ruchlemer R, Catovsky D, Matutes E, Bunker CB. Cutaneous findings in chronic lymphocytic leukaemia. *Br J Dermatol* 2004;**150**:1129–1135.

6. Cerroni L, Zenahlik P, Kerl H. Specific infiltrates of B-cell chronic lymphocytic leukemia (B-CLL) arising at sites of herpes simplex and herpes zoster scars. *Cancer* 1995;**76**:26–31.

7. Winkelmann RK, Connolly SM, Yiannias JA, Muenter MD, Harmon CB. Postzoster eruptions: granuloma annulare, granulomatous vasculitis and pseudolymphoma. *Eur J Dermatol* 1995; **5**:470–476.

8. Roo E, Villegas C, Lopez-Bran E, Jimenez E, Valle P, Sanchez-Yus E. Postzoster cutaneous pseudolymphoma. *Arch Dermatol* 1994;**130**:661–663.

9. Cerroni L. Pseudolymphoma? *Arch Dermatol* 1995;**131**:226.

10. Cerroni L, Höfler G, Bäck B, Wolf P, Maier G, Kerl H. Specific cutaneous infiltrates of B-cell chronic lymphocytic leukemia (B-CLL) at sites typical for *Borrelia burgdorferi* infection. *J Cutan Pathol* 2002;**29**:142–147.

11. Smoller BR, Warnke RA. Cutaneous infiltrate of chronic lymphocytic leukemia and relationship to primary cutaneous epithelial neoplasms. *J Cutan Pathol* 1998;**25**:160–164.

12. Hull PR, Saxena A. Mycosis fungoides and chronic lymphocytic leukaemia – composite T-cell and B-cell lymphomas presenting in the skin. *Br J Dermatol* 2000;**143**:439–444.

13. Porter WM, Sidwell RU, Catovsky D, Bunker CB. Cutaneous presentation of chronic lymphatic leukaemia and response to ultraviolet B phototherapy. *Br J Dermatol* 2001;**144**:1092–1094.

14. Robak E, Góra-Tybor J, Kordek R *et al.* Richter syndrome first manifesting as cutaneous B-cell lymphoma clonally distinct from primary B-cell chronic lymphocytic leukemia. *Br J Dermatol* 2005;**153**:833–837.

15. Grey M. Efficacy of alemtuzumab in cutaneous chronic lymphocytic leukaemia involving facial skin. *Br J Haematol* 2008;**142**:1.

16. Kazakov DV, Belousova IE, Michaelis S, Palmedo G, Samtsov AV, Kempf W. Unusual manifestation of specific cutaneous involvement by B-cell chronic lymphocytic leukemia: spontaneous regression with scar formation. *Dermatology* 2003;**207**:111–115.

17. Robertson LE, Pugh W, O'Brien S *et al.* Richter's syndrome: a report on 39 patients. *J Clin Oncol* 1993;**11**:1985–1989.

18. Ratnavel RC, Dunn-Walters DK, Boursier L *et al.* B-cell lymphoma associated with chronic lymphatic lekaemia: two cases with contrasting aggressive and indolent behaviour. *Br J Dermatol* 1999;**140**:708–714.

19. Yamazaki ML, Lum CA, Izumi AK. Primary cutaneous Richter syndrome: prognostic implications and review of the literature. *J Am Acad Dermatol* 2009;**60**:157–161.

Cutaneous manifestations of myelogenous leukemia

Myelogenous leukemias are a spectrum of diseases encompassing chronic myeloproliferative diseases, myelodysplastic disorders and acute myeloid leukemias and related disorders. The classification of these neoplasms has been considerably changed in the last years, and the new World Health Organization (WHO) classification of tumors of hematopoietic and lymphoid tissues takes into consideration genetic features along with conventional clinical, histopathologic and phenotypic aspects (Table 19.1) [1]. However, most reports on skin involvement predate the new classification, so the frequency of cutaneous involvement in the different subtypes is not known. Skin manifestations are more common in patients with more mature forms of subtypes of it, but can be observed in all forms of acute myeloid leukemia, as well as in a small percentage of patients with chronic myelogenous leukemia and also in those with myelodysplastic syndromes [2–13]. In these last two groups of patients, skin involvement usually is related to transformation or progression of the chronic myeloid or myelodysplastic disorder. Recently, specific skin involvement has also been observed in the context of therapy-related myeloid leukemia [14].

Cases showing isolated extramedullary tumors with myeloid differentiation have been referred to as chloroma or granulocytic sarcoma in the past, but are currently referred to as myeloid sarcomas [15–18]. Myeloid sarcoma may precede or be concomitant with myelogenous leukemia. In the last few years, some publications dealing with blastic plasmacytoid dendritic cell neoplasms showed that in some patients a relationship between this entity and myelogenous leukemia exists (see Chapter 16). Indeed, in the WHO classification blastic plasmacytoid dendritic cell neoplasm is mentioned in the chapter on acute myeloid leukemia and related precursor neoplasms (see Table 19.1) [19].

Table 19.1 WHO classification of acute myeloid leukemias and related precursor neoplasms [1].

Acute myeloid leukemia with recurrent genetic abnormalities
AML with t(8;21)(q22;q22); *RUNX1-RUNX1T1*
AML with inv(16)(p13.1;q22) or t(16;16)(p13.1;q22); *CBFB-MYH11*
APL with t(15;17)(q22;q12); *PML-RARA*
AML with t(9;11)(p22;q23); *MLLT3-MLL*
AML with t(6;9)(p23;q34); *DEK-NUP214*
AML with inv(3)(q21;q26.2) or t(3;3)(q21;q26.2); *RPN1-EVI1*
AML (megakaryoblastic) with t(1;22)(p13;q13); *RBM15-MKL1*
Provisional entity: AML with mutated *NPM1*
Provisional entity: AML with mutated *CEBPA*

Acute myeloid leukemia with myelodysplasia-related changes

Therapy-related myeloid neoplasms

Acute myeloid leukemia, not otherwise specified
AML with minimal differentiation
AML without maturation
AML with maturation
Acute myelomonocytic leukemia
Acute monoblastic/monocytic leukemia
Acute erythroid leukemia
Acute megakaryoblastic leukemia
Acute basophilic leukemia
Acute panmyelosis with myelofibrosis

Myeloid sarcoma

Myeloid proliferations related to Down syndrome
Transient abnormal myelopoiesis
Myeloid leukemia associated with Down syndrome

Blastic plasmacytoid dendritic cell neoplasm

Clinical features

The majority of patients are adults who present with multiple, localized or generalized papules, plaques and nodules with a characteristic reddish-brown or violaceous color in the context of a known leukemia (Fig. 19.1) [1]. Cases have been reported in children and even neonates [20,21]. Interestingly, a neonate with typical "blueberry muffin"

Skin Lymphoma: The Illustrated Guide. By L. Cerroni, K. Gatter and H. Kerl. Published 2009 Blackwell Publishing, ISBN: 978-1-4051-8554-7.

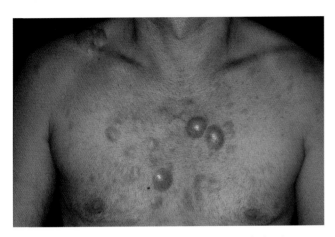

Figure 19.1 Cutaneous manifestations of myelogenous leukemia. Large tumors on the chest in a 40-year-old patient without a leukemic picture who developed overt leukemia 2 months after the onset of skin lesions ("aleukemic leukemia cutis").

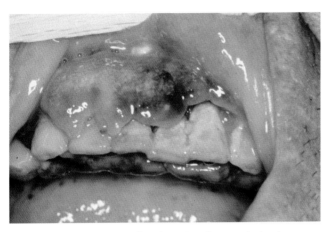

Figure 19.2 Cutaneous manifestations of myelogenous leukemia. Involvement of the gingiva with characteristic violaceous plaques.

clinical presentation and skin infiltrates of myelomonocytic leukemia did not have any other manifestations at staging, suggesting that "aleukemic" leukemia cutis may be observed in newborns, too [22]. Involvement of the mucosal regions is common (Fig. 19.2). Diagnosis of specific cutaneous infiltrates may be difficult in cases presenting with unusual clinical features such as solitary skin nodules, maculopapular eruptions clinically resembling drug or viral eruptions or other uncommon presentations [2,23,24].

Spontaneous regression of skin lesions without treatment has been observed in congenital myelogenous leukemia [25].

As for other types of leukemia, specific manifestations have been observed at the site of cutaneous inflammation [26,27]. This phenomenon seems to be more frequent for lesions of Sweet's syndrome, but has been observed also at sites of psoriasis, basal cell carcinoma, and infusion of gabexate mesilate that had leaked from the vein, suggesting that there may be a predilection for sites of cutaneous inflammation in some cases [28–30].

In a distinct proportion of patients specific skin infiltrates represent the first clinical manifestation of the disease, preceding blood and/or bone marrow changes by weeks or even months ("aleukemic" leukemia cutis) [31,32]. These patients should not be managed in a different way from others with cutaneous manifestations of known myelogenous leukemia.

Histopathology, immunophenotype and molecular genetics

Histopathology

There are no differences in the histopathologic features of skin involvement by acute or chronic myelogenous leukemia [2]. Specific cutaneous lesions show mild, moderate or dense, diffuse or nodular dermal infiltrates, often with perivascular and periadnexal accentuation and sparing of the upper papillary dermis. Involvement of the subcutis is common. In most cases the infiltrate is composed of medium-sized, round to oval cells with a slightly eosinophilic cytoplasm and distinct, sometimes indented, bilobular or kidney-shaped basophilic nuclei (atypical monocytoid cells) (Fig. 19.3). Large cells may also be seen. Different morphologic features may be observed in different subtypes of acute myeloid leukemia. Variable numbers of mitotic figures (including atypical mitoses) and apoptotic cells can be found. Reactive cells (e.g. lymphocytes, mast cells) are present in some cases. A granulomatous reaction may also be observed [2,31,33,34].

Prominent single files of neoplastic cells between collagen bundles can be observed in the majority of cases ("Indian filing") (Fig. 19.4). A distinctive "figurate" pattern characterized by concentric layering of neoplastic cells around blood vessels and adnexal structures is frequently found (Fig. 19.5).

Cutaneous lesions of myeloid sarcoma present with large cutaneous-subcutaneous tumors composed of myeloblasts or monoblasts.

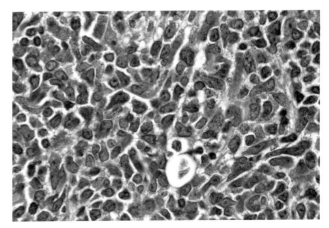

Figure 19.3 Cutaneous manifestations of myelogenous leukemia. Monomorphous infiltrate of atypical monocytoid cells.

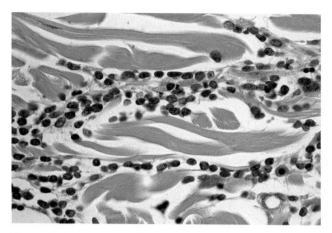

Figure 19.4 Cutaneous manifestations of myelogenous leukemia. Linear arrangement of neoplastic cells ("Indian filing").

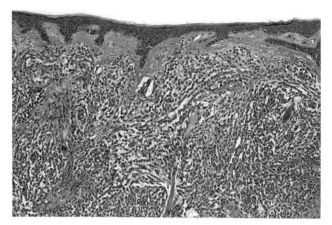

Figure 19.5 Cutaneous manifestations of myelogenous leukemia. Typical disposition of neoplastic cells with "layering" around vessels and adnexal structures ("figurate" pattern).

Immunophenotype

The phenotype of cutaneous lesions of myelogenous leukemia depends on the type of myeloid leukemia. Markers that are usually expressed by neoplastic cells include lysozyme, myeloperoxidase, CD13, CD14, CD15, CD33, CD43, CD45, CD68, and CD117 (Fig. 19.6), but some cases may show positivity for only a few of these antigens. All these markers are available for study on formalin-fixed, paraffin-embedded sections of tissue, thus allowing phenotypization of routine material. Staining for naphtol-ASD-chloracetate-esterase (NASDCl, Leder stain) is positive mainly in cases with a more mature phenotype, but tends to be negative in more immature cells. Staining for CD56 is positive in a minority of cases only; however, as positive cases exist, this marker cannot be used for reliable differentiation from lesions of blastic plasmacytoid dendritic cell neoplasm [2,6,35]. As skin lesions of myelogenous leukemia are commonly positive for CD4 and rarely for CD123, distinction between these two entities may

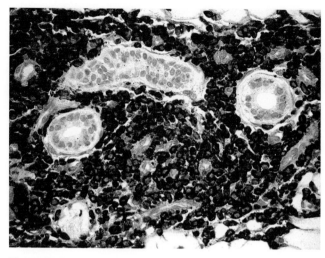

Figure 19.6 Cutaneous manifestations of myelogenous leukemia. Positive staining of neoplastic cells for myeloperoxidase.

be very difficult (for a detailed discussion of differential diagnostic features see Chapter 16) [36,37]. Neoplastic cells in some cases may be positive for S100 protein, thus representing a pitfall in the differential diagnosis with histiocytic disorders (e.g., Langerhans cell histiocytosis) if complete phenotypic analyses are not carried out.

There seems to be no clear-cut correlation between features seen in specific skin infiltrates and the subtype of the underlying myelogenous leukemia. In addition, a recent study demonstrated that the phenotype may be different in bone marrow and skin lesions of patients with acute myeloid leukemia involving the skin [38].

Molecular genetics

The same t(15;17)(q22;q12) rearrangement has been detected in bone marrow and skin lesions of a case of acute promyelocytic leukemia, suggesting that fluorescence *in situ* hybridization (FISH) may be an adjunctive tool for specific diagnosis of cutaneous infiltrates [39]. In most reported cases of cutaneous manifestations of myelogenous leukemia, however, molecular investigations were not carried out.

Treatment and prognosis

The skin manifestations are managed by treating the underlying myelogenous leukemia. Patients with "aleukemic leukemia cutis" should be managed in the same way as patients with blood and/or bone marrow involvement, as the disease inevitably progresses over short periods of time (usually less than 1 year, rarely longer) [40].

There seems to be no difference in survival between patients with specific skin manifestations of acute or chronic myelogenous leukemia. The course is aggressive, and survival is usually of a few months only.

Résumé		
Clinical	Adults. Generalized cutaneous papules, plaques and tumors. Common involvement of mucosal regions (gingival hypertrophy).	
Morphology	Nodular or diffuse infiltrates characterized by predominance of atypical myeloid cells. "Indian filing", "figurate" pattern.	
Immunology	Myeloperoxidase	+(−)
	NASDCL	+(−)
	CD13, CD14, CD15, CD33, CD68, CD117	+(−)
	CD56	−/+
	CD4	+
	CD123	−(+)
Treatment guidelines	Systemic chemotherapy; bone marrow transplantation.	

TEACHING CASE

This 55-year-old man presented with scattered livid papules on the trunk and extremities (Fig. 19.7a, b). He had a history of acute myeloid leukemia (M5 according to the FAB classification system, acute monocytic leukemia according to the WHO 2008 scheme) in complete remission after bone marrow transplantation. A bone marrow biopsy at time of onset of skin lesions did not show signs of recurrent disease. Biopsy of a cutaneous papule revealed a sparse infiltrate composed mainly of myeloid cells (Fig. 19.7c, d) that were positive for CD68 (Fig. 19.7e) and CD117. A diagnosis of cutaneous relapse of the myeloid leukemia was made. A second bone marrow transplantation was attempted, but the patient succumbed to sepsis.

Comment: This case illustrates the difficulties in establishing a diagnosis of specific cutaneous manifestations of myeloid leukemia in early lesions of the disease. Although the infiltrate may mimic that of an inflammatory skin disorder, morphology of the cells and phenotype allow one to make the correct diagnosis. The case also shows the possibility that a relapse may be diagnosed in the skin without evident bone marrow involvement (aleukemic leukemia cutis), underlining the need for proper evaluation of cutaneous lesions in these patients.

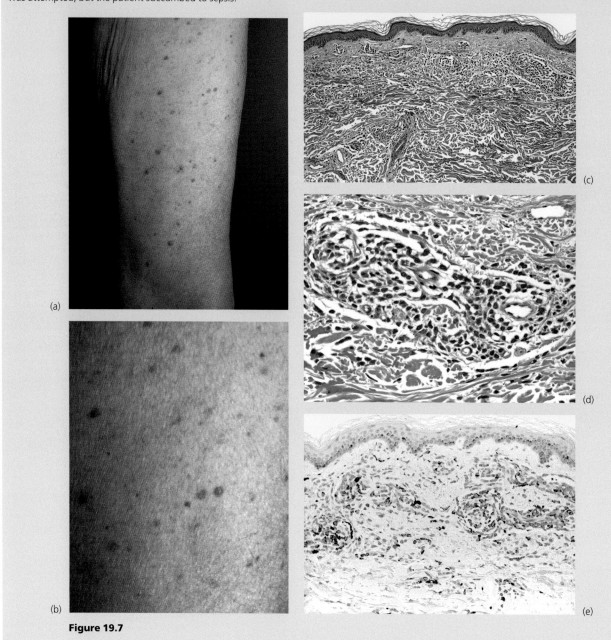

Figure 19.7

References

1. Swerdlow SH, Campo E, Harris NL *et al.*, eds. *WHO Classification of Tumours of Haematopoietic and Lymphoid Tissues*. Lyon: IARC Press, 2008: 109–144.
2. Kaddu S, Zenahlik P, Beham-Schmid C, Kerl H, Cerroni L. Specific cutaneous infiltrates in patients with myelogenous leukemia: a clinicopathologic study of 26 patients with assessment of diagnostic criteria. *J Am Acad Dermatol* 1999;**40**:966–978.
3. Desch JK, Smoller BR. The spectrum of cutaneous disease in leukemias. *J Cutan Pathol* 1993;**20**:407–410.
4. Janier M, Raynaud E, Blanche P, Daniel F, Herreman G. Leukaemia cutis and erythroleukaemia. *Br J Dermatol* 1999;**141**: 372–373.
5. Kaiserling E, Horny HP, Geerts ML, Schmid U. Skin involvement in myelogenous leukemia: morphologic and immunophenotypic heterogeneity of skin infiltrates. *Mod Pathol* 1994; **7**: 771–779.
6. Kuwabara H, Nagai M, Yamaoka G, Ohnishi H, Kawakami K. Specific skin manifestations in CD56 positive acute myeloid leukemia. *J Cutan Pathol* 1999;**26**:1–5.
7. Nagao K, Kikuchi A, Kawai Y *et al.* Skin infiltration in acute promyelocytic leukemia. *Dermatology* 1997;**194**:168–171.
8. Namba Y, Koizumi H, Nakamura H *et al.* Specific cutaneous lesions of the scalp in myelodysplastic syndrome with deletion of 20q. *J Dermatol* 1999;**26**:220–224.
9. Sepp N, Radaszkiewicz T, Meijer CJLM *et al.* Specific skin manifestations in acute leukemia with monocytic differentiation: a morphologic and immunohistochemical study of 11 cases. *Cancer* 1993;**71**:124–132.
10. Stawiski MA. Skin manifestations of leukemias and lymphomas. *Cutis* 1978;**21**:814–818.
11. Ueda K, Kume A, Furukawa Y, Higashi N. Cutaneous infiltration in acute promyelocytic leukemia. *J Am Acad Dermatol* 1997;**36**: 104–106.
12. Kajisawa C, Matsui C, Morohashi M. A specific cutaneous lesion revealing myelodysplastic syndrome. *Eur J Dermatol* 1998;**8**: 517–518.
13. Cho-Vega JH, Medeiros LJ, Prieto VG, Vega F. Leukemia cutis. *Am J Clin Pathol* 2008;**129**:130–142.
14. Weinel S, Malone J, Jain D, Callen JP. Therapy-related leukaemia cutis: a review. *Australas J Dermatol* 2008;**49**:187–190.
15. Traweek ST, Arber DA, Rappaport H, Brynes RK. Extramedullary myeloid cell tumors: an immunohistochemical and morphologic study of 28 cases. *Am J Surg Pathol* 1993; **17**: 1011–1019.
16. Sisack MJ, Dunsmore K, Sidhu-Malik N. Granulocytic sarcoma in the absence of myeloid leukemia. *J Am Acad Dermatol* 1997; **37**:308–311.
17. Dreizen S, McCredie KB, Keating MJ. Mucocutaneous granulocytic sarcomas of the head and neck. *J Oral Pathol* 1987;**16**: 57–60.
18. Pileri SA, Orazi A, Falini B. Myeloid sarcoma. In: Swerdlow SH, Campo E, Harris NL *et al.*, eds. *WHO Classification of Tumours of Haematopoietic and Lymphoid Tissues*. Lyon: IARC Press, 2008: 140–141.
19. Facchetti F, Jones DM, Petrella T. Blastic plasmacytoid dendritic cell neoplasm. In: Swerdlow SH, Campo E, Harris NL *et al.*, eds. *WHO Classification of Tumours of Haematopoietic and Lymphoid Tissues*. Lyon: IARC Press, 2008:145–147.
20. Husak R, Blume-Peytaki U, Orfanos CE. Aleukemic leukemia cutis in an adolescent boy. *N Engl J Med* 1999; **340**: 893–894.
21. Canioni D, Fraitag S, Thomas C *et al.* Skin lesions revealing neonatal acute leukemias with monocytic differentiation: a report of 3 cases. *J Cutan Pathol* 1996;**23**:254–258.
22. Torrelo A, Madero L, Mediero IG, Bano A, Zambrano A. Aleukemic congenital leukemia cutis. *Ped Dermatol* 2004;**21**:458–461.
23. Benez A, Metzger S, Metzler G, Fierlbeck G. Aleukemic leukemia cutis presenting as benign-appearing exanthema. *Acta Derm Venereol (Stockh)* 2001;**81**:45–47.
24. Chang HY, Wong KM, Bosenberg M, McKee PH, Haynes HA. Myelogenous leukemia cutis resembling stasis dermatitis. *J Am Acad Dermatol* 2003;**49**:128–129.
25. Landers MC, Malempati S, Tilford D, Gatter K, White C, Schroeder TL. Spontaneous regression of aleukemia congenital leukemia cutis. *Ped Dermatol* 2005;**22**:26–30.
26. Metzler G, Cerroni L, Schmidt H *et al.* Leukemic cells within skin lesions of psoriasis in a patient with acute myelogenous leukemia. *J Cutan Pathol* 1997;**24**:445–448.
27. Diaz-Cascajo C, Bloedern-Schlicht N. Cutaneous infiltrates of myelogenous leukemia in association with pre-existing skin diseases. *J Cutan Pathol* 1998;**25**:185–186.
28. Urano Y, Miyaoka Y, Kosaka M *et al.* Sweet's syndrome associated with chronic myelogenous leukemia: demonstration of leukemic cells within a skin lesion. *J Am Acad Dermatol* 1999;**40**: 275–279.
29. Deguchi M, Tsunoda T, Yuda F, Tagami H. Sweet's syndrome in acute myelogenous leukemia showing dermal infiltration of leukemic cells. *Dermatology* 1997;**194**:182–184.
30. Miyakura T, Yamamoto T, Kurashige Y *et al.* Leukemia cutis originating in the extravasation site of i.v. gabexate mesilate infusion. *J Dermatol* 2008;**35**:29–32.
31. Ohno S, Yokoo T, Ohta M *et al.* Aleukemic leukemia cutis. *J Am Acad Dermatol* 1990;**22**:374–377.
32. Okun MM, Fitzgibbon J, Nahass GT, Forsman K. Aleukemic leukemia cutis, myeloid subtype. *Eur J Dermatol* 1995;**5**:290–293.
33. Baksh FK, Nathan D, Richardson W, Kestenbaum T, Woodroof J. Leukemia cutis with prominent giant cell reaction. *Am J Dermatopathol* 1998;**20**:48–52.
34. Tomasini C, Quaglino P, Novelli M, Fierro MT. "Aleukemic" granulomatous leukemia cutis. *Am J Dermatopathol* 1998;**20**: 417–421.
35. Kaddu S, Beham-Schmid C, Zenahlik P, Kerl H, Cerroni L. CD56 blastic transformation of chronic myeloid leukemia involving the skin. *J Cutan Pathol* 1999;**26**:497–503.
36. Cibull TL, Thomas AB, O'Malley DP, Billings SD. Myeloid leukemia cutis: a histologic and immunohistochemical review. *J Cutan Pathol* 2008;**35**:180–185.
37. Hejmadi RK, Thompson D, Shah F, Naresh KN. Cutaneous presentation of aleukemic monoblastic leukemia cutis – a case report and review of literature with focus on immunohistochemistry. *J Cutan Pathol* 2008;**3**(suppl. 1):46–49.

38. Sachdev R, George TI, Sundram UN. Discordant immuno-phenotypic profiles in acute myeloid leukaemia involving bone marrow and skin (leukaemia cutis). *J Haematopathol* 2008;**1**: 164.

39. Wrede JE, Sundram U, Kohler S, Cherry AM, Arber DA, George TI. Fluorescence in situ hybridization investigation of cutaneous lesions in acute promyelocytic leukemia. *Mod Pathol* 2005;**18**: 1569–1576.

40. Chang H, Shih LY, Kuo TT. Primary aleukemic myeloid leukemia cutis treated successfully with combination chemotherapy: report of a case and review of the literature. *Ann Hematol* 2003; **82**:435–439.

20 Cutaneous manifestations of other leukemias

Besides B-cell chronic lymphocytic leukemia (B-CLL) and myelogenous leukemias (see Chapters 18 and 19), the skin may be the site of specific manifestations in other types of leukemia. In most cases the leukemia is already known and cutaneous lesions are not biopsied, as the diagnosis is already established. Thus, these patients are seldom sent to dermatologic departments, and the exact incidence of skin lesions in various types of leukemia is unknown.

Most cases of skin involvement by different types of leukemia present with papules, plaques and nodules that retain, at least in part, the histopathologic and phenotypic features of the original disease. Some leukemias described in the following paragraphs present with peculiar manifestations that pose problems in the differential diagnosis and are worth a brief description.

Interestingly, similar to what may be observed in B-CLL and myelogenous leukemias, in other types of leukemia specific skin manifestations have also been found at sites of cutaneous inflammation, suggesting that this mechanism of skin infiltration is common to several types of leukemia, irrespective of the specific classification [1]. In this context, we have observed patients with Sézary syndrome or with late leukemic manifestations of mycosis fungoides who developed specific skin manifestations at the site of drug eruptions, probably following a mechanism similar to that observed in leukemic infiltrates at sites of skin inflammation.

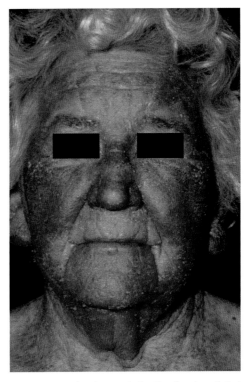

Figure 20.1 Cutaneous involvement in T-cell prolymphocytic leukemia. Erythematous scaly lesions on the face in a patient with erythroderma. The clinical picture is indistinguishable from that of Sézary syndrome.

T-CELL PROLYMPHOCYTIC LEUKEMIA

T-cell prolymphocytic leukemia (T-PLL) is a rare hematologic disease [2]. Cutaneous involvement occurs in up to one-third of patients and is characterized by papules, plaques or tumors often indistinguishable from those of mycosis fungoides/ Sézary syndrome. Erythroderma may develop (Fig. 20.1). Skin manifestations may be the first sign of the disease [3].

Histology reveals a monomorphous infiltrate of small lymphocytes, sometimes with epidermotropism (Fig. 20.2).

Immunohistology shows an α/β T-helper phenotype (βF1$^+$, CD2$^+$, CD3$^+$, CD4$^+$, CD7$^+$, CD8$^-$) in the majority of lesions, but co-expression of CD4 and CD8 is found in about one-fourth of cases. CD52 is strongly expressed. Markers of T-lymphoblastic leukemia/lymphoma (TdT, CD1a) are negative.

The T-cell receptor (TCR) genes are monoclonally rearranged. The most frequent chromosomal aberration is inversion of chromosome 14 with breakpoints in the long arm at q11 and q32 [2].

The disease usually runs an aggressive course and prognosis is poor. Recently treatment with anti-CD52 antibody (Campath) has shown promising results [4]. The rationale for the treatment is provided by the CD52 positivity of neoplastic cells.

Skin Lymphoma: The Illustrated Guide. By L. Cerroni, K. Gatter and H. Kerl. Published 2009 Blackwell Publishing, ISBN: 978-1-4051-8554-7.

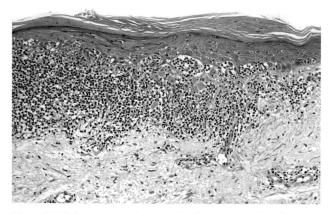

Figure 20.2 Cutaneous involvement in T-cell prolymphocytic leukemia. Dense band-like infiltrate of lymphocytes with epidermotropism. The histopathologic features are indistinguishable from those of mycosis fungoides and Sézary syndrome.

It is interesting to note that a recent report described a patient with a previous "lymphomatoid contact dermatitis" who in follow-up developed a T-PLL, once more showing the difficulties in diagnosis and differential diagnosis of cutaneous lymphoproliferative diseases [5].

Differentiation of cutaneous manifestations of T-PLL from Sézary syndrome may be extremely difficult on clinicopathologic grounds alone.

Résumé

T-cell prolymphocytic leukemia

Clinical	Adults. Generalized papules, plaques and tumors. Erythroderma may develop.
Morphology	Histopathologic features similar to those of mycosis fungoides/Sézary syndrome.
Immunology	CD2, 3, 4, 5, 7 + CD52 + CD8 – (about 25% of cases CD4+/CD8+) βF1 +
Genetics	Monoclonal rearrangement of the TCR genes detected in the majority of cases. Inversion of chromosome 14 with breakpoints in the long arm at q11 and q32.
Treatment guidelines	Systemic chemotherapy; Campath.

AGGRESSIVE NATURAL KILLER CELL LEUKEMIA

Aggressive natural killer (NK) cell leukemia is characterized by a proliferation of NK cells, observed predominantly in young Asian patients [6]. There is a strong association with Epstein–Barr virus (EBV) infection, and a distinct overlap with extranodal NK cell lymphoma, nasal type. It has been suggested that this disease represents the leukemic form of extranodal NK/T-cell lymphoma, nasal type (see Chapter 6).

The skin may be involved, usually concurrently with blood and bone marrow manifestations. Liver and spleen are also frequently affected.

Neoplastic cells present variable morphology (Fig. 20.3) and have a phenotype identical to extranodal NK-cell lymphoma, nasal type, characterized by expression of CD2, CD56 and cytotoxic proteins, negativity for CD3, and positivity for CD3ε. *In situ* hybridization for EBV is positive as a rule (Fig. 20.4). TCR genes are in germline configuration.

The prognosis is very poor, as the disease usually runs a fulminant course. Treatment should be administered in a hematologic setting.

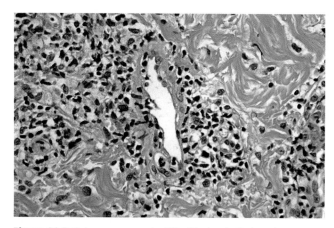

Figure 20.3 Cutaneous aggressive NK cell leukemia. Perivascular infiltrates of small- and medium-sized cells admixed with a few large cells.

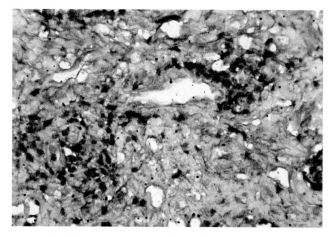

Figure 20.4 Cutaneous aggressive NK cell leukemia. Positive signal upon *in situ* hybridization for EBV (EBER-1).

Résumé

Aggressive NK cell leukemia

Clinical	Adolescents, young adults; mostly Asian patients. Generalized papules, plaques and tumors.
Morphology	Histopathologic features similar to those of extranodal NK/T-cell lymphoma, nasal type.
Immunology	CD2, 56 + CD3 − CD3ε + EBER-1 +
Genetics	TCR genes in germline configuration.
Treatment guidelines	Systemic chemotherapy, bone marrow transplantation (usually fulminant course in spite of treatment).

References

1. Kim JE, Kim MY, Kim HO, Park YM. Plasma cell leukaemia cutis preferentially localized to recent puncture sites. *Br J Dermatol* 2004;**151**:237–238.
2. Catovsky D, Müller-Hermelink HK, Ralfkiaer E. T-cell prolymphocytic leukaemia. In: Swerdlow SH, Campo E, Harris NL *et al.*, eds. *WHO Classification of Tumours of Haematopoietic and Lymphoid Tissues.* Lyon: IARC Press, 2008: 270–271.
3. Serra A, Estrach MT, Marti R, Villamor N, Rafel M. Cutaneous involvement as the first manifestation in a case of T-cell prolymphocytic leukaemia. *Acta Derm Venereol (Stockh)* 1998;**78**:198–200.
4. Pawson R, Dyer MJ, Barge R *et al.* Treatment of T-cell prolymphocytic leukemia with human CD52 antibody. *J Clin Oncol* 1997;**15**:2667–2672.
5. Abraham S, Braun RP, Matthes T, Saurat JH, Braun RPA. Follow-up: previously reported apparent lymphomatoid contact dermatitis, now followed by T-cell prolymphocytic leukaemia. *Br J Dermatol* 2006;**155**:633–634.
6. Chan JKC, Jaffe ES, Ralfkiaer E, Ko YH. Aggressive NK-cell leukaemia. In: Swerdlow SH, Campo E, Harris NL *et al.*, eds. *WHO Classification of Tumours of Haematopoietic and Lymphoid Tissues.* Lyon: IARC Press, 2008: 276–277.

Section 6: Cutaneous manifestations of Hodgkin lymphoma

21 Cutaneous manifestations of Hodgkin lymphoma

Hodgkin lymphoma is regarded as a distinct malignant lymphoma characterized by the presence of neoplastic Reed–Sternberg cells in association with different patterns of reactive cells. It is now accepted that more than 90% of cases of Hodgkin lymphoma represent variants of B-cell lymphomas. A viral etiology is possible because the Epstein–Barr virus (EBV) genome has been detected frequently.

Skin manifestations of nodal Hodgkin lymphoma were not uncommon in the past [1–8]. Modern treatment modalities have resulted in a dramatic decrease in cutaneous involvement, although occasional cases are still reported [9–14]. Rare cases of Hodgkin lymphoma presenting as primary disease in the skin have also been described [15–17]. It should be noted that some authors consider these to be examples of cutaneous anaplastic large cell lymphoma or lymphomatoid papulosis rather than true cases of primary cutaneous Hodgkin lymphoma. However, in rare cases complete phenotypic analyses revealed features that are indeed supporting the diagnosis of Hodgkin lymphoma, and it may be that in exceptional cases Hodgkin lymphoma arises primary in the skin without concomitant extracutaneous disease.

It is not possible to classify skin lesions according to the histopathologic subtypes seen in lymph nodes and recognized in the World Health Organization (WHO) classification of tumors of hematopoietic and lymphoid tissues (nodular lymphocyte-predominant Hodgkin lymphoma, nodular sclerosis classic Hodgkin lymphoma, mixed cellularity classic Hodgkin lymphoma, lymphocyte-rich classic Hodgkin lymphoma, and lymphocyte-depleted classic Hodgkin lymphoma) [18].

Besides specific involvement by neoplastic cells, as in all systemic lymphomas the skin may be the site of non-specific cutaneous manifestations including non-specific dermatitis and pruritus sine materia, among others [19]. This last condition is a characteristic (albeit not pathognomonic) sign of the disease, and the diagnosis of Hodgkin lymphoma should always be considered in these patients.

Nodal Hodgkin lymphoma may be preceded by, concomitant with or followed by other cutaneous lymphoproliferative disorders including mycosis fungoides, lymphomatoid papulosis and anaplastic large cell lymphoma (see also Chapters 2 and 4) [19–27]. Cases of Hodgkin lymphoma associated with granulomatous slack skin have also been described [28,29]. These may represent examples of mycosis fungoides-associated granulomatous slack skin in patients with Hodgkin lymphoma rather than true specific cutaneous manifestations of the Hodgkin lymphoma. Similarly, the patient reported as having "follicular mucinosis" in association with Hodgkin lymphoma [30] may perhaps have had co-existent mycosis fungoides-associated follicular mucinosis.

The onset of cutaneous manifestations of Hodgkin lymphoma has been observed in an HIV-infected patient [31], and nodal Hodgkin lymphoma may arise in the setting of immune suppression (see Chapter 15).

Clinical features

Clinically, skin lesions in Hodgkin lymphoma are usually confined to the drainage area of affected lymph nodes (retrograde lymphatic spread) [8,32]. Papules, plaques and tumors may all be observed (Figs 21.1, 21.2) [32,33]. Ulceration is not uncommon. In some cases lesions are generalized.

As already mentioned, rare patients with primary cutaneous Hodgkin lymphoma have been described, some of whom have developed nodal specific manifestations of the disease after variable periods of time (sometimes several years) [15–17,34].

Histopathology, immunophenotype and molecular genetics

Histology shows the typical features of Hodgkin lymphoma with Reed–Sternberg and Hodgkin cells on a background of small lymphocytes, histiocytes, eosinophils and plasma cells (Figs 21.3, 21.4) [32]. Reed–Sternberg cells may be absent in some cutaneous lesions. It should be noted that Hodgkin and Reed–Sternberg-like cells may be found in a variety of other conditions including mainly lymphomatoid papulosis and cutaneous anaplastic large cell lymphoma.

Skin Lymphoma: The Illustrated Guide. By L. Cerroni, K. Gatter and H. Kerl. Published 2009 Blackwell Publishing, ISBN: 978-1-4051-8554-7.

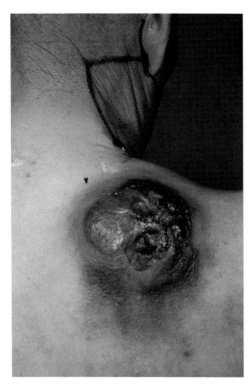

Figure 21.1 Cutaneous Hodgkin lymphoma. Large ulcerated tumor on the right shoulder.

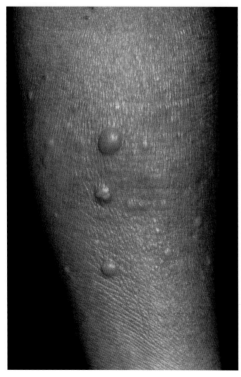

Figure 21.2 Cutaneous Hodgkin lymphoma. Papules and small nodules on the arm.

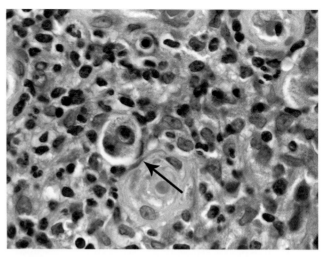

Figure 21.3 Cutaneous Hodgkin lymphoma. Reed–Sternberg cell (*arrow*) on the background of small lymphocytes, histiocytes and eosinophils.

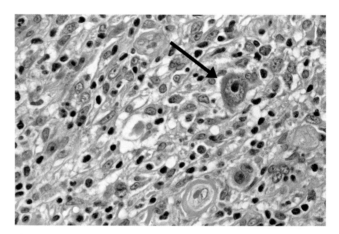

Figure 21.4 Cutaneous Hodgkin lymphoma. Large Hodgkin cell with eosinophilic nucleolus (*arrow*) admixed with small lymphocytes, histiocytes and eosinophils.

Immunohistology reveals in most cases a CD30⁺, CD15⁺ phenotype of Reed–Sternberg and Hodgkin cells, although CD15 may be negative in some cases [32,35]. The small lymphocytes are of both B- and T-cell lineages.

In the lymph nodes, neoplastic cells in nodular lymphocyte-predominant Hodgkin lymphoma are positive for CD45, CD20, CD79a, and Bcl-6. CD30 and CD15 are usually negative in this subtype. In the classic Hodgkin lymphoma subtypes, in the lymph nodes neoplastic cells are always positive for CD30, and only rarely positive for CD20 or CD79a. CD15 is usually positive in a proportion of the cells. PAX5 is almost always positive in these subtypes, and confirms the differentiation toward the B-cell lineage.

There are no molecular data on specific cutaneous manifestations of Hodgkin lymphoma.

Treatment and prognosis

Patients with specific cutaneous manifestations of Hodgkin lymphoma should be treated in a hematologic setting according to schemes tailored for the underlying disease. In the past, the prognosis for patients with skin manifestations of nodal Hodgkin lymphoma was poor in spite of aggressive treatment. Modern treatment modalities have resulted in a steady decline in the onset of specific skin manifestations. Because only occasional patients present with cutaneous involvement, there is little information on which to base both prognostic evaluation and therapeutic options. However, cutaneous Hodgkin lymphoma usually represents advanced (stage IV) disease and carries a bad prognosis.

Résumé	
Clinical	Adults. Solitary, grouped or, rarely, generalized cutaneous papules, plaques and tumors. Lesions are commonly located at the drainage area of affected lymph nodes.
Morphology	Nodular or diffuse infiltrates characterized by presence of Reed–Sternberg and Hodgkin cells on a background of small lymphocytes, histiocytes and eosinophils.
Immunology	CD30 + CD15 + (−)
Genetics	Data on genetic features of specific skin manifestations are not available.
Treatment guidelines	Treatment planned on the basis of the underlying disease. Radiotherapy of isolated skin tumors.

References

1. Gordon RA, Lookingbill DP, Abt AB. Skin infiltration in Hodgkin's disease. *Arch Dermatol* 1980;**116**:1038–1040.
2. Heyd J, Weissberg N, Gottschalk S. Hodgkin's disease of the skin: a case report. *Cancer* 1989;**63**:924–929.
3. O'Bryan-Tear CG, Burke M, Coulson IH, Marsden RA. Hodgkin's disease presenting in the skin. *Clin Exp Dermatol* 1987;**12**:69–71.
4. Silverman CL, Strayer DS, Wasserman TH. Cutaneous Hodgkin's disease. *Arch Dermatol* 1982;**118**:918–921.
5. Smith JL, Butler JJ. Skin involvement in Hodgkin's disease. *Cancer* 1980;**45**:354–361.
6. Torne R, Umbert P. Hodgkin's disease presenting with superficial lymph nodes and tumors of the scalp. *Dermatologica* 1986;**172**: 225–228.
7. White RM, Patterson JW. Cutaneous involvement in Hodgkin's disease. *Cancer* 1985;**55**:1136–1145.
8. Benninghoff DL, Medina A, Alexander LL, Camiel MR. The mode of spread of Hodgkin's disease to the skin. *Cancer* 1970;**26**: 1135–1140.
9. Derrick EK, Deutsch GP, Price ML. Cutaneous extension of Hodgkin's disease. *J R Soc Med* 1991;**84**:684–685.
10. Nelson MC, Petrik JH, Lack EE *et al.* Lymphocyte-predominant Hodgkin disease manifested as a subcutaneous arm mass. *Am J Radiol* 1990;**155**:658–659.
11. Tassies D, Sierra J, Montserrat E *et al.* Specific cutaneous involvement in Hodgkin's disease. *Hematol Oncol* 1992;**10**:75–79.
12. Takagawa S, Maruyama R, Yokozeki H *et al.* Skin invasion of Hodgkin's disease mimicking scrofuloderma. *Dermatology* 1999; **199**:268–270.
13. Introcaso CE, Kantor J, Porter DL, Junkins-Hopkins JM. Cutaneous Hodgkin's disease. *J Am Acad Dermatol* 2008;**58**:295–298.
14. Garcia-Morales I, Herrera-Saval A, Rios JJ, Camacho F. Zosteriform cutaneous metastases from Hodgkin's lymphoma in a patient with scrofuloderma and nodal tuberculosis. *Br J Dermatol* 2004;**151**:722–724.
15. Sioutos N, Kerl H, Murphy SB, Kadin ME. Primary cutaneous Hodgkin disease: unique clinical, morphologic and immunophenotypic findings. *Am J Dermatopathol* 1994;**16**:2–8.
16. Kumar S, Kingma DW, Weiss WB, Raffeld M, Jaffe ES. Primary cutaneous Hodgkin's disease with evolution to systemic disease: association with Epstein–Barr virus. *Am J Surg Pathol* 1996; **20**:754–759.
17. Guitart J, Fretzin D. Skin as the primary site of Hodgkin's disease: a case report of primary cutaneous Hodgkin's disease and review of its relationship with non-Hodgkin's lymphoma. *Am J Dermatopathol* 1998;**20**:218–222.
18. Swerdlow SH, Campo E, Harris NL *et al.*, eds. *WHO Classification of Tumours of Haematopoietic and Lymphoid Tissues.* Lyon: IARC Press, 2008: 321–334.
19. Rubenstein M, Duvic M. Cutaneous manifestations of Hodgkin's disease. *Int J Dermatol* 2006;**45**:251–256.
20. Caya JG, Choi H, Tieu TM, Wollenberg NJ, Almagro UA. Hodgkin's disease followed by mycosis fungoides in the same patient: case report and review of the literature. *Cancer* 1984;**53**:463–467.
21. Clement M, Bhakri H, Monk B *et al.* Mycosis fungoides and Hodgkin's disease. *J R Soc Med* 1984;**77**:1037–1038.
22. Davis TH, Morton CC, Miller-Cassman R, Balk SP, Kadin ME. Hodgkin's disease, lymphomatoid papulosis, and cutaneous T-cell lymphoma derived from a common T-cell clone. *N Engl J Med* 1992;**326**:1115–1122.
23. Hawkins KA, Schinella R, Schwartz M *et al.* Simultaneous occurrence of mycosis fungoides and Hodgkin disease. *Am J Hematol* 1983;**14**:355–362.
24. Kadin ME. Lymphomatoid papulosis and associated lymphomas: how are they related? *Arch Dermatol* 1993;**129**:351–353.
25. Kamarashev J, Dummer R, Hess Schmid M *et al.* Primary cutaneous T-cell-rich B-cell lymphoma and Hodgkin's disease in a patient with Gardner's syndrome. *Dermatology* 2000;**201**: 362–365.
26. Simrell CR, Boccia RV, Longo DL, Jaffe ES. Coexisting Hodgkin's disease and mycosis fungoides. *Arch Pathol Lab Med* 1986;**110**: 1029–1034.
27. Weinman VF, Ackerman AB. Lymphomatoid papulosis: a critical review and new findings. *Am J Dermatopathol* 1981;**3**:129–162.

28. DeGregorio R, Fenske NA, Glass LF. Granulomatous slack skin: a possible precursor of Hodgkin's disease. *J Am Acad Dermatol* 1995;**33**:1044–1047.

29. Noto G, Pravatà G, Miceli S, Aricò M. Granulomatous slack skin: report of a case associated with Hodgkin's disease and a review of the literature. *Br J Dermatol* 1994;**131**:275–279.

30. Stewart M, Smoller BR. Follicular mucinosis in Hodgkin's disease: a poor prognostic sign? *J Am Acad Dermatol* 1991;**24**: 784–785.

31. Shaw MT, Jacobs SR. Cutaneous Hodgkin's disease in a patient with human immunodeficiency virus infection. *Cancer* 1989;**64**: 2585–2587.

32. Cerroni L, Beham-Schmid C, Kerl H. Cutaneous Hodgkin's disease: an immunohistochemical analysis. *J Cutan Pathol* 1995;**22**: 229–235.

33. Hayes TG, Rabin VR, Rosen T, Zubler MA. Hodgkin's disease presenting in the skin: case report and review of the literature. *J Am Acad Dermatol* 1990;**22**:944–947.

34. Jurisic V, Bogunovic M, Colovic N, Colovic M. Indolent course of the cutaneous Hodgkin's disease. *J Cutan Pathol* 2005;**32**: 176–178.

35. Moretti S, Pimpinelli N, Di Lollo S, Vallecchi C, Bosi A. *In situ* immunologic characterization of cutaneous involvement in Hodgkin's disease. *Cancer* 1989;**63**:661–666.

Section 7: Pseudolymphomas of the skin

22 Pseudolymphomas of the skin

Pseudolymphomas of the skin are benign lymphocytic proliferations that simulate cutaneous malignant lymphomas clinically and/or histopathologically [1–6]. The term pseudolymphoma is not specific but merely descriptive, as it encompasses reactive skin conditions with different etiologies, pathogeneses, clinicopathologic presentations and behaviors. Cutaneous pseudolymphomas are traditionally divided into T- and B-cell pseudolymphomas according to the histopathologic and immunophenotypical features [7], although in many conditions this distinction is artificial. For example, pseudolymphomas induced by drugs may present with either a T- or a B-cell pattern, and the same drug may induce different patterns in different patients. Thus, in what follows we classify cutaneous pseudolymphomas according to specific clinicopathologic entities (Table 22.1).

In recent years, many reactive skin diseases have been added to the list of cutaneous pseudolymphomas, mainly because of the presence of histopathologic features similar to those observed in malignant lymphomas of the skin. On the other hand, several entities classified in the past as cutaneous pseudolymphomas have been reclassified as low-grade malignant lymphomas, based on clinicopathologic and genetic features as well as on follow-up data. Nevertheless, most of the diseases reported as "pseudolymphoma" in the past are benign reactive skin disorders and need to be clearly separated from cutaneous malignant lymphomas. In this context, the introduction of the concept of "clonal dermatoses," that is, reactive skin conditions with monoclonal populations of T or B lymphocytes showing a possible evolution into clear-cut cutaneous malignant lymphoma, has brought confusion to an already confused field [8–10]. True "progression" from a clear-cut cutaneous pseudolymphoma into a malignant lymphoma of the skin is exceptional, if it occurs at all.

There are no exact data concerning the incidence, prevalence and geographic distribution of cutaneous pseudolymphomas.

Cutaneous pseudolymphomas associated with infectious organisms (such as *Borrelia burgdorferi* lymphocytoma) commonly arise in regions with endemic *B. burgdorferi* infection. There has also been a rise in the number of cases of *Borrelia* lymphocytoma in countries where *Borrelia* species are absent, in patients returning from travels in endemic regions. It should be remembered that *Borrelia* infection has been convincingly linked to some cases of cutaneous B-cell lymphoma as well, so detection of *Borrelia* DNA is not equivalent with a diagnosis of benignancy (see Chapter 11).

The clinical manifestations of cutaneous pseudolymphomas are protean. The lesions are often solitary although they may be regionally clustered or generalized in distribution. Cutaneous pseudolymphomas may also show the features of generalized erythroderma. The course of pseudolymphomas varies considerably. The lesions may persist for weeks, months or even years; they may resolve spontaneously and they may recur unpredictably.

Histologic criteria for the diagnosis of cutaneous pseudolymphomas include two main features: (i) the architectural pattern of the infiltrates; and (ii) the cellular composition of those infiltrates, which frequently show a mixed character. These histologic features need to be integrated carefully with the immunophenotypical data [11–13]. The introduction of polymerase chain reaction (PCR) analysis of the rearrangement of the T-cell receptor (TCR) and immunoglobulin heavy-chain (J_H) genes allows the clonality of cutaneous T- and B-cell infiltrates to be established [14–17]. Although, as a rule, malignant lymphomas reveal a monoclonal population of lymphocytes whereas pseudolymphomas show a polyclonal infiltrate, it must be underlined that demonstration of monoclonality may be lacking in true malignant lymphomas, and that a distinct proportion of cutaneous pseudolymphomas harbor a monoclonal T- or B-cell population. In addition, pseudoclonality represents a pitfall in cutaneous infiltrates (see Chapter 1), particularly when results are interpreted without knowledge of other data [18]. In this context, it must be clearly stated that differentiation of benign from malignant lymphoid infiltrates of the skin is possible only after careful synthesis and integration of the clinical, histopathologic, immunophenotypical and molecular features. In some cases, the true diagnosis will be revealed only at follow-up.

Skin Lymphoma: The Illustrated Guide. By L. Cerroni, K. Gatter and H. Kerl. Published 2009 Blackwell Publishing, ISBN: 978-1-4051-8554-7.

Table 22.1 Classification of cutaneous pseudolymphomas

Clinicopathologic entity	Simulated malignant lymphoma
Actinic reticuloid	Mycosis fungoides/Sézary syndrome
Lymphomatoid contact dermatitis	
Solitary T-cell pseudolymphoma (superficial type)	
Lichenoid ("lymphomatoid") keratosis	
Lichenoid pigmented purpuric dermatitis (including lichen aureus)	
Lichen sclerosus et atrophicus	
Vitiligo (inflammatory stages)	
Annular lichenoid dermatitis of youth (*exact nosology yet unclear*)	
CD8+ cutaneous infiltrates in HIV-infected patients	
Lymphomatoid drug reaction, T-cell type	
Pseudolymphomas in tattoos, T-cell type	
Pseudolymphomas at sites of vaccination, T-cell type	
Mycosis fungoides-like infiltrates in regressing malignant epithelial and melanocytic tumors	
Pseudolymphomas in herpes simplex or herpes zoster infections	Cytotoxic NK/T-cell lymphomas *or* Lymphomatoid papulosis/cutaneous
PLEVA, including the febrile ulceronecrotic variant	anaplastic large cell lymphoma
Atypical lymphoid infiltrates (CD30+) associated with: orf, milker's nodule, molluscum contagiosum and other infectious disorders	Lymphomatoid papulosis/cutaneous anaplastic large cell lymphoma
Persistent arthropod bite reactions (including nodular scabies)	
Drug eruptions with clusters of CD30+ lymphocytes	
Other reactive infiltrates with CD30+ cells	
Lupus panniculitis	Subcutaneous "panniculitis-like" T-cell lymphoma
Lymphocytoma cutis	Follicle center lymphoma
	Marginal zone B-cell lymphoma
	Diffuse large B-cell lymphoma
Lymphomatoid drug reaction, B-cell type	Follicle center lymphoma
Pseudolymphoma after vaccination, B-cell type	
Pseudolymphoma in tattoos, B-cell type	Marginal zone B-cell lymphoma
Morphea, inflammatory stage	
Syphilis (secondary)	
"Acral pseudolymphomatous angiokeratoma" (small papular pseudolymphoma)	
Inflammatory pseudotumor (plasma cell granuloma)	Marginal zone B-cell lymphoma, plasmacytic variant
Cutaneous plasmacytosis	
Lymphocytic infiltration of the skin (Jessner–Kanof)	Cutaneous manifestations of B-cell chronic lymphocytic leukemia
Cutaneous extramedullary hematopoiesis	Cutaneous manifestations of myeloid leukemia
Reactive angio-endotheliomatosis/intravascular histiocytosis	Intravascular diffuse large cell lymphoma
Benign intravascular proliferation of lymphoid blasts	

Actinic reticuloid

The concept of chronic actinic dermatitis encompasses four chronic photodermatoses: persistent light reactivity, photo-sensitivity dermatitis, photosensitive eczema and actinic reticuloid [19–22]. Actinic reticuloid is a severe persistent photodermatitis that usually affects older men. The disease is characterized by extreme photosensitivity to a broad spectrum of UV radiation [23]. Clinically and histologically,

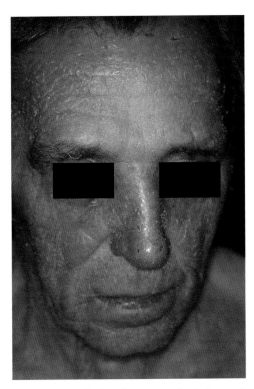

Figure 22.1 Actinic reticuloid. Erythematous scaling lesions on the face.

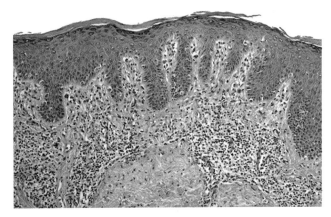

Figure 22.2 Actinic reticuloid. Psoriasiform epidermal hyperplasia with band-like infiltrate of lymphocytes in the upper dermis. Note focal exocytosis of solitary lymphocytes.

it has many of the features of mycosis fungoides and Sézary syndrome. The patients present in the early stages with erythemas on the face and neck and on the back of the hands (Fig. 22.1). Ectropion may be present. As the eruption progresses, it becomes lichenified as a consequence of chronic scratching, and scaly plaques may develop. In some areas, the lesions may consist of lichenoid papules. Recurrent erythroderma is common in these patients [24]. A "leonine" face with deep furrowing of markedly thickened skin as well as diffuse alopecia can also be seen. Pruritus is generally severe and intractable and may lead to attempts at suicide. The disease is chronic and shows no tendency to spontaneous remission [25]. Although "progression" into T-cell lymphoma has been reported, it seems more likely that these cases represented examples of mycosis fungoides from the onset, and that actinic reticuloid is not a potential precursor of cutaneous T-cell lymphoma [26,27].

Histologic examination reveals dense, superficial or deep perivascular mixed-cell infiltrates of lymphocytes, histiocytes, plasma cells and eosinophils as well as some atypical mononuclear cells with hyperchromatic lobulated nuclei (Fig. 22.2). In the upper part of the dermis the infiltrate is band-like or patchy. The papillary dermis is usually thickened. Stellate and multinucleated fibroblasts are present. Exocytosis of lymphocytes within the hyperplastic epidermis can be found. When present, the features of lichen simplex chronicus superimposed upon an inflammatory process are helpful in distinguishing actinic reticuloid from mycosis fungoides and

Sézary syndrome. Immunohistology is characterized by the predominance of CD8+ T cells [28–30].

The clinical differentiation of actinic reticuloid from cutaneous T-cell lymphomas (mycosis fungoides and Sézary syndrome) can be difficult because circulating Sézary cells may be found in the peripheral blood of patients with actinic reticuloid [31]. A low helper:suppressor ratio in the peripheral blood has been found in patients with erythrodermic actinic reticuloid, as opposed to the high ratio commonly observed in patients with Sézary syndrome [32]. Unlike patients with mycosis fungoides and Sézary syndrome, on phototesting, patients with chronic actinic dermatitis are sensitive to UV-B, UV-A and, in most instances, to visible light. Fluorescent light may lead to an exacerbation of the disease. In patients with actinic reticuloid, the minimal erythema dose is lower than normal.

Treatment of chronic actinic dermatitis is difficult and numerous therapeutic approaches have been proposed [33]. Photoprotection is crucial. Any relevant associated contact or photocontact allergens have to be identified and avoided. Some patients have been reported to respond to corticosteroids, photochemotherapy with psoralen and UV-A (PUVA), interferon-α or a combination treatment with azathioprine, hydroxychloroquine and prednisone. Ciclosporin (sometimes combined with bath PUVA) or topical tacrolimus ointment (especially for facial lesions) also appears to be effective [34–36].

Lymphomatoid contact dermatitis

The term lymphomatoid contact dermatitis was coined by Gomez Orbaneja *et al.* in 1976 [37]. These authors described four patients with persistent allergic contact dermatitis proved by patch tests. The clinical picture and histologic features in their patients were highly suggestive of mycosis fungoides. Clinically, lymphomatoid contact dermatitis is characterized by pruritic erythematous plaques (Fig. 22.3). Generalized

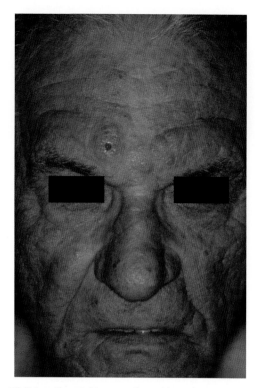

Figure 22.3 Lymphomatoid contact dermatitis. Erythematous papules and small plaques on the forehead.

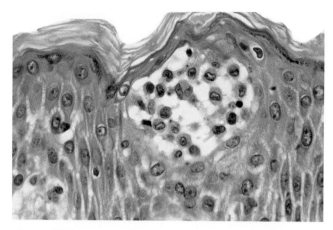

Figure 22.5 Lymphomatoid contact dermatitis. Spongiotic vesicle with Langerhans cells, keratinocytes and a few lymphocytes simulating "Darier's nests" ("Pautrier's microabscesses").

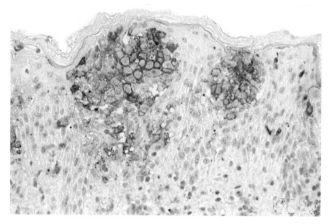

Figure 22.6 Lymphomatoid contact dermatitis. Staining for CD1a reveals large numbers of Langerhans cells within the intraepidermal nests.

plaques or exfoliative erythroderma can be observed rarely. The lesions undergo phases of exacerbation and remission.

Histologically, lymphomatoid contact dermatitis resembles mycosis fungoides (Fig. 22.4) [38]. The differentiation is determined mainly on the basis of changes within the epidermis. In lymphomatoid contact dermatitis, there are usually only a few intraepidermal atypical lymphocytes that have no tendency to form "Darier's nests" ("Pautrier's microabscesses"). Small intraepidermal collections of keratinocytes admixed with Langerhans cells and a few lymphocytes are common, and should not be misinterpreted as true "Darier's nests" (Fig. 22.5). Staining for CD1a highlights Langerhans cells in

these intraepidermal collections (Fig. 22.6). Analysis of TCR gene rearrangement commonly shows a polyclonal population of T lymphocytes in the skin lesions of lymphomatoid contact dermatitis. However, in the majority of patch test lesions in patients with "conventional" contact dermatitis, monoclonality can be observed by Southern blotting, demonstrating that the finding of a clonal population of T lymphocytes in such patients does not have any diagnostic implications [39].

Patch tests for a variety of common antigens can give a positive reaction in lymphomatoid contact dermatitis, and the diagnosis should be reserved for patients in whom the lymphomatoid skin lesions are caused by a positively reacting antigen. Although lymphomatoid contact dermatitis has been reported to evolve into true malignant lymphoma, it is more likely that such patients had malignant lymphoma from the outset. For the management of patients, a thorough search for antigens is necessary in order to interrupt the process. When contact with the responsible allergens is avoided, the lesions heal in a relatively short time.

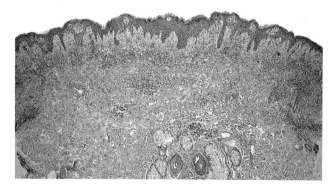

Figure 22.4 Lymphomatoid contact dermatitis. Band-like infiltrate in the superficial dermis with focal spongiosis and intraepidermal collections of cells.

Solitary T-cell pseudolymphoma

This is probably one of the most controversial types of pseudolymphoma, as definition and differential diagnostic criteria are not clear, lesions with different clinicopathologic features have been included in different reports, and many overlaps with cutaneous small/medium pleomorphic T-cell lymphoma exist (see Chapter 8). In short, the literature is confusing, as similar cases were included in different diagnostic categories.

At least two different conditions have been described in the literature as solitary T-cell pseudolymphoma. One is characterized by superficial lesions with clinicopathologic features similar to those observed in mycosis fungoides, and arises in patients who are not obviously taking any drug (thus ruling out the diagnosis of lymphomatoid drug eruption; see corresponding section in this chapter) [40,41]. There may be an overlap between this variant of solitary T-cell pseudolymphoma and so-called lichenoid keratosis (see below). The lesions are frequently located on the breasts of adult women (Fig. 22.7). Histology reveals a band-like infiltrate in an expanded papillary dermis, sometimes with exocytosis of lymphocytes within the epidermis (Figs 22.8, 22.9). In several patients, a monoclonal rearrangement of the TCR genes has been reported. Some of the cases reported in the past as "unilesional" or "solitary" mycosis fungoides may represent examples of solitary T-cell pseudolymphoma, but at present it is not possible to establish with certainty whether they are wholly benign monoclonal lymphoid proliferations or represent a variant of cutaneous T-cell lymphoma with a very favorable course [42]. Surgical excision results in complete remission; recurrences are uncommon.

The second type presents with nodular lesions and reveals overlapping features with cutaneous small/medium pleomorphic T-cell lymphoma, and it is currently unclear whether these lesions represent a reactive process or a low-grade malignant T-cell lymphoma [43–45]. A detailed discussion

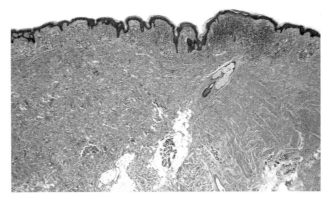

Figure 22.8 Solitary T-cell pseudolymphoma. Dense band-like infiltrate in the upper dermis.

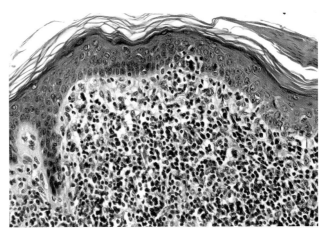

Figure 22.9 Solitary T-cell pseudolymphoma. Note focal epidermotropism of lymphocytes (detail of Fig. 22.8).

of nomenclature, clinicopathologic features and differential diagnosis of these cases is provided in Chapter 8.

Lichenoid (lymphomatoid) keratosis

Lichenoid (lymphomatoid) keratosis is a benign epithelial neoplasm, related in some cases to seborrheic keratosis and lentigo actinica (Fig. 22.10) [46–48]. Patients are elderly adults with small scaly plaques located usually on the trunk. The histopathologic features with dense band-like inflammatory lymphoid infiltrates and often epidermotropism of lymphocytes may be indistinguishable from those of mycosis fungoides (Fig. 22.11) [49]. Moreover, clonality of T lymphocytes can sometimes be found in these lesions. In many cases, on the edge of the inflammatory infiltrate there are small rests of an epithelial neoplasm (seborrheic keratosis, lentigo actinica) that underwent regression. Accurate clinicopathologic correlation is crucial to establish a correct diagnosis.

Differentiation of lichenoid (lymphomatoid) keratosis from one variant of solitary T-cell pseudolymphoma may be impossible in cases that do not show clear-cut features of an

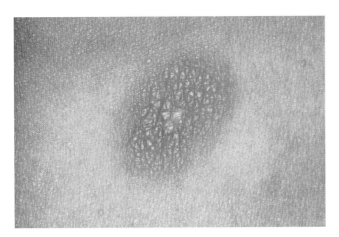

Figure 22.7 Solitary T-cell pseudolymphoma. Solitary plaque on the breast.

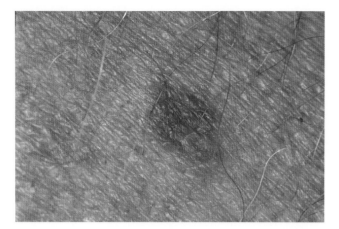

Figure 22.10 Lichenoid (lymphomatoid) keratosis. Small scaly plaque on the breast.

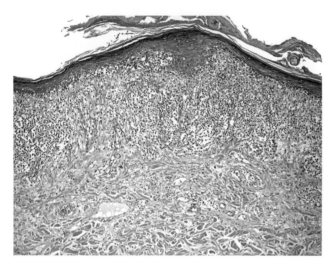

Figure 22.11 Lichenoid (lymphomatoid) keratosis. Band-like infiltrate of lymphocytes with exocytosis in the lower layers of the epidermis.

epithelial neoplasm, and the two conditions may be strictly related (see above).

Lichen aureus/lichenoid pigmented purpuric dermatitis

Lichen aureus is a benign skin condition characterized by asymmetric persistent purpuric skin macules and thin plaques with a typical golden-brown color clinically (Fig. 22.12), and by a band-like lymphocytic infiltrate that may simulate mycosis fungoides histopathologically (Fig. 22.13) [50]. Patients are usually adults with asymmetric, solitary or, more commonly, localized lesions. Molecular analyses may reveal T-lymphocyte clonality in some cases [50]. Accurate clinicopathologic correlation is crucial to establish a correct diagnosis. Local steroid ointments or PUVA therapy can be used to treat lichen aureus.

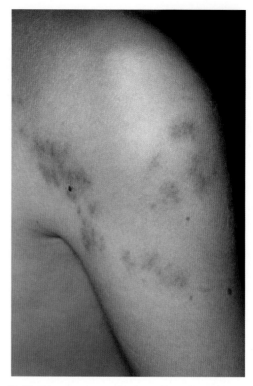

Figure 22.12 Lichen aureus. Localized macules with characteristic brown-orange color.

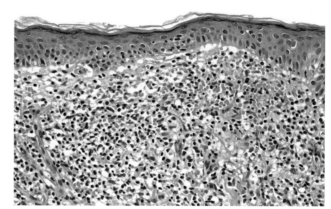

Figure 22.13 Lichen aureus. Dense infiltrate of lymphocytes with prominent extravasation of erythrocytes and vacuolar changes of the basal keratinocytes.

A relationship between lichen aureus or lichenoid pigmented purpuric dermatitis and mycosis fungoides has been postulated (see also Chapter 2) [50–53]. In a large group of patients with long follow-up data, however, we could not observe any progression from conventional lichen aureus to mycosis fungoides [54]. On the other hand, some patients showed persistent lesions with clonal populations of T lymphocytes after many years of follow-up, suggesting that lichen aureus may belong to a spectrum of clonal dermatoses. Nonetheless, we believe that lichen aureus is a benign inflammatory disorder, and that cases of mycosis fungoides preceded by pigmented pur-puric dermatitis probably represented examples of mycosis fungoides from the outset [55]. Evaluation of the literature, however, is complicated by the inclusion in this group of patients with different clinicopathologic features, including some with clear-cut features of mycosis fungoides [56].

Lichen sclerosus

Sometimes, cases of lichen sclerosus on genital skin reveal histopathologic features characterized by dense band-like lymphoid infiltrates and epidermotropism of lymphocytes that may be indistinguishable from those of mycosis fungoides (Figs 22.14, 22.15) [57]. Immunohistochemical stainings may reveal many intraepidermal T lymphocytes (Fig. 22.16). Moreover, T-lymphocyte clonality can be found in some of these cases [57–59]. The finding of the typical hyalinization of the collagen is a useful clue for the diagnosis of lichen sclerosus but it may be missing, especially in small biopsies. Accurate clinicopathologic correlation is required to establish

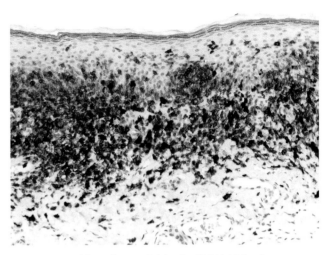

Figure 22.16 Lichen sclerosus. Staining for CD3 highlights the intraepidermal T lymphocytes.

a correct diagnosis. In this context, a diagnosis of mycosis fungoides on genital skin should never be made without a precise correlation between histopathologic and clinical fea-tures, even in cases that show monoclonality of the infiltrate. More specifically, we have never come across patients with solitary mycosis fungoides located on the genital skin.

Vitiligo

A lichenoid inflammation can be observed in the early (inflammatory) stage of vitiligo [60]. Some of these cases present with clinical and histopathologic features mimick-ing those of mycosis fungoides (Fig. 22.17) [61]. Clinically there are erythematous, scaly patches, whereas typical acromic lesions of vitiligo are missing. Even when depigmenta-tion occurs, the differential diagnosis with hypopigmented mycosis fungoides can be very difficult. Histopathologically,

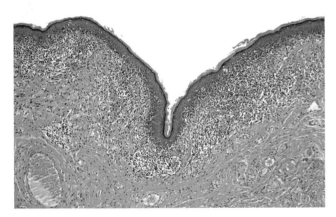

Figure 22.14 Lichen sclerosus. Dense band-like infiltrate of lymphocytes with exocytosis within the lower layers of the epidermis.

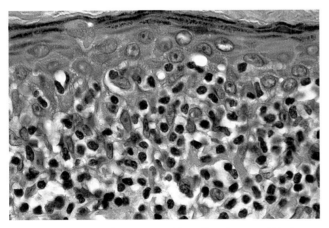

Figure 22.15 Lichen sclerosus. Intraepidermal lymphocytes within the lower layers of the epidermis. Note some lymphocytes with perinuclear halo ("haloed lymphocytes") mimicking mycosis fungoides (detail of Fig. 22.14).

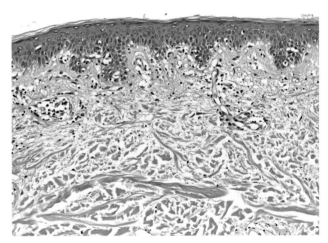

Figure 22.17 Vitiligo, inflammatory stage. Superficial infiltrate with exocytosis of lymphocytes within the lower part of the epidermis.

pseudolymphomatous lesions of vitiligo show dense, band-like infiltrates of lymphocytes with exocytosis of cells within the lower part of the epidermis. Most cells are CD8+ cytotoxic lymphocytes, thus mimicking the hypopigmented variant of mycosis fungoides observed frequently in children. The onset of conventional lesions of vitiligo during follow-up allow the correct diagnosis in these cases. In this context, it should be underlined that a diagnosis of mycosis fungoides should be established only upon compelling clinicopathologic evidence, and that a delay of a few months in the diagnosis of early mycosis fungoides is probably better than a wrong diagnosis of "cancer," particularly in children.

The treatment of the inflammatory stage of vitiligo has never been investigated in detail, as in many cases the diagnosis is established only retrospectively.

Annular lichenoid dermatitis of youth

A condition termed "annular lichenoid dermatitis of youth" has been reported recently as a simulator of mycosis fungoides [62–64]. Patients are children and adolescents who present with annular erythematous macules that evolve into round or oval annular patches with elevated erythematous borders and central depigmentation. Lesions occur mostly on the trunk. Histology reveals a band-like lymphocytic infiltrate with vacuolar alterations at the dermoepidermal junction and many necrotic keratinocytes at the tip of the rete ridges (the rete ridges are "squared off" by the lichenoid infiltrate) (Fig. 22.18). Although this condition has been described as a simulator of mycosis fungoides, in our opinion definitive proof of its benignancy is still lacking, and patients should be carefully followed up. In fact, a similar presentation has been termed "lymphomatoid annular erythema" [65], and has been considered a variant of mycosis fungoides in young patients.

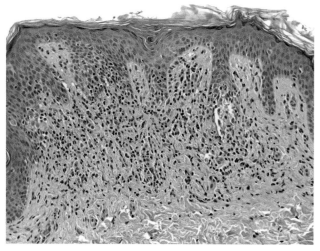

Figure 22.18 "Annular lichenoid dermatitis of youth." Dense lichenoid infiltrate with prominent necrosis of keratinocytes at the tip of rete ridges.

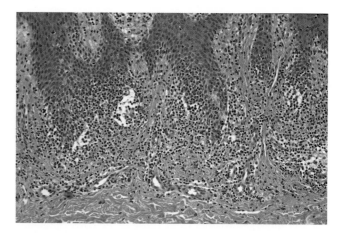

Figure 22.19 Mycosis fungoides in an adult patient simulating the histopathologic presentation of "annular lichenoid dermatitis of youth" (see text).

Interestingly, in adults with history of mycosis fungoides we have observed rarely onset of lesions with histopathologic features similar to those described in so-called annular lichenoid dermatitis of youth (Fig. 22.19).

CD8+ cutaneous infiltrates in human immunodeficiency virus (HIV)-infected patients

The onset of aggressive non-Hodgkin lymphomas, including skin lymphomas, has been described in patients with advanced HIV infection (see Chapter 15). Besides true lymphomas, in some patients a cutaneous eruption clinically and histopathologically similar to mycosis fungoides, but characterized by a predominance of CD8+ T lymphocytes has been observed [66,67]. The lymphocytes in these cases are polyclonal, indicating that this eruption is a cutaneous pseudolymphoma rather than a true T-cell lymphoma of the skin. CD8+ cutaneous infiltrates arise usually in HIV-infected patients with a profound CD4 lymphopenia and are considered as a bad prognostic sign for the underlying disease (the bad prognosis, however, may be linked to the very low CD4 count rather than to the skin lesions *per se*). PUVA, topical steroids and even chemotherapy have been used for the treatment of this uncommon condition [66]. Regression upon antiviral triple treatment has been observed [68]. A similar condition, but with monoclonal CD8+ T lymphocytes, has been observed in common variable immunodeficiency.

CD30+ T-cell pseudolymphomas

In recent years, the presence of CD30+ large blasts has been described in the skin in several reactive conditions. The most frequent causes are infections, particularly viral ones (orf,

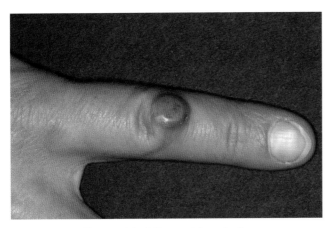

Figure 22.20 Milker's nodule. Solitary nodule on the finger.

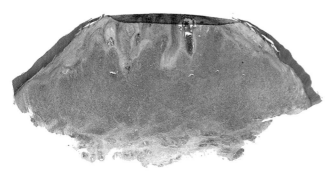

Figure 22.21 Milker's nodule. Epidermal hyperplasia, large telangiectatic vessels and dense infiltrate of lymphocytes.

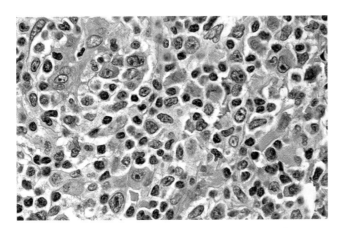

Figure 22.22 Milker's nodule. Note presence of large blastic cells (detail of Fig. 22.21).

milker's nodule, molluscum contagiosum, viral warts, herpes simplex, and herpes zoster among others), as well as arthropod reactions, scabies and drug eruptions (Figs 22.20–22.24) (see also specific sections) [69–74]. CD30+ cells have also been observed occasionally in many other cutaneous conditions, including among others hidradenitis, rhynophyma, and cysts, as well as at the sites of cutaneous abscess or of injury caused by red sea coral. We have rarely observed the presence of

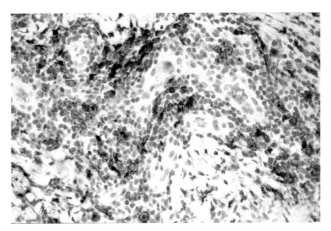

Figure 22.23 Milker's nodule. Positivity of the larger cells for CD30 (same case as Figs 22.21, 22.22).

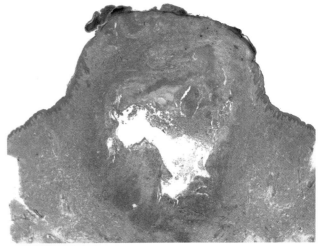

(a)

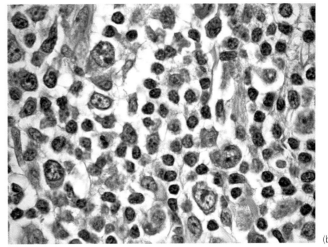

(b)

Figure 22.24 Molluscum contagiosum. (a) Cystic cavity with dense inflammatory reaction. (b) Note several large, activated lymphocytes (same case as Fig. 22.25).

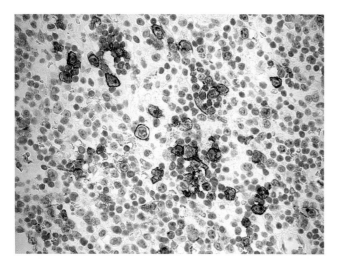

Figure 22.25 Molluscum contagiosum. Positivity for CD30 in several cells, partly arranged in small clusters (same case as Fig. 22.24).

dense lymphoid infiltrates with scattered CD30+ cells in skin lesions of mycotic infections as well. In fact, any reactive condition showing large, activated lymphoid cells may reveal positivity of the latter for CD30. The finding may be related, at least in part, to improved methods of antigen demasking and immunohistochemical staining of routinely fixed, paraffin-embedded sections of tissue (see Chapter 1).

Besides the presence of large atypical CD30+ cells, the histology in these lesions reveals the typical changes of the specific underlying disorder. Moreover, in these reactive conditions CD30+ lymphocytes are scattered throughout the infiltrate and are usually not arranged in clusters or sheets as observed in lymphomatoid papulosis or cutaneous anaplastic large cell lymphoma. However, in some cases clusters of large CD30+ lymphocytes may be observed, and differentiation may be very difficult or even impossible (Fig. 22.25). Unlike the situation in lymphomatoid papulosis and cutaneous anaplastic large cell lymphoma, gene rearrangement studies in CD30+ pseudolymphomas reveal the presence of a polyclonal population of T lymphocytes.

The therapy of CD30+ pseudolymphomas depends on the specific diagnosis and includes surgical excision, cryotherapy and antiviral treatment.

Pseudolymphomas in herpes simplex and herpes zoster infections

We have seen in consultation several cases of herpes simplex or herpes zoster infection that had been previously diagnosed as cutaneous lymphoma, usually aggressive cytotoxic NK/T-cell lymphoma or cutaneous CD30+ lymphoproliferative disorders (see previous section) [75]. Similar cases have been reported in the literature, particularly in immunocompromised patients [76–78]. As mentioned in the previous section, in

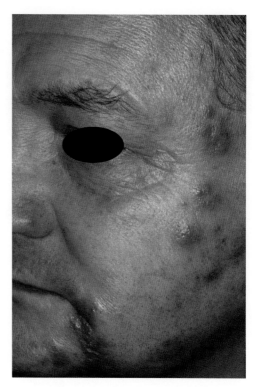

Figure 22.26 Herpes zoster presenting with follicular papules without vesiculation.

many of these cases a variable population of large CD30+ cells can be observed.

Clinical features may deviate from conventional presentation of herpes simplex or herpes zoster, as lesions may be papules rather than vesicles, and in immunocompromised patients may be vegetating, thus simulating a neoplastic process (Fig. 22.26). Histology may also be misleading, as in a proportion of cases typical cytopathic changes are missing or present only focally, particularly in lesions involving only the follicles or other adnexal structures (Fig. 22.27) [75,79]. Reassuring histopathologic features are represented by the presence of different cell types other than the large blastic elements (mixed cell infiltrate). Prominent necrosis may be observed. Immunohistologic investigations are less sensitive than molecular ones in confirming the viral etiology, and at present only antibodies for herpes simplex 1/2 are available, but not for the varicella zoster virus.

In the context of the discussion on cutaneous pseudolymphomas arising at the site of herpes simplex or herpes zoster infection, we would like to underline that most of the cases reported in the past as pseudolymphoma at the site of herpes zoster scar in patients with B-cell chronic lymphocytic leukemia (B-CLL) actually represent specific infiltrates of B-CLL at sites of previous herpes infections (see also Chapter 18).

Treatment of pseudolymphomas arising at sites of herpes simplex or herpes zoster infection should be achieved with conventional antiviral strategies used for these infections.

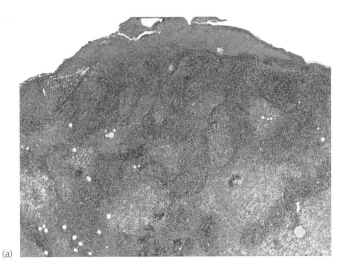

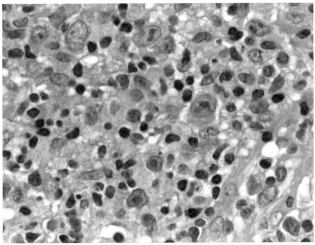

Figure 22.27 Herpes simplex. (a) Ulcerated lesion with dense lymphoid infiltrates. (b) Note several large, activated lymphocytes.

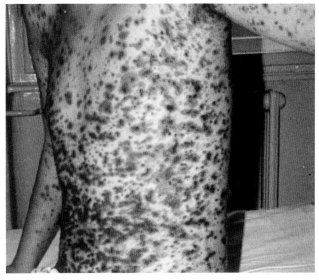

Figure 22.28 Pityriasis lichenoides et varioliformis acuta, ulceronecrotic variant. Confluent hemorrhagic, partly ulcerated lesions on the entire body.

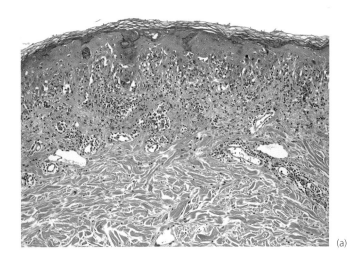

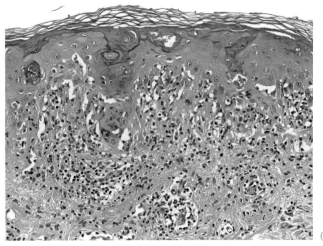

Figure 22.29 Pityriasis lichenoides et varioliformis acuta, ulceronecrotic variant. (a) Acute lesion with several necrotic keratinocytes and superficial lymphoid infiltrates. (b) Note exocytosis of lymphocytes.

Pityriasis lichenoides

The exact nosology of pityriasis lichenoides et varioliformis acuta (PLEVA) (Mucha–Habermann disease) has been the source of considerable debate [80–83]. Many reports demonstrated that in some cases the T lymphocytes of PLEVA are monoclonally rearranged [80–84]. Evolution of PLEVA into cytotoxic mycosis fungoides has been documented, and some authors suggested that the disease may represent yet another variant of the cutaneous T-cell lymphomas [85]. On the other hand, in some reports of "atypical" PLEVA the exact diagnosis and classification of the cases were questionable (see Chapter 4) [86,87]. It has been suggested that at least one variant of PLEVA, the so-called febrile ulceronecrotic type, may be related to the cutaneous cytotoxic lymphomas (Figs 22.28, 22.29) [88–90]. In fact, patients may die of this disease (although not from lymphoma-specific causes), and the clinicopathologic features resemble those of other cytotoxic lymphomas (although the infiltrates are never as dense or as deep, nor is cytomorphology as atypical). Transition between "conventional" PLEVA and the febrile ulceronecrotic form has been reported [90]. A definitive conclusion cannot be reached at present. In this context, patients with classic PLEVA should not be overdiagnosed nor treated as having a cutaneous T-cell lymphoma, as the disease is most likely of an inflammatory (or infectious) nature and behaves in a benign fashion. In contrast, patients with the febrile ulceronecrotic variant of PLEVA should be monitored carefully and require more aggressive treatment, such as methotrexate. One case has been successfully treated with oral ciclosporin [91]. Death from complications may ensue in these patients in spite of aggressive, early treatment.

The presence of CD30+ cells within lesions of PLEVA or variants has been the source of debate, as this immunohistochemical staining is considered a valid tool for the differential diagnosis of PLEVA from lymphomatoid papulosis. Although some of these cases probably represented genuine manifestations of lymphomatoid papulosis [86,87], some convincing cases of CD30+ PLEVA have been published [92]. If compelling clinicopathologic features of PLEVA are present, the presence of a few CD30+ cells within the infiltrate should not be a reason for changing the diagnosis.

Atypical forms of PLEVA in children should be treated with great caution, as in some patients progression to typical mycosis fungoides has been documented (see also section on mycosis fungoides in children in Chapter 2). In these cases the PLEVA-like manifestations probably represented a clinicopathologic variant of mycosis fungoides from the outset.

Lupus panniculitis

Patients with lupus erythematosus may rarely present with prominent involvement of the subcutaneous tissues, a condition that has been termed lupus panniculitis or lupus profundus. Lupus panniculitis reveals subcutaneous plaques and indurations, mostly located on the extremities, which can simulate clinically and histopathologically those observed in subcutaneous "panniculitis-like" T-cell lymphoma (see Chapter 5) (Fig. 22.30) [93,94]. Antinuclear antibodies (ANA) and other clinical and/or serologic criteria for the diagnosis of systemic lupus erythematosus are absent in many of these cases. Histology shows a predominantly lobular panniculitis, often with concomitant presence of broadened fibrotic septa. Necrosis may be a prominent feature. A useful characteristic for the differentiation of subcutaneous "panniculitis-like" T-cell lymphoma from lupus panniculitis is the presence in the former of so-called "rimming" of fat cells by pleomorphic, atypical T lymphocytes that are positive for proliferation markers. In this context, it must be remembered that rimming of fat lobuli by lymphocytes is not a diagnostic feature *per se*, as it can be observed in several benign and malignant

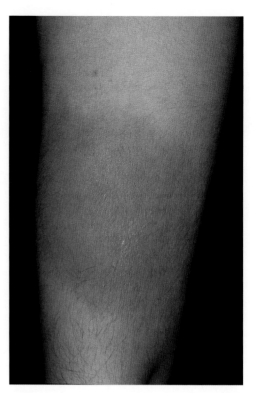

Figure 22.30 Lupus panniculitis. Erythematous infiltrated plaque on the leg.

lymphoid infiltrates with involvement of the subcutaneous fat [95].

In contrast to subcutaneous "panniculitis-like" T-cell lymphoma, B cells, plasma cells and germinal centers are usually a prominent feature in lupus panniculitis (Figs 22.31, 22.32). The B cells are typically arranged in nodules (with or without germinal centers) located at the periphery of the lobules (Fig. 22.33). For practical purposes, the finding of such clusters of B lymphocytes rules out the diagnosis of subcutaneous "panniculitis-like" T-cell lymphoma. The proliferation rate is low and proliferating cells are not arranged around the adipocytes (Fig. 22.34). In lupus panniculitis the dermoepidermal junction may show features of lupus erythematosus (interface dermatitis). Analysis of TCR gene rearrangement reveals polyclonal populations of T lymphocytes in lupus panniculitis, in contrast to subcutaneous "panniculitis-like" T-cell lymphoma where monoclonality of T lymphocytes is found in most cases.

Although lupus panniculitis and subcutaneous "panniculitis-like" T-cell lymphoma can be differentiated in most cases, we have come across patients who presented with clinical features suggestive of lupus erythematosus (e.g. positivity of ANA and/or subsets, features of lupus erythematosus in organs other than the skin such as lupus nephritis, etc.) and at the same time lesions diagnostic of subcutaneous "panniculitis-like" T-cell lymphoma. These patients present formidable difficulties in diagnosis, as features of both diseases

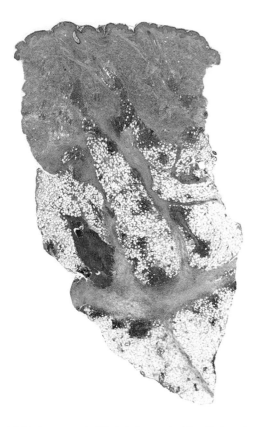

Figure 22.31 Lupus panniculitis. Lobular panniculitis with dense lymphoid infiltrates and fibrotic septa.

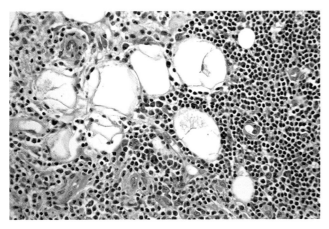

Figure 22.32 Lupus panniculitis. Note mixed-cell infiltrate with lymphocytes, histiocytes, neutrophils and several plasma cells (detail of Fig. 22.31).

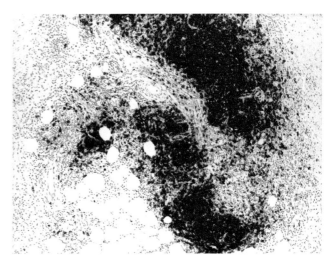

Figure 22.33 Lupus panniculitis. Large clusters of CD20$^+$ B lymphocytes.

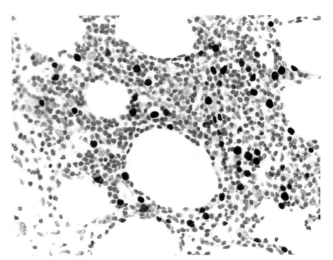

Figure 22.34 Lupus panniculitis. Staining for Ki67 shows proliferation of a minority of the cells. Note absence of "rimming" of proliferating cells around the adipocytes.

Lymphomatoid drug reactions

A pseudolymphoma syndrome characterized by generalized lymphadenopathy, hepatosplenomegaly, leukocytosis, fever, malaise, arthralgia, severe edema of the face and cutaneous lesions such as erythematous pruritic macules, papules and nodules has been described in patients treated with anticonvulsants, particularly hydantoin derivatives [96,97]. Many other drugs may induce lymphoid infiltrates in the skin that simulate malignant lymphoma clinically and/or histopathologically [41,98–100]. The external use of etheric plant oils may also cause lymphoproliferative reactions that mimic malignant lymphomas, clinically and histologically.

Lymphomatoid drug eruptions may present with a T- or B-cell pattern, simulating either mycosis fungoides, Sézary syndrome, follicle center lymphoma or marginal zone B-cell

are present concomitantly. We believe that a subset of patients with lupus erythematosus may develop specific infiltrates of subcutaneous "panniculitis-like" T-cell lymphoma, but the exact frequency of this association is yet unclear (see also Chapter 5).

Treatment of lupus panniculitis is similar to that of other variants of lupus erythematosus. The lesions respond well to systemic steroids but recurrences are the rule.

lymphoma [101–107]. A rare type of lymphomatoid drug eruption with many CD30+ cells may simulate the CD30+ cutaneous lymphoproliferative disorders [70]. It should be noted that the same drug may be responsible for cutaneous lesions with different histopathologic features and phenotypes in different patients.

Clinically, patients present with generalized papules, plaques or nodules (Fig. 22.35) or even erythroderma [108]. A digitate dermatitis-like pattern has also been observed [106]. Accentuation of skin changes in sun-exposed areas may occur.

Histopathologically, pseudolymphomatous drug eruptions are characterized by dense band-like nodular or diffuse infiltrates of lymphocytes, sometimes with atypical cells, revealing a T- or B-cell pattern (Figs 22.36, 22.37). Eosinophils may or may not be present. In some cases, the histopathologic changes may be those of lymphadenosis benigna cutis with formation of reactive germinal centers (Fig. 22.38). Cases presenting with band-like infiltrates and simulating mycosis fungoides histopathologically usually show higher degrees of atypia than genuine examples of patch-stage mycosis fungoides ("too atypical to be early mycosis fungoides"). Clinicopathologic correlation is diagnostic in most such cases. Molecular analysis of J_H and TCR genes usually shows a polyclonal pattern.

Lymphomatoid drug reactions invariably regress when the offending drug is withdrawn and recur if the same or a similar compound is reintroduced.

Rarely, the development of a true cutaneous lymphoma has been recorded in relation to the use of drugs that commonly

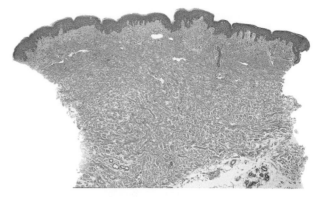

Figure 22.36 Lymphomatoid drug eruption, T-cell type. Patchy lichenoid infiltrate of lymphocytes without epidermotropism within the superficial dermis.

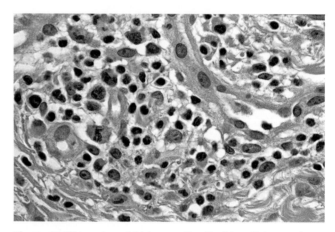

Figure 22.37 Lymphomatoid drug eruption, T-cell type. Note several atypical lymphocytes and one mitotic figure (detail of Fig. 22.36).

induce lymphomatoid drug eruptions [109]. In these cases, the skin lesions do not regress upon discontinuation of the drug.

It should be noted that we have observed drug eruptions characterized by a remarkable nuclear atypia and high proliferation of the cells (>80%). On the other hand, patients with systemic leukemias/lymphomas (or cutaneous lymphomas in advanced stages) may present with drug eruptions characterized by colonization of the skin lesions by neoplastic cells. In short, the interplay between the immune system (in both normal and neoplastic conditions) and drugs that induce immune reactions is probably much more complicated than the dichotomy benign/malignant implies, and we routinely evaluate patients with markedly atypical lymphomatoid drug eruptions in order to exclude the presence of an occult hematologic disease.

Lymphocytoma cutis

Several synonyms have been used for lymphocytoma cutis including lymphadenosis benigna cutis, cutaneous lymphoplasia, cutaneous lymphoid hyperplasia and pseudolymphoma

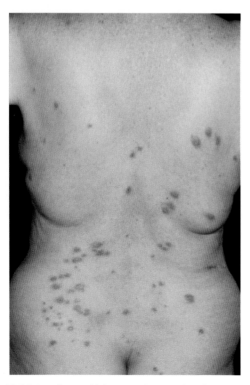

Figure 22.35 Lymphomatoid drug eruption. Papules, plaques and nodules on the back.

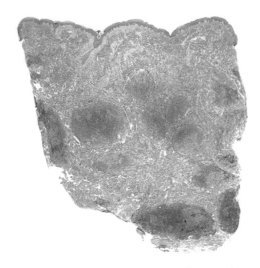

Figure 22.38 Lymphomatoid drug eruption, B-cell type. Nodular infiltrates of lymphocytes with reactive germinal centers. (Courtesy of Dr Dieter Metze, Münster, Germany.)

of Spiegler-Fendt. Various antigenic stimuli can induce these lesions: insect bites, drugs, vaccinations, acupuncture, wearing of gold pierced earrings, medicinal leech therapy and tattoos [110–112]. One of the most common associations, particularly in endemic countries, is found with the spirochete *B. burgdorferi* [13,113].

Women are affected more commonly than men. There are numerous clinical presentations of lymphocytoma cutis.

Frequently, a firm solitary lesion can be observed although lesions may be clustered in a region or, rarely, be scattered widely. There is usually a nodule or tumor although papules or plaques may also be observed, sometimes with a symmetric distribution [114]. The color varies from reddish brown to reddish purple. Scaling and ulceration are absent.

Involvement of particular body sites (earlobe, nipple, scrotum) is almost pathognomonic of *B. burgdorferi*-associated lymphocytoma cutis (Figs 22.39, 22.40) [113]. The *B. burgdorferi*-associated type of lymphocytoma cutis often occurs in children and is the most frequent pseudolymphoma in this age group in regions with endemic *B. burgdorferi* infection.

Histologic examination shows dense, nodular, mixed-cell infiltrates, often with the formation of lymphoid follicles (Fig. 22.41). Although the infiltrates may be "top-heavy," in *B. burgdorferi*-associated lymphocytoma cutis there are frequently dense, diffuse lymphoid infiltrates involving the entire dermis and superficial subcutaneous fat (Fig. 22.42). In addition, in these lesions the reactive germinal centers are commonly devoid of mantle zones and may show confluence,

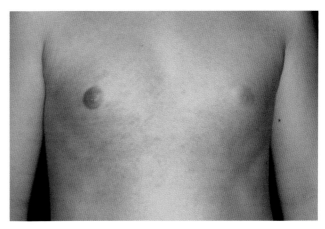

Figure 22.40 Lymphocytoma cutis associated with infection by *Borrelia burgdorferi*. Erythematous nodule on the right nipple.

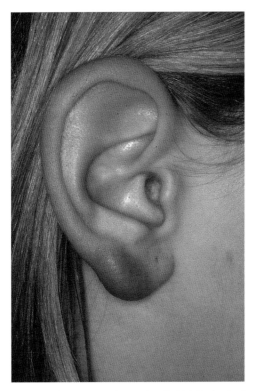

Figure 22.39 Lymphocytoma cutis associated with infection by *Borrelia burgdorferi*. Erythematous nodule on the right earlobe.

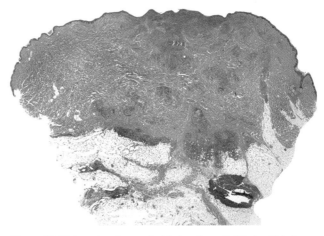

Figure 22.41 Lymphocytoma cutis. Wedge-shaped infiltrate within the entire dermis. Note small regular germinal centers.

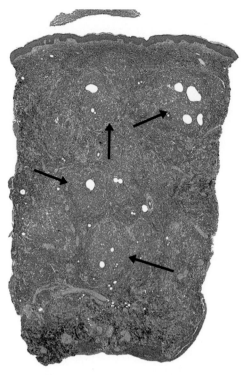

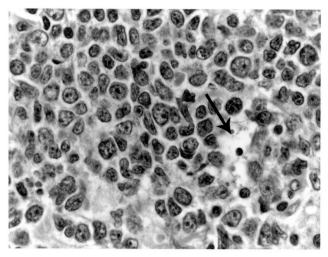

Figure 22.43 Lymphocytoma cutis associated with infection by *Borrelia burgdorferi*. Large blastic cells (centroblasts, large centrocytes) admixed with "tingible body" macrophages characterized by large empty spaces with nests of apoptotic cells (*arrow*).

Figure 22.42 Lymphocytoma cutis associated with infection by *Borrelia burgdorferi*. Dense diffuse lymphoid infiltrate with prominent follicular structures devoid of a mantle (*arrows*).

simulating the picture of a large B-cell lymphoma (Fig. 22.43) [113,115]. Plasma cells and eosinophils are found in almost all cases as well as a distinct population of T lymphocytes, features that represent useful clues for the differential diagnosis.

Immunohistology reveals a normal phenotype of germinal center cells (CD20+, CD10+, Bcl-6+, Bcl-2−), normal (high) proliferation, and polytypical expression of immunoglobulin

light-chains (Figs 22.44, 22.45). A regular network of follicular dendritic cells can be highlighted with stainings for CD21 or CD35. A prominent population of reactive T lymphocytes is always present. Molecular analysis of the J_H gene rearrangement shows a polyclonal pattern in most (but not all) cases [13].

Lymphocytoma cutis may resolve spontaneously in several months or years. Small nodules can be removed by surgical excision, and local injection of corticosteroids or interferon-α may result in regression. Cryosurgery and topical tacrolimus have also been applied with success [116,117]. Patients with lesions of lymphocytoma cutis and evidence of *B. burgdorferi* (detection of serum antibodies by enzyme-linked immunosorbent assay (ELISA) or immunoblotting or of *Borrelia* DNA

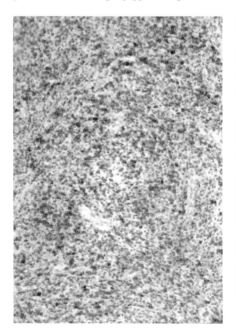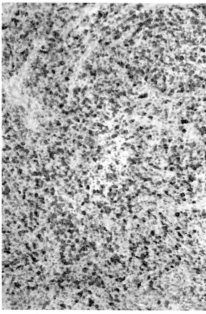

Figure 22.44 Lymphocytoma cutis associated with infection by *Borrelia burgdorferi*. Polyclonal expression of immunoglobulin light-chains κ and λ.

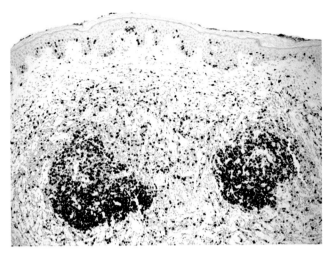

Figure 22.45 Lymphocytoma cutis associated with infection by *Borrelia burgdorferi*. Germinal centers with normal (high) proliferation rate. Note absence of mantle and polarization of the staining reflecting the presence of normal dark and light areas within the germinal centers.

by PCR) can be treated with doxycycline, erythromycin or ceftriaxone. In refractory lesions, a very effective treatment method is radiotherapy.

Rarely *B. burgdorferi* may be the cause of a systemic pseudolymphomatous syndrome that recedes after antibiotic treatment [118].

Persistent nodular arthropod bite reactions and nodular scabies

The most typical example of this group of lymphomatoid infiltrates is nodular scabies, but many other arthropods can induce skin lesions that may simulate malignant lymphoma histopathologically. Clinically, in nodular scabies, elevated

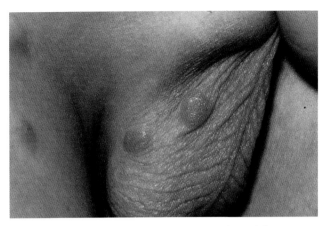

Figure 22.46 Typical lesions of nodular scabies on the genital area.

round or oval bright reddish papules and nodules occur most frequently on the genitalia, elbows and in the axillae (Fig. 22.46). The lesions are found in approximately 7% of patients with scabies. The nodules are very pruritic and may persist for many months.

The mite and its parts are seldom identified in the long-standing papules or nodules of scabies. The clinical differential diagnosis includes prurigo nodularis and malignant lymphoma; some lesions of secondary syphilis may be diagnosed incorrectly as a pseudolymphoma of this type.

Histopathologically, dense superficial and deep perivascular lymphohistiocytic infiltrates with plasma cells and varying numbers of eosinophils are seen (Figs 22.47, 22.48) [119]. Eosinophils are also scattered among collagen bundles. Prominent vessels with thickened walls lined by plump endothelial cells are nearly always found. The epidermis may be slightly spongiotic, hyperplastic and hyperkeratotic. Large atypical lymphocytes can be observed. The histologic features of nodular scabies may mimic those of mycosis fungoides, lymphomatoid papulosis or Hodgkin lymphoma. Occasionally,

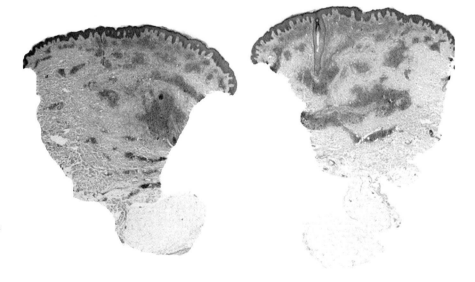

Figure 22.47 The nodular lesions of scabies infiltrate deeply into the dermis and are composed of a mixture of lymphocytes, macrophages, plasma cells and eosinophils.

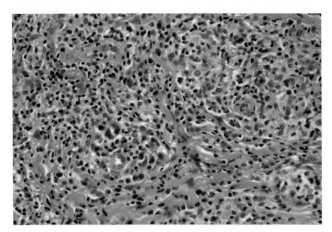

Figure 22.48 Nodular scabies. Note some atypical lymphocytes and many eosinophils (detail of Fig. 22.47).

a B-cell pattern analogous to lymphocytoma cutis can be recognized in persistent nodular arthropod bite reactions.

Immunohistologic investigations reveal that T lymphocytes predominate in nodular scabies. Although previous reports claimed that the use of antibodies for CD30 differentiated the skin lesions of persistent arthropod bites from those of lymphomatoid papulosis, because the first are negative while the latter are positive [120], in truth in most (if not all) cases of scabies, as well as in other arthropod bite reactions, the CD30 antigen is expressed by the large lymphoid cells.

Antiscabietic therapy is usually ineffective in cases caused by *Sarcoptes scabiei*. Large nodules may be excised surgically. Intralesional injection of corticosteroids may be helpful. Spontaneous resolution in time is the rule for all persistent arthropod bite reactions.

Pseudolymphomas at sites of vaccination

Rarely, a florid inflammatory reaction develops at sites of vaccinations [121]. Clinically, lesions may show either superficial papules or nodules, or subcutaneous tumors [111,121]. The histopathologic pattern may be lichenoid, simulating that seen in mycosis fungoides, or nodular with the formation of germinal centers, simulating a follicle center lymphoma (Fig. 22.49) [122]. The germinal centers, however, display reactive features (well-formed mantle zone, presence of tingible body macrophages and of polarization, high proliferation). In contrast to follicle center lymphoma, Bcl-6$^+$ germinal center cells are not observed outside the germinal centers. Other characteristic histopathologic features are represented by the presence of areas of degeneration and fibrosis surrounded by a histiocytic reaction characterized by macrophages with granular basophilic cytoplasm (Fig. 22.50) [121]. The presence of macrophages with these peculiar features strongly suggests the causative role of aluminum-adsorbed vaccines in the occurrence of this type of pseudolymphoma [122].

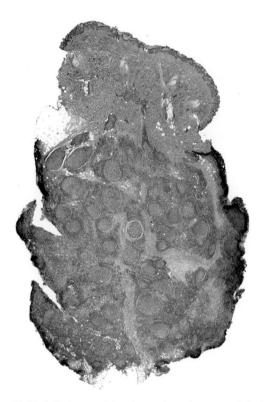

Figure 22.49 Follicular pseudolymphoma after subcutaneous injection of vaccine. Dense nodular infiltrate of lymphocytes with follicular pattern.

It is believed that pseudolymphomas after vaccination represent a form of local reactive hyperplasia or a persisting delayed hypersensitivity reaction to a vaccine constituent. Lesions may arise after injection of different vaccines, including those used for allergen hyposensitization [123]. We have observed the onset of bilateral lesions of lymphocytoma cutis at the skin sites of different injections of early summer meningoencephalitis ("Früh Sommer Meningo-Encephalitis" – FSME) vaccinations performed after an interval of over 1 year [121].

Lesions tend to persist unchanged for months or years. Intralesional steroids may be ineffective.

Pseudolymphomas in tattoos

Besides granulomatous infiltrates, inflammatory reactions to tattoos may sometimes reveal lymphoid follicular structures or a mycosis fungoides-like pattern (Figs 22.51, 22.52) [113,124–126]. Red tattoo pigment (cinnabar) is most frequently (but not always) responsible for the lymphomatoid infiltrate. The presence of pigment suggests the correct diagnosis. A well-documented case of cutaneous lymphoma arising in a tattoo has been reported, so careful follow-up of these lesions is necessary [127]. The management of pseudolymphomas in tattoos can be very difficult because of the large areas of skin involved in some patients. Intralesional

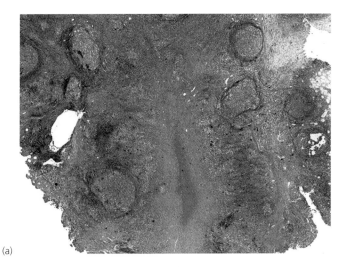

(a)

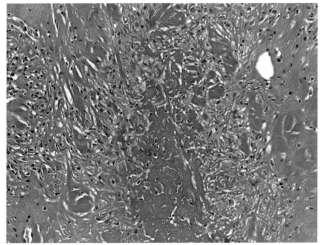

(b)

Figure 22.50 Pseudolymphoma after vaccination. (a) Central area of necrosis surrounded by reactive germinal centers. (b) Detail of necrotic area with several macrophages with basophilic granular cytoplasm (see text).

steroid injections, laser vaporization or surgical excision of small lesions may be used for treatment.

Acral pseudolymphomatous angiokeratoma (small papular pseudolymphoma)

Acral pseudolymphomatous angiokeratoma (termed originally "acral pseudolymphomatous angiokeratoma in children" – APACHE) is characterized by unilateral, clustered, red-violaceous papules and small nodules usually located on the hands and feet of children [128–132]. The etiology is unknown. Histopathologic investigations reveal a dense nodular lymphoid infiltrate with occasional plasma cells and eosinophils (Fig. 22.53). A proliferation of capillaries can be observed. The term angiokeratoma is misleading; based on the distinctive clinicopathologic features the more correct (but non-specific) designation "small papular pseudolymphoma"

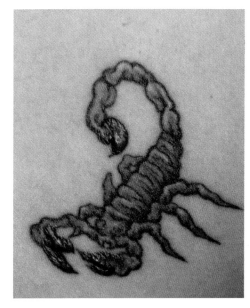

Figure 22.51 Pseudolymphoma within a tattoo. Onset of several papules and small plaques in the red pigmented areas of the tattoo.

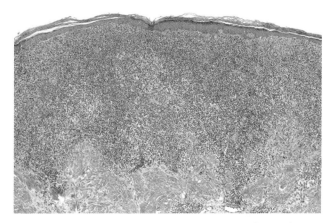

Figure 22.52 Pseudolymphoma within a tattoo. Dense infiltrate of lymphocytes simulating a cutaneous lymphoma.

has been suggested for this benign lymphoproliferative disease [129]. There may be some overlap with solitary T-cell pseudolymphomas (see above) but a variable amount of B lymphocytes, sometimes predominating over the T cells, is found within the inflammatory infiltrate [133]. Lesions can be treated by cryotherapy, surgical excision or laser vaporization.

Localized scleroderma/morphea

In the inflammatory stage of connective tissue diseases, especially in localized scleroderma, dense lymphoid infiltrates may be observed, simulating cutaneous lymphomas (particularly cutaneous marginal zone B-cell lymphoma) histopathologically (Fig. 22.54) [134,135]. Plasma cells are almost invariably present and reveal a polyclonal pattern of immunoglobulin

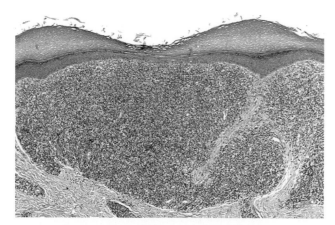

Figure 22.53 Acral pseudolymphomatous angiokeratoma (small papular pseudolymphoma). Nodular lymphoid infiltrate in the superficial and mid-dermis of acral skin.

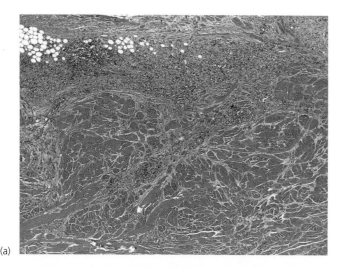

(a)

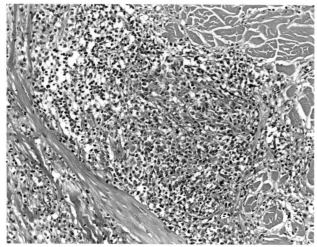

(b)

Figure 22.54 Morphea, inflammatory stage. (a) Sclerosis of the collagen fibers and dense lymphoid infiltrates. (b) Details of lymphoid infiltrates with several plasma cells.

light-chain expression. Sclerosis of the collagen bundles may not be prominent in the early stages of morphea, thus causing problems in the differential diagnosis. Correlation with the clinical picture confirms the diagnosis. Treatment does not differ from the conventional therapy of the disease.

Secondary syphilis

Rarely, cutaneous lesions in secondary syphilis may show dense lymphoplasmacellular infiltrates simulating histopathologically the picture of a cutaneous marginal zone B-cell lymphoma (Figs 22.55, 22.56) [136–138]. Two histopathological patterns in particular should raise suspicion of a possible pseudolymphomatous syphilis: the first is characterized by features of interface/lichenoid dermatitis in conjunction with presence of dense lymphoid infiltrates admixed with plasma cells; the second shows granulomatous features associated with dense inflammatory infiltrates with plasma cells. These plasma cells always reveal a polyclonal pattern of immunoglobulin light-chain expression, and immunohistologic staining for *Treponema pallidum* reveals variable numbers of microorganisms. Positivity of serologic tests for syphilis confirms the diagnosis, and antibiotic treatment leads to a rapid resolution of the lesions. In addition to histopathologic pitfalls, secondary

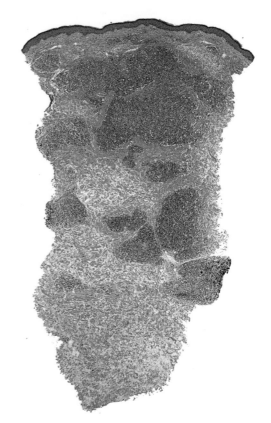

Figure 22.55 Pseudolymphoma in secondary syphilis. Dense nodular lymphoid infiltrates throughout the entire dermis.

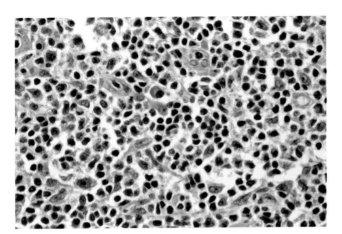

Figure 22.56 Pseudolymphoma in secondary syphilis. Lymphocytes and histiocytes admixed with several plasma cells (detail of Fig. 22.55).

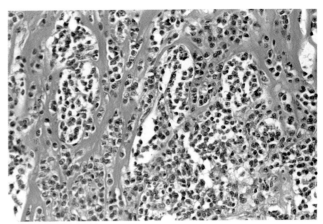

Figure 22.57 Inflammatory pseudotumor of the skin (plasma cell granuloma). Fibrotic areas with numerous plasma cells.

syphilis may rarely present with nodular infiltrates simulating a lymphoma clinically. A case published recently showed the clinical presentation of so-called "facies leonina," similar to what can be observed in specific manifestations of B-cell chronic lymphocytic leukemia (B-CLL) (see Chapter 18) [139].

Although the vast majority of cases of pseudolymphoma in syphilis occur in the secondary stage of the disease, in the past we have observed pseudolymphomatous infiltrates in late (tertiary) manifestations of it (gumma syphilitica with dense sheets of lymphocytes admixed with plasma cells), and recently in primary syphilis on the genital skin. In these last cases the histopathologic features simulated those of a CD30+ cutaneous lymphoproliferative disease (spectrum lymphomatoid papulosis/anaplastic large cell lymphoma). Cases of so-called "malignant syphilis", too, can simulate the picture of a cutaneous aggressive cytotoxic lymphoma. In such cases usually the diagnosis has not been suspected clinically (hence the biopsy), and staining with antibodies for *Treponema pallidum* helps establishing the correct diagnosis.

Cutaneous inflammatory pseudotumor (plasma cell granuloma)

Cutaneous inflammatory pseudotumor is a term that in previous years encompassed at least two main entities: plasma cell granuloma and inflammatory myofibroblastic tumor [140,141]. However, these two diseases should not be lumped within the same diagnostic group, as inflammatory myofibroblastic tumor is a neoplasm of intermediate biologic potential that frequently recurs and rarely can metastasize [142], whereas plasma cell granuloma is a fully benign condition. In this section we will only mention cutaneous plasma cell granuloma, as cutaneous myofibroblastic tumor is not a histopathologic simulator of malignant lymphomas.

Plasma cell granuloma can simulate the histopathologic picture of the plasmacytic variant of marginal zone B-cell

lymphoma or of secondary skin manifestations of multiple myeloma [143]. Some cases of plasma cell granuloma may represent postinfective reactions to different micro-organisms (Epstein–Barr virus, *B. burgdorferi*, mycobacteria, human herpesvirus (HHV)-8).

Clinically, patients with plasma cell granuloma present with firm cutaneous or subcutaneous nodules of long duration. On histopathologic examination, circumscribed nodules with thick hyalinized collagen bundles and a dense inflammatory infiltrate with lymphocytes, sheets of plasma cells and occasionally germinal centers can be observed (Fig. 22.57). Immunohistology reveals polyclonal expression of immunoglobulin light-chains. Molecular analyses do not reveal monoclonality of the infiltrate.

Surgical excision of the lesions results in cure.

Cutaneous plasmacytosis

Cutaneous plasmacytosis is a condition reported almost exclusively in Japan or rarely other Asiatic countries and associated with polyclonal plasma cell infiltrates in the skin [144–146]. If extracutaneous involvement is observed, then the disease is classified as systemic plasmacytosis, a syndrome characterized by a benign plasma cell proliferation with polyclonal hypogammaglobulinemia, cutaneous lesions, generalized lymphadenopathy, systemic symptoms such as fever, fatigue and weight loss, and possible involvement of other organs including the spleen, liver, retroperitoneum, and lung. Clinically, cutaneous plasmacytosis is characterized by multiple red-brown plaques and nodules located mainly on the trunk. The lesions are asymptomatic. Histopathologically, the lesions show variably dense superficial and deep infiltrates composed mostly of mature plasma cells without atypical features (Fig. 22.58). The plasma cells reveal a polyclonal pattern of immunoglobulin light-chain expression. Cutaneous marginal zone B-cell lymphoma, plasmacytic

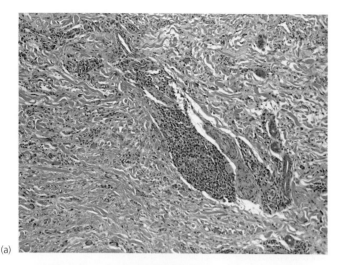

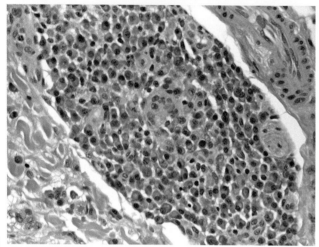

Figure 22.58 Cutaneous plasmacytosis. (a) Dense perivascular infiltrates of plasma cells. (b) Normal plasma cells without atypical features.

variant, may be a differential diagnostic concern in these cases, but the absence of immunoglobulin light-chain restriction is a helpful clue for the correct diagnosis.

The exact nosology of cutaneous plasmacytosis is still unclear. It has been suggested that the disease may represent a particular variant of plasma cell-type multicentric Castleman disease involving the skin. [147]. In this context, it is interesting to note that elevated serum levels of interleukin-6 have been found in patients with cutaneous plasmacytosis, similar to what can be observed in multicentric Castleman disease. In contrast to Castleman disease, however, presence of HHV-8 was not demonstrated in lesions of cutaneous plasmacytosis (however, in this study only immunohistologic stainings were performed) [145].

Treatment of cutaneous plasmacytosis has been described only in anecdotal reports. Successful results have been obtained with topical PUVA therapy, melphalan, a combination of prednisone and cyclophosphamide [148], and intralesional steroids, as well as with new drugs such as topical pimecrolimus [149].

Lymphocytic infiltration of the skin/lupus tumidus

Lymphocytic infiltration of the skin (Jessner–Kanof) can be confused histopathologically mainly with specific skin manifestations of B-CLL (Fig. 22.59a). The co-expression of CD20, CD5 and CD43 by the B cells of B-CLL as well as the detection of a monoclonal rearrangement of the J_H gene, in contrast to the predominance of polyclonal T lymphocytes in lymphocytic infiltration of the skin, helps to clearly distinguish these diseases. Clusters of CD123$^+$ plasmacytoid monocytes are present in lymphocytic infiltration of the skin but not in cutaneous lesions of B-CLL (Fig. 22.59b).

Interestingly, at the 2008 meeting of the Swiss Dermatologic Society a case of lymphocytic infiltration progressing to cutaneous marginal zone B-cell lymphoma was presented, drawing attention to the CD123$^+$ plasmacytoid dendritic

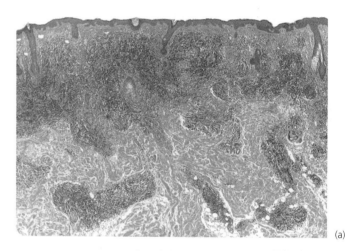

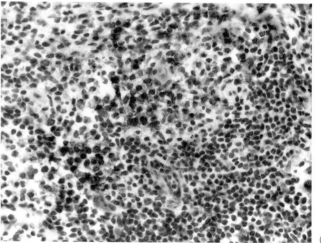

Figure 22.59 Lupus erythematosus, tumidus type (so-called lymphocytic infiltration of Jessner–Kanof). (a) Note dense infiltrates around the vessels and appendageal structures in the entire dermis. (b) Staining for CD123 highlights clusters of plasmacytoid dendritic cells.

cells, that are present in both diseases, as a possible common denominator between the two entities. We must underline, however, that we have never observed a similar case, and that the association may have been fortuitous.

It has been proposed that lymphocytic infiltration of the skin and lupus erythematosus tumidus represent one and the same disease [150], an interpretation that we fully share. Atypical lymphoid infiltrates can be observed also in patients with chronic discoid lupus erythematosus, but other features of lupus dermatitis allow one to make the correct diagnosis. In these cases, the presence of clusters of CD123+ plasmacytoid dendritic cells is a helpful clue for the diagnosis of lupus dermatitis.

Cutaneous extramedullary hematopoiesis

The skin may rarely be the site of onset of extramedullary hematopoiesis, a disorder caused by abnormal hematopoiesis in the bone marrow often due to chronic myeloproliferative or myelodysplastic disorders, particularly chronic idiopathic myelofibrosis [151]. Both the clinical and the histopathologic presentations may simulate cutaneous manifestations of myeloid leukemia. Clinically there are red-livid papules, plaques or even tumors on the entire body. Histology shows in the dermis the presence of bone marrow precursor cells deriving from all three lineages (erythroblasts, megakaryoblasts, and myeloid precursors) (Fig. 22.60). In contrast to leukemic infiltrates, these cells usually do not form sheets or large nodules, and are found scattered between the collagen bundles. Immunohistologic stainings for CD41, CD42b or CD61 allows identification of the megakaryoblasts, whereas erythroblasts may be stained by antibodies against hemoglobin or glycophorin [152]. Myeloid precursors can be identified by markers such as CD68, myeloperoxidase, lysozyme, CD14, CD34, CD117 and CD163; differentiation from myeloid

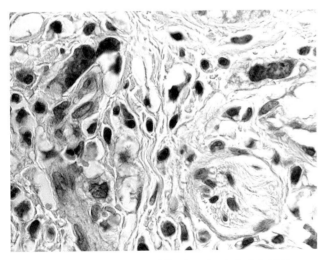

Figure 22.60 Cutaneous extramedullary hematopoiesis. Note large megakaryoblast and other immature cells.

leukemia can be achieved only by comparing the morphology with the phenotype of the cells and integrating it with clinical data, as neoplastic cells of myeloid leukemias may express similar antigens.

Extramedullary hematopoiesis (usually restricted to one lineage only) has also been observed in the background of cutaneous pilomatricoma, involuting congenital hemangioma, pyogenic granuloma, and leg ulcers in otherwise healthy individuals. The prognosis of cutaneous trilineage extramedullary hematopoiesis is usually poor. Patients have been managed with radiation therapy, but treatment of the underlying condition is often difficult.

Reactive angio-endotheliomatosis/ intravascular histiocytosis

In rare cases, an intravascular proliferation of endothelial cells and/or histiocytes may mimic the histopathologic picture of intravascular large cell lymphoma (reactive angio-endotheliomatosis, intravascular histiocytosis) (see also Chapter 14) (Fig. 22.61) [153,154]. Lesions may arise on the background of disparate conditions including chronic cutaneous infections, autoimmune disorders or other systemic diseases [155,156]. Immunohistologic and molecular analyses allow a clear-cut distinction from intravascular large cell lymphomas (Fig. 22.62). Management of the lesions is dependent on the associated disorder but sometimes skin lesions do not show improvement upon successful treatment of the background condition [155].

Benign intravascular proliferation of lymphoid blasts

Two unique cases of intravascular proliferation of large lymphoid cells simulating the picture of intravascular large cell lymphoma have been published recently [157,158]. One case was characterized by strong positivity of the intravascular cells for CD30. The lesions were considered benign because of the lack of other signs of intravascular large cell lymphoma, the favorable course at follow-up, the unusual clinical presentation (at the site of trauma on the arm in one case, within an endometrial polyp in the second), and the lack of clonal T-cell rearrangement. Prof. Facchetti (Brescia, Italy) recently showed to one of us (LC) a similar case arising within a granuloma pyogenicum, demonstrating that this phenomenon may be less rare than previously thought (Ardighieri L. *et al.*, *J Cut Pathol*, in press). We must admit that definitive proof of benignancy in these cases is lacking, as it is well known that intravascular lymphoma may arise within both hemangiomas and capillaries of solid tumors. High proliferative activity, found in the original case published by Bryant *et al.* [157] as well as in the one that we reviewed, adds uncertainty to the exact classification of these lesions. In the case that we reviewed, unlike typical intravascular large cell lymphoma, the proliferation of large cells was confined almost exclusively

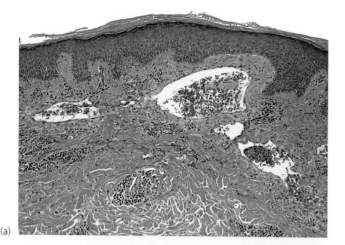

(a)

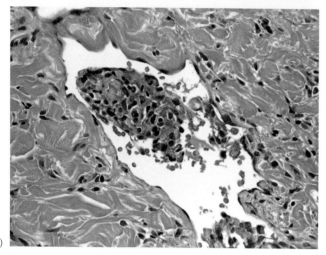

(b)

Figure 22.61 Intravascular histiocytosis. (a) Large intravascular clusters of cells. (b) Detail showing intravascular mid-sized cells with abundant cytoplasm admixed with small lymphocytes (same case as Fig. 22.62).

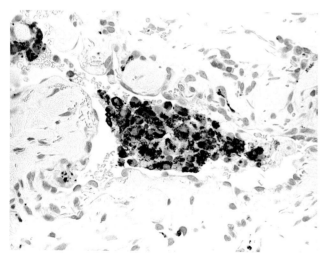

Figure 22.62 Intravascular histiocytosis. Positivity of the intravascular cells for CD68 confirms their histiocytic differentiation (same case as Fig. 22.61).

to podoplanine-positive lymphatic vessels, whereas blood vessels were not involved.

Other cutaneous pseudolymphomas

In addition to the cutaneous pseudolymphomas discussed in the previous paragraphs, the occurrence of other skin conditions clinically and/or histopathologically simulating cutaneous lymphomas has been reported sporadically, particularly in infectious disorders. Besides lymphocytoma cutis, infection by *Borrelia burgdorferi* may cause pseudolymphomatous infiltrates (mimicking cutaneous marginal zone B-cell lymphoma) in patients with acrodermatitis chronica atrophicans. The lesions clinically resemble those observed in the lymphoplasmacytoid variant of marginal zone B-cell lymphoma, being characterized by irregular plaques and flat tumors located mainly on the distal lower extremities. Histology shows sheets of plasma cells that reveal a polyclonal expression of the immunoglobulin light-chains κ and λ.

We and others [159] have observed cases of cutaneous leishmaniasis that deviated from the conventional presentation by showing a pseudolymphomatous infiltrate with several CD30+ large cells. Careful scrutiny of the histopathologic sections reveals the presence of typical intracellular micro-organisms within some of the histiocytes.

Cases of eruption of lymphocyte recovery with histopathologic features mimicking those of mycosis fungoides have been observed [160].

It should also be remembered that molecular analyses have demonstrated on many occasions that a monoclonal population of lymphocytes can be detected in several benign skin conditions besides cutaneous lymphomas – lichen planus for example [84]. It is crucial to keep in mind this possibility when evaluating molecular analyses of TCR and J_H gene rearrangement in skin infiltrates. In addition, pseudoclones may be the source of false-positive molecular reports. Pseudoclones may be due to the presence of small numbers of T or B lymphocytes that reveal an oligoclonal or monoclonal pattern of TCR or J_H gene rearrangement. Careful correlation with the morphologic and phenotypic features is crucial in order to avoid this pitfall.

"Malignant" pseudolymphomas

Although the definition of cutaneous pseudolymphoma is that of a benign condition which simulates a malignant lymphoma clinically and/or histopathologically, there are rare examples of non-lymphoid malignancies that may be misinterpreted as true malignant lymphomas, with consequences as catastrophic as those of an erroneous diagnosis of lymphoma in a reactive infiltrate. For these conditions we use the working term of "malignant" pseudolymphomas, although we are well aware of the semantic contradiction implied by the use of this term. On the other hand, this oxymoron helps to remind us that not all simulators of cutaneous lymphomas are benign conditions.

One of the lesions of this group that has been best characterized is the lymphoepithelial-like carcinoma of the skin, a variant of cutaneous squamous cell carcinoma with prominent lymphoid infiltrates. We have seen cases characterized by a prominent follicular reaction with large germinal centers that, together with the nodules of large keratino-cytes surrounded by lymphoid infiltrates, simulated the picture of a cutaneous follicle center lymphoma. Complete phenotypic analyses, of course, reveal the epithelial origin of the neoplastic cells in these cases, thus allowing a precise diagnosis. Cutaneous cases of lymphoepithelial-like carcinoma are not associated with EBV infection, and are not related to the true lymphoepithelial carcinoma. The treatment and prognosis are similar to those of other cutaneous squamous cell carcinomas.

Cutaneous angiosarcomas may present with heavy inflammatory infiltrates, simulating the picture of a cutaneous T- or B-cell lymphoma [161]. The clinical presentation is usually that of a conventional cutaneous angiosarcoma (either on the head and neck in the elderly, or associated with chronic lymphedema), but histology shows dense lymphoid infiltrates intermingled with sheets of atypical endothelial cells that resemble diffuse areas of large cell lymphoma (Fig. 22.63). As germinal centers are often present as well, the erroneous diagnosis of cutaneous follicle center lymphoma may be suggested. Again, complete phenotypic investigations allow the correct diagnosis to be made (Fig. 22.64). It has been suggested that the presence of a pseudolymphomatous reaction is related to a better prognosis in cutaneous angiosarcoma.

Complete regression of malignant epithelial tumors may sometimes show histopathologically a band-like lymphoid infiltrate with some exocytosis of lymphocytes, thus posing differential diagnostic problems with mycosis fungoides. This

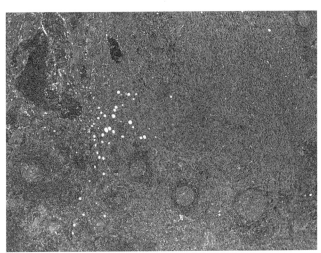

(a)

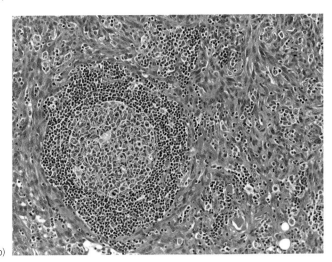

(b)

Figure 22.63 Pseudolymphomatous angiosarcoma. (a) Sheets of cells with reactive germinal centers. (b) Detail of sheets of large epithelioid cells admixed with small lymphocytes; note a reactive germinal center (same case as Fig. 22.64).

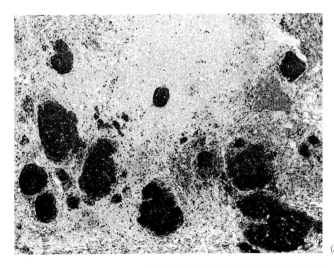

(a)

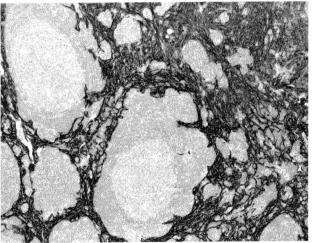

(b)

Figure 22.64 Pseudolymphomatous angiosarcoma. (a) Staining for CD20 shows many large nodules of B cells. (b) Staining for podoplanine confirms that the epithelioid cells are endothelial cells (same case as Fig. 22.63).

pattern is similar to what is observed in lichenoid keratoses, a pathologic process that represents for the most part regression of a seborrheic keratosis or of a solar lentigo (see earlier). Recently, a pseudolymphomatous infiltrate simulating mycosis fungoides has also been described in a case of melanoma with

almost complete regression [162]. Especially when pigmentation is present in the papillary dermis, immunohistologic stainings for melanocytes should be used together with other phenotypic markers for the precise characterization of the cases.

TEACHING CASE

A biopsy specimen from a 9-year-old boy was sent in consultation to one of us (LC). The boy presented with an erythematous patch on the right shoulder (Fig. 22.65a). Histology revealed a dense, band-like infiltrate with epidermotropic lymphocytes (Fig. 22.65b,c). Immunohistology showed that the lymphocytes expressed a T-cytotoxic

phenotype (Fig. 22.65d, staining for CD8). A provisional diagnosis of mycosis fungoides was made.

A few months later the family came to Graz for clinicopathologic correlation, bringing pictures taken during the summertime (Fig. 22.65e). The picture clearly documented the evolution of the lesion toward a conventional macule of vitiligo. A second small macule appeared close to the first one. The boy had no other sign of mycosis fungoides, and the diagnosis was revised to vitiligo.

Comment: The inflammatory stage of vitiligo bears close histopathologic resemblance to mycosis fungoides, and at times can be indistinguishable from it. The band-like infiltrate with intraepidermal cytotoxic lymphocytes was erroneously interpreted as a patch of cytotoxic mycosis fungoides, a variant that happens to be relatively frequent in children. However, follow-up clearly showed that the patient had vitiligo, once again underlining that, particularly in children, a diagnosis of mycosis fungoides should be made only upon compelling clinicopathologic evidence.

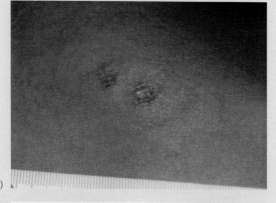
(a)
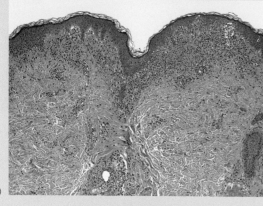
(b)
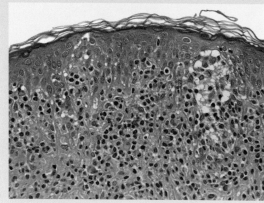
(c)
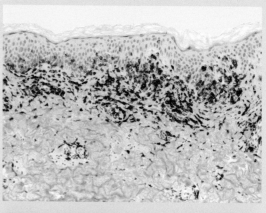
(d)
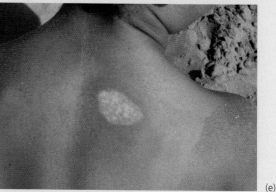
(e)

Figure 22.65

TEACHING CASE

This 49–year-old woman complained of sudden onset of exanthematic, confluent erythematous, partly livid macules and papules (Fig. 22.66a). A biopsy specimen revealed dense patchy-lichenoid infiltrates in the superficial dermis with prominent atypical features (Fig. 22.66b,c). The cells revealed a T-helper phenotype and showed a proliferation rate of >80% (Fig. 22.66d, staining for MIB-1/Ki67).

Accurate history taking revealed that the eruption started under therapy with thiamazol, a compound used to treat hyperthyreosis. After discontinuation of the drug and systemic steroid therapy, the eruption resolved completely.

Comment: This case shows that pseudolymphomatous drug eruptions can present with markedly atypical lymphoid infiltrates, even with remarkably high proliferation rate, thus representing a pitfall in the differential diagnosis with lymphoma. However, the clinical picture, symmetric distribution, sudden onset, and clinical history all suggested a diagnosis of drug eruption, confirmed by follow-up examination.

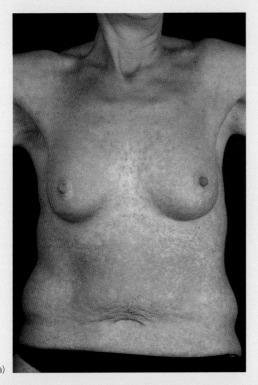
(a)

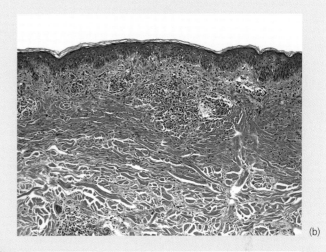
(b)

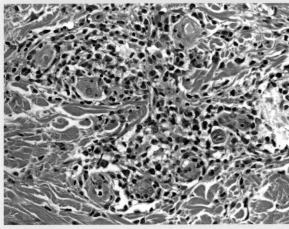
(c)

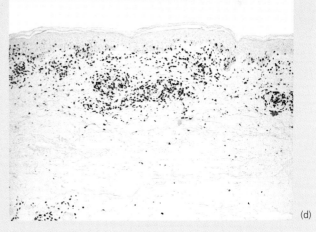
(d)

Figure 22.66

References

1. Clark WH, Mihm MC, Reed RJ, Ainsworth AM. The lympho-cytic infiltrates of the skin. *Hum Pathol* 1974;**5**:25–43.

2. Connors RC, Ackerman AB. Histologic pseudomalignancies of the skin. *Arch Dermatol* 1976;**112**:1767–1780.

3. LeBoit PE. Cutaneous lymphomas and their histopathologic imitators. *Semin Dermatol* 1986;**5**:322–333.

4. Kerl H, Ackerman AB. Inflammatory diseases that simulate lymphomas: cutaneous pseudolymphomas. In: Fitzpatrick TB, Eisen AZ, Wolff K *et al.*, eds. *Dermatology in General Medicine*, 4th edn. New York: McGraw-Hill, 1993:1315–1327.

5. Caro WA, Helwig EB. Cutaneous lymphoid hyperplasia. *Cancer* 1969;**24**:487–502.

6. Kerl H, Cerroni L. Pseudolymphomas of the skin. In: Rigel DS, Friedman RJ, Dzubow LM *et al.*, eds. *Cancer of the Skin*. Philadelphia: Elsevier Saunders, 2005:411–422.

7. Smolle J, Torne R, Soyer HP, Kerl H. Immunohistochemical classification of cutaneous pseudolymphomas: delineation of distinct patterns. *J Cutan Pathol* 1990;**17**:149–159.

8. Siddiqui J, Hardman DL, Misra M, Wood GS. Clonal dermatitis: a potential precursor of cutaneous T-cell lymphomas with varied clinical manifestations. *J Invest Dermatol* 1997;**108**:584.

9. Wood GS, Ngan BY, Tung R *et al.* Clonal rearrangements of immunoglobulin genes and progression to B-cell lymphoma in cutaneous lymphoid hyperplasia. *Am J Pathol* 1989;**135**:13–19.

10. Nihal M, Mikkola D, Horvath N *et al.* Cutaneous lymphoid hyper-plasia: a lymphoproliferative continuum with lymphomatous potential. *Hum Pathol* 2003;**34**:617–622.

11. Cerroni L, Kerl H. Diagnostic immunohistology: cutaneous lymphomas and pseudolymphomas. *Semin Cutan Med Surg* 1999;**18**:64–70.

12. Cerroni L, Goteri G. Differential diagnosis between cutaneous lymphoma and pseudolymphoma. *Anal Quant Cytol Histol* 2003;**25**:191–198.

13. Leinweber B, Colli C, Chott A, Kerl H, Cerroni L. Differential diagnosis of cutaneous infiltrates of B lymphocytes with folli-cular growth pattern. *Am J Dermatopathol* 2004;**26**:4–13.

14. Wood GS. T-cell receptor and immunoglobulin gene re-arrangements in diagnosing skin disease. *Arch Dermatol* 2001;**137**:1503–1506.

15. Bakels V, van Oostveen JW, van der Putte SCJ, Meijer CJLM, Willemze R. Immunophenotyping and gene rearrangement analysis provide additional criteria to differentiate between cutaneous T-cell lymphomas and pseudo-T-cell lymphomas. *Am J Pathol* 1997;**150**:1941–1949.

16. Medeiros LJ, Picker LJ, Abel EA *et al.* Cutaneous lymphoid hyperplasia: immunologic characteristics and assessment of criteria recently proposed as diagnostic of malignant lymphoma. *J Am Acad Dermatol* 1989;**21**:929–942.

17. Rijlaarsdam JU, Bakels V, van Oostveen JW *et al.* Demon-stration of clonal immunoglobulin gene rearrangements in cutaneous B-cell lymphomas and pseudo-B-cell lymphomas: differential diagnostic and pathogenetic aspects. *J Invest Dermatol* 1992;**99**:749–754.

18. Böer A, Tirumalae R, Bresch M, Falk TM. Pseudoclonality in cutaneous pseudolymphomas: a pitfall in interpretation of rearrangement studies. *Br J Dermatol* 2008;**159**:394–402.

19. Ive FA, Magnus IA, Warin RP, Wilson Jones E. "Actinic reticuloid": a chronic dermatosis associated with severe photosensitivity and the histological resemblance to lymphoma. *Br J Dermatol* 1969;**81**:469–485.

20. Norris PG, Hawk JLM. Chronic actinic dermatitis: a unifying concept. *Arch Dermatol* 1990;**126**:376–378.

21. Lim HW, Morison WL, Kamide R *et al.* Chronic actinic dermatitis: an analysis of 51 patients evaluated in the United States and Japan. *Arch Dermatol* 1994;**130**:1284–1289.

22. Toonstra J. Actinic reticuloid. *Semin Diagn Pathol* 1991;**8**:109–116.

23. Giannelli F, Botcherby PK, Marimo B, Magnus IA. Cellular hypersensitivity to UV-1: a clue to the aetiology of actinic retic-uloid? *Lancet* 1983;**321**:88–91.

24. Toonstra J, Wildschut A, Boer J *et al.* Actinic reticuloid. *J Am Acad Dermatol* 1989;**21**:205–214.

25. Dawe RS, Crombie IK, Ferguson J. The natural history of chronic actinic dermatitis. *Arch Dermatol* 2000;**136**:1215–1220.

26. Bilsland D, Crombie IK, Ferguson J. The photosensitivity der-matitis and actinic reticuloid syndrome: no association with lymphoreticular malignancy. *Br J Dermatol* 1994;**131**:209–214.

27. Jensen NE, Sneddon IB. Actinic reticuloid with lymphoma. *Br J Dermatol* 1970;**82**:287–291.

28. Heller P, Wieczorek R, Waldo E *et al.* Chronic actinic dermatitis: an immunohistochemical study of its T-cell antigenic profile, with comparison to cutaneous T-cell lymphoma. *Am J Dermatopathol* 1994;**16**:510–516.

29. Toonstra J, van der Putte SCJ, van Wichen DF *et al.* Actinic reticuloid: immunohistochemical analysis of the cutaneous infiltrate in 13 patients. *Br J Dermatol* 1989;**120**:779–786.

30. Reddy K, Bhawan J. Histologic mimickers of mycosis fungoides: a review. *J Cutan Pathol* 2007;**34**:519–525.

31. Neild VS, Hawk JLM, Eady RAJ, Cream JJ. Actinic reticuloid with Sézary cells. *Clin Exp Dermatol* 1982;**7**:143–148.

32. Chu AC, Robinson D, Hawk JLM *et al.* Immunologic differ-entiation of the Sézary syndrome due to cutaneous T-cell lymphoma and chronic actinic dermatitis. *J Invest Dermatol* 1986;**86**:134–137.

33. Ferguson J. The management of the photosensitivity dermatitis and actinic reticuloid (PD/AR) syndrome. *J Dermatol Treat* 1990;**1**:143–145.

34. Granlund H, Reitamo S. Cyclosporin A in the treatment of chronic actinic dermatitis. *Eur J Dermatol* 1992;**2**:237–241.

35. Uetsu N, Okamoto H, Fujii K, Doi R, Horio T. Treatment of chronic actinic dermatitis with tacrolimus ointment. *J Am Acad Dermatol* 2002;**47**:881–884.

36. Gröne D, Kunz M, Zimmermann R, Gross G. Successful treat-ment of nodular actinic reticuloid with tacrolimus ointment. *Dermatology* 2006;**212**:377–380.

37. Gomez Orbaneja J, Iglesias Diez L, Sanchez Lozano JL, Conde Salazar L. Lymphomatoid contact dermatitis. *Contact Dermatitis* 1976;**2**:139–143.

38. Ackerman AB, Breza TS, Capland L. Spongiotic simulants of mycosis fungoides. *Arch Dermatol* 1974;**109**:216–220.

39. Wolff-Sneedorff A, Thomsen K, Secher L, Lange Vejlsgaard G. Gene rearrangement in positive patch tests. *Exp Dermatol* 1995;**4**:322–326.

40. van der Putte SCJ, Toonstra J, Felten PC, van Vloten WA. Solitary non-epidermotropic T cell pseudolymphoma of the skin. *J Am Acad Dermatol* 1986;**14**:444–453.

41. Rijlaarsdam JU, Willemze R. Cutaneous pseudo-T-cell lymphomas. *Semin Diagn Pathol* 1991;**8**:102–108.

42. Cerroni L, Fink-Puches R, El-Shabrawi-Caelen L *et al.* Solitary skin lesions with histopathologic features of early mycosis fungoides. *Am J Dermatopathol* 1999;**21**:518–524.

43. Bergman R, Khamaysi Z, Sahar D, Ben-Arieh Y. Cutaneous lymphoid hyperplasia presenting as a solitary facial nodule. *Arch Dermatol* 2006;**142**:1561–1566.

44. Arai E, Shimizu M, Hirose T. A review of 55 cases of cutaneous lymphoid hyperplasia: reassessment of the histopathologic findings leading to reclassification of 4 lesions as cutaneous marginal zone lymphoma and 19 as pseudolymphomatous folliculitis. *Hum Pathol* 2005;**36**:505–511.

45. Setyadi HG, Nash JW, Duvic M. The solitary lymphomatoid papule, nodule, or tumor. *J Am Acad Dermatol* 2007;**57**:1072–1083.

46. Al-Hoqail I, Crawford RI. Benign lichenoid keratoses with histologic features of mycosis fungoides: clinicopathologic description of a clinically significant histologic pattern. *J Cutan Pathol* 2002;**29**:291–294.

47. Glaun RS, Dutta B, Helm KF. A proposed new classification system for lichenoid keratosis. *J Am Acad Dermatol* 1996;**35**:772–774.

48. Arai E, Shimizu M, Tsuchida T, Izaki S, Ogawa F, Hirose T. Lymphomatoid keratosis. An epidermotropic type of cutaneous lymphoid hyperplasia: clinicopathological, immunohistochemical, and molecular biological study of 6 cases. *Arch Dermatol* 2007;**143**:53–59.

49. Kossard S. Unilesional mycosis fungoides or lymphomatoid keratosis? *Arch Dermatol* 1997;**133**:1312–1313.

50. Boyd AS, Vnencak-Jones CL. T-cell clonality in lichenoid purpura: a clinical and molecular evaluation of seven patients. *Histopathology* 2003;**43**:302–303.

51. Barnhill RL, Braverman IM. Progression of pigmented purpura-like eruptions to mycosis fungoides: report of three cases. *J Am Acad Dermatol* 1988;**19**:25–31.

52. Crowson AN, Magro CM, Zahorchak R. Atypical pigmentary purpura: a clinical, histopathologic, and genotypic study. *Hum Pathol* 1999;**30**:1004–1012.

53. Toro JR, Sander CA, LeBoit PE. Persistent pigmented purpuric dermatitis and mycosis fungoides: simulant, precursor, or both? A study by light microscopy and molecular methods. *Am J Dermatopathol* 1997;**19**:108–118.

54. Fink-Puches R, Wolf P, Kerl H, Cerroni L. Lichen aureus. Clinicopathologic features, natural history, and relationship to mycosis fungoides. *Arch Dermatol* 2008;**144**:1169–1173.

55. Viseux V, Schoenlaub P, Cnudde F *et al.* Pigmented purpuric dermatitis preceding the diagnosis of mycosis fungoides by 24 years. *Dermatology* 2003;**207**:331–332.

56. Magro CM, Schaefer JT, Crowson AN, Li J, Morrison C. Pigmented purpuric dermatosis. Classification by phenotypic and molecular profiles. *Am J Clin Pathol* 2007;**128**:218–229.

57. Citarella L, Massone C, Kerl H, Cerroni L. Lichen sclerosus with histopathologic features simulating early mycosis fungoides. *Am J Dermatopathol* 2003;**25**:463–465.

58. Lukowsky A, Muche JM, Sterry W, Audring H. Detection of expanded T cell clones in skin biopsy samples of patients with lichen sclerosus et atrophicus by T cell receptor-γ polymerase chain reaction assays. *J Invest Dermatol* 2000;**115**:254–259.

59. Regauer S, Beham-Schmid C. Detailed analysis of the T-cell lymphocytic infiltrate in penile lichen sclerosus: an immunohistochemical and molecular investigation. *Histopathology* 2006;**48**:730–735.

60. Attili VR, Attili SK. Lichenoid inflammation in vitiligo – a clinical and histopathologic review of 210 cases. *Int J Dermatol* 2008;**47**:663–669.

61. Petit T, Cribier B, Bagot M, Wechsler J. Inflammatory vitiligo-like macules that simulate hypopigmented mycosis fungoides. *Eur J Dermatol* 2003;**13**:410–412.

62. Annessi G, Paradisi M, Angelo C *et al.* Annular lichenoid dermatitis of youth. *J Am Acad Dermatol* 2003;**49**:1029–1036.

63. Durdu M, Akyilmaz M, Tuncer I. Annular lichenoid dermatitis of youth. *Ped Dermatol* 2007;**24**:582–584.

64. Kleikamp S, Kutzner H, Frosch PJ. Anuläre lichenoide Dermatose der Kindheit – ein weiterer Fall bei einem 12-jährigen Mädchen. *J Deutsch Dermatol Ges* 2008;**8**:653–656.

65. Cogrel O, Boralevi F, Lepreux S *et al.* Lymphomatoid annular erythema: a new form of juvenile mycosis fungoides. *Br J Dermatol* 2005;**152**:565–566.

66. Guitart J, Variakojis D, Kuzel T, Rosen S. Cutaneous CD8+ T cell infiltrates in advanced HIV infection. *J Am Acad Dermatol* 1999;**41**:722–727.

67. Zhang P, Chiriboga L, Jacobson M *et al.* Mycosis fungoides-like T-cell cutaneous lymphoid infiltrates in patients with HIV infection. *Am J Dermatopathol* 1995;**17**:29–35.

68. Schartz NEC, De la Blanchardiere A, Alaoui S *et al.* Regression of CD8+ pseudolymphoma after HIV antiviral triple therapy. *J Am Acad Dermatol* 2003;**49**:139–141.

69. Gallardo F, Barranco C, Toll A, Pujol RM. CD30 antigen expression in cutaneous inflammatory infiltrates of scabies: a dynamic immunophenotypic pattern that should be distinguished from lymphomatoid papulosis. *J Cutan Pathol* 2002;**29**:368–373.

70. Nathan DL, Belsito DV. Carbamazepine-induced pseudolymphoma with CD-30 positive cells. *J Am Acad Dermatol* 1998;**38**:806–809.

71. Rose C, Starostik P, Bröcker EB. Infection with parapoxvirus induces CD30-positive cutaneous infiltrates in humans. *J Cutan Pathol* 1999;**26**:520–522.

72. Kim KJ, Lee MW, Choi JH *et al.* CD30-positive T-cell-rich pseudolymphoma induced by gold acupuncture. *Br J Dermatol* 2002;**146**:882–884.

73. Moreno-Ramirez D, Garcia-Escudero A, Rios-Martin JJ, Herrera-Saval A, Camacho F. Cutaneous pseudolymphoma in association with molluscum contagiosum in an elderly patient. *J Cutan Pathol* 2003;**30**:473–475.

74. Werner B, Massone C, Kerl H, Cerroni L. Large CD30–positive cells in benign, atypical lymphoid infiltrates of the skin. *J Cutan Pathol* 2008;**35**(2):1100–1107.

75. Leinweber B, Kerl H, Cerroni L. Histopathologic features of cutaneous herpes virus infections (herpes simplex, herpes varicella/zoster). A broad spectrum of presentations with common pseudolymphomatous aspects. *Am J Surg Pathol* 2006;**30**:50–58.

76. Wolff HH, Wendt V, Winzer M. Cutaneous pseudolymphoma at the site of prior herpes zoster eruption. *Arch Dermatol Res* 1987;**279**:S52–S4.

77. Wain EM, Antony F, Appleton MAC, Whittaker SJ, Robson A. Genital herpes masquerading as a cutaneous T-cell lymphoma: a report of two cases. *J Cutan Pathol* 2008;**35**:770–773.

78. Aram G, Rohwedder A, Nazeer T, Shoss R, Fisher A, Carlson JA. Varicella-Zoster-virus folliculitis promoted clonal cutaneous lymphoid hyperplasia. *Am J Dermatopathol* 2005;**27**:411–417.

79. Böer A, Herder N, Winter K, Falk T. Herpes folliculitis: clinical, histopathological, and molecular pathologic observations. *Br J Dermatol* 2006;**154**:743–746.

80. Dereure O, Levi E, Kadin ME. T-cell clonality in pityriasis lichenoides et varioliformis acuta: a heteroduplex analysis of 20 cases. *Arch Dermatol* 2000;**136**:1483–1486.

81. Kadin ME. T-cell clonality in pityriasis lichenoides. Evidence for a premalignant or reactive immune disorder? *Arch Dermatol* 2002;**138**:1089–1090.

82. Magro C, Crowson AN, Kovatich A, Burns F. Pityriasis lichenoides: a clonal T-cell lymphoproliferative disorder. *Hum Pathol* 2002;**33**:788–795.

83. Bowers S, Warshaw EM. Pityriasis lichenoides and its subtypes. *J Am Acad Dermatol* 2006;**55**:557–572.

84. Schiller PI, Flaig MJ, Puchta U, Kind P, Sander CA. Detection of clonal T-cells in lichen planus. *Arch Dermatol Res* 2000;**292**:568–569.

85. Tomasini D, Zampatti C, Palmedo G, Bonfacini V, Sangalli G, Kutzner H. Cytotoxic mycosis fungoides evolving from pityriasis lichenoides chronica in a seventeen-year-old girl. *Dermatology* 2002;**205**:176–179.

86. Panhans A, Bodemer C, Macinthyre E, Fraitag S, Paul C, de Prost Y. Pityriasis lichenoides of childhood with atypical CD30-positive cells and clonal T-cell receptor gene rearrangements. *J Am Acad Dermatol* 1996;**35**:489–490.

87. Cerroni L. Lymphomatoid papulosis, pityriasis lichenoides et varioliformis acuta, and anaplastic large cell (Ki-1+) lymphoma. *J Am Acad Dermatol* 1997;**37**:287.

88. Fink-Puches R, Soyer HP, Kerl H. Febrile ulceronecrotic pityriasis lichenoides et varioliformis acuta. *J Am Acad Dermatol* 1994;**30**:261–263.

89. Rivera R, Ortiz P, Rodriguez-Peralto JL, Vanaclocha F, Iglesias L. Febrile ulceronecrotic pityriasis lichenoides et varioliformis acuta with atypical cells. *Int J Dermatol* 2003;**42**:26–28.

90. Sotiriou E, Patsatsi A, Tsorova C, Lazaridou E, Sotiriadis D. Febrile ulceronecrotic Mucha-Habermann disease: a case report and review of the literature. *Acta Derm Venereol (Stockh)* 2008;**88**:350–355.

91. Kim HS, Yu DS, Kim JW. A case of febrile ulceronecrotic Mucha-Habermann's disease successfully treated with oral cyclosporin. *J Eur Acad Dermatol Venereol* 2007;**21**:272–273.

92. Herron MD, Bohnsack JF, Vanderhooft SL. Septic, CD-30 positive febrile ulceronecrotic pityriasis lichenoides et varioliformis acuta. *Ped Dermatol* 2005;**22**:360–365.

93. Magro CM, Crowson AN, Kovatich AJ, Burns F. Lupus profundus, indeterminate lymphocytic lobular panniculitis and subcutaneous T-cell lymphoma: a spectrum of subcuticular T-cell lymphoid dyscrasia. *J Cutan Pathol* 2001;**28**:235–247.

94. Massone C, Kodama K, Salmhofer W *et al.* Lupus erythematosus panniculitis (lupus profundus): clinical, histopathological, and molecular analysis of nine cases. *J Cutan Pathol* 2005;**32**:396–404.

95. Lozzi GP, Massone C, Citarella L, Kerl H, Cerroni L. Rimming of adipocytes by neoplastic lymphocytes. A histopathologic feature not restricted to subcutaneous T-cell lymphoma. *Am J Dermatopathol* 2006;**28**:9–12.

96. Choi TS, Doh KS, Kim SH *et al.* Clinicopathological and genotypic aspects of anticonvulsant-induced pseudolymphoma syndrome. *Br J Dermatol* 2003;**148**:730–736.

97. Schreiber MM, McGregor JG. Pseudolymphoma syndrome: a sensitivity to anticonvulsant drugs. *Arch Dermatol* 1968;**97**:297–300.

98. Magro CM, Crowson AN, Kovatich AJ, Burns F. Drug-induced reversible lymphoid dyscrasia: a clonal lymphomatoid dermatitis of memory and activated T cells. *Hum Pathol* 2003;**34**:119–129.

99. Ploysangam T, Breneman DL, Mutasim DF. Cutaneous pseudolymphomas. *J Am Acad Dermatol* 1998;**38**:877–905.

100. Crowson AN, Magro CM. Antidepressant therapy: a possible cause of atypical cutaneous lymphoid hyperplasia. *Arch Dermatol* 1995;**131**:925–929.

101. Aguilar JL, Barcelo CM, Martin-Urda MT *et al.* Generalized cutaneous B-cell pseudolymphoma induced by neuroleptics. *Arch Dermatol* 1992;**128**:121–123.

102. Kardaun SH, Scheffer E, Vermeer BJ. Drug-induced pseudolymphomatous skin reactions. *Br J Dermatol* 1988;**118**:545–552.

103. Magro CM, Crowson AN. Drugs with antihistaminic properties as a cause of atypical cutaneous lymphoid hyperplasia. *J Am Acad Dermatol* 1995;**32**:419–428.

104. Rosenthal CJ, Noguera CA, Coppola A, Kapelner SN. Pseudolymphoma with mycosis fungoides manifestations, hyperresponsiveness to diphenylhydantoin, and lymphocyte dysregulation. *Cancer* 1982;**49**:2305–2314.

105. Rijlaarsdam JU, Scheffer E, Meijer CJLM, Kruyswijk MRJ, Willemze R. Mycosis fungoides-like lesions associated with phenytoin and carbamazepine therapy. *J Am Acad Dermatol* 1991;**24**:216–220.

106. Mutasim DF. Lymphomatoid drug eruption mimicking digitate dermatosis: cross reactivity between two drugs that suppress angiotensin II function. *Am J Dermatopathol* 2003;**25**:331–334.

107. Paley C, Geskin LJ, Zirwas MJ. Cutaneous B-cell pseudolymphoma due to paraphenylenediamine. *Am J Dermatopathol* 2006;**28**:438–441.

108. Wolf IH, Smolle J, Cerroni L, Kerl H. Erythroderma with lichenoid granulomatous features induced by erythropoietin. *J Cutan Pathol* 2005;**32**:371–374.

109. Sangueza OP, Cohen DE, Calciano A, Lee M, Stiller MJ. Mycosis fungoides induced by phenytoin. *Eur J Dermatol* 1993;**3**:474–477.

110. Stavrianeas NG, Katoulis AC, Kanelleas A, Hatziolou E, Georgala S. Papulonodular lichenoid and pseudolymphomatous reaction at the injection site of hepatitis B virus vaccination. *Dermatology* 2002;**205**:166–168.

111. Smolle J, Cerroni L, Kerl H. Multiple pseudolymphomas caused by Hirudo medicinalis therapy. *J Am Acad Dermatol* 2000;**43**:867–869.

112. Rijlaarsdam JU, Bruynzeel DP, Vos W, Meijer CJLM, Willemze R. Immunohistochemical studies of lymphadenosis benigna cutis occurring in a tattoo. *Am J Dermatopathol* 1988;**10**:518–523.

113. Colli C, Leinweber B, Müllegger R *et al.* Borrelia burgdorferi associated lymphocytoma cutis: clinicopathologic, immunophenotypic, and molecular study of 106 cases. *J Cutan Pathol* 2004;**31**:232–240.

114. Emberger M, Laimer M, Lanschuetzer CM, Selhofer S, Cerroni L. Symmetrical reddish swelling of the eyebrows in a 12-year-old girl – symmetrical Borrelia burgdorferi-associated lymphocytoma cutis of the eyebrows. *Arch Dermatol* 2008;**144**:673–678.

115. Grange F, Wechsler J, Guillaume JC et al. Borrelia burgdorferi associated lymphocytoma cutis simulating a primary cutaneous large B-cell lymphoma. J Am Acad Dermatol 2002;47: 530–534.

116. Kuflik AS, Schwartz RA. Lymphocytoma cutis: a series of five patients successfully treated with cryosurgery. J Am Acad Dermatol 1992;26:449–452.

117. El-Dars LD, Statham BN, Blackford S, Williams N. Lymphocytoma cutis treated with topical tacrolimus. Clin Exp Dermatol 2005;30:305–307.

118. Aigelsreiter A, Pump A, Buchhäusl W et al. Successful antibiotic treatment of Borreliosis associated pseudolymphomatous systemic infiltrates. J Infect 2005;51:203–206.

119. Fernandez N, Torres A, Ackerman AB. Pathologic findings in human scabies. Arch Dermatol 1977;113:320–324.

120. Smoller BR, Longacre TA, Warnke RA. Ki-1 (CD30) expression in differentiation of lymphomatoid papulosis from arthropod bite reactions. Mod Pathol 1992;5:492–496.

121. Cerroni L, Borroni RG, Massone C, Chott A, Kerl H. Cutaneous B-cell pseudolymphoma at the site of vaccination. Am J Dermatopathol 2007;29:538–542.

122. Chong H, Brady K, Metze D, Calonje E. Persistent nodules at injection sites (aluminium granuloma)-clinicopathological study of 14 cases with a diverse range of histological reaction patterns. Histopathology 2006;48:182–188.

123. Goerdt S, Spieker T, Wölffer LU et al. Multiple cutaneous B-cell pseudolymphomas after allergen injections. J Am Acad Dermatol 1996;34:1072–1074.

124. Kahofer P, El-Shabrawi-Caelen L, Horn M, Kern T, Smolle J. Pseudolymphoma occurring in a tattoo. Eur J Dermatol 2003; 13:209–212.

125. Amann U, Luger T, Metze D. Lichenoid-pseudolymphomatöse Tätowierungsreaktion. Hautarzt 1997;48:410–413.

126. Di Landro A, Marchesi L, Valsecchi R, Motta T, Locati F. Pseudolymphomatous reaction to a red pigment in tattoo. Eur J Dermatol 1997;7:235–237.

127. Sangueza OP, Yadav S, White CR Jr, Braziel RM. Evolution of B-cell lymphoma from pseudolymphoma: a multidisciplinary approach using histology, immunohistochemistry, and Southern blot analysis. Am J Dermatopathol 1992;14:408–413.

128. Hara M, Matsunaga J, Tagami H. Acral pseudolymphomatous angiokeratoma of children (APACHE): a case report and immunohistologic study. Br J Dermatol 1991;124:387–388.

129. Kaddu S, Cerroni L, Pilatti A, Soyer HP, Kerl H. Acral pseudolymphomatous angiokeratoma. Am J Dermatopathol 1994;16: 130–133.

130. Marukami T, Ohtsuki M, Nakagawa H. Acral pseudolymphomatous angiokeratoma of children: a pseudolymphoma rather than an angiokeratoma. Br J Dermatol 2001;145:512–514.

131. Ramsay B, Dahl MCG, Malcom AJ, Wilson Jones E. Acral pseudolymphomatous angiokeratoma of children. Arch Dermatol 1990;126:1524–1525.

132. Lee MW, Choi JH, Sung KJ, Moon KC, Koh JK. Acral pseudolymphomatous angiokeratoma of children (APACHE). Ped Dermatol 2003;20:457–458.

133. Okuyama R, Masu T, Mizuashi M, Watanabe M, Tagami H, Aiba S. Pseudolymphomatous angiokeratoma: report of three cases and an immunohistological study. Clin Exp Dermatol 2009; 34:161–165.

134. Magro CM, Crowson AN, Harrist TJ. Atypical lymphoid infiltrates arising in cutaneous lesions of connective tissue disease. Am J Dermatopathol 1997;19:446–455.

135. Brazzelli V, Vassallo C, Ardigo M, Rosso R, Borroni G. Unusual histologic presentation of morphea. Am J Dermatopathol 2000;22:359.

136. Hodak E, David M, Rothem A, Bialowance M, Sandbank M. Nodular secondary syphilis mimicking cutaneous lymphoreticular process. J Am Acad Dermatol 1987;17:914–917.

137. McComb ME, Telang GH, Vonderheid EC. Secondary syphilis presenting as pseudolymphoma of the skin. J Am Acad Dermatol 2003;49:S174–176.

138. Tsai KY, Brenn T, Werchniak AE. Nodular presentation of secondary syphilis. J Am Acad Dermatol 2007;57:s57–s58.

139. Battistella M, Le Cleach L, Lacert A, Perrin P. Extensive nodular secondary syphilis with prozone phenomenon. Arch Dermatol 2008;144:1078–1079.

140. El Shabrawi-Caelen L, Kerl K, Cerroni L, Soyer HP, Kerl H. Cutaneous inflammatory pseudotumor – a spectrum of various diseases? J Cutan Pathol 2004;31:605–611.

141. Kerl H, Cerroni L. The morphologic spectrum of cutaneous inflammatory pseudotumors. Am J Dermatopathol 2001;23: 545–546.

142. Coffin CM, Hornik JL, Fletcher CDM. Inflammatory myofibroblastic tumor: comparison of clinicopathologic, histologic, and immunohistochemical features including ALK expression in atypical and aggressive cases. Am J Surg Pathol 2007;31:509–520.

143. Hurt MA, Santa Cruz DJ. Cutaneous inflammatory pseudotumor: lesions resembling "inflammatory pseudotumors" or "plasma cell granulomas" of extracutaneous sites. Am J Surg Pathol 1990;14:764–773.

144. Uhara H, Saida T, Ikegawa S et al. Primary cutaneous plasmacytosis: report of three cases and review of the literature. Dermatology 1994;189:251–255.

145. Jayaraman AG, Cesca C, Kohler S. Cutaneous plasmacytosis. A report of five cases with immunohistochemical evaluation for HHV-8 expression. Am J Dermatopathol 2006;28:93–98.

146. Leonard AL, Meehan SA, Ramsey D, Brown L, Sen F. Cutaneous and systemic plasmacytosis. J Am Acad Dermatol 2007;56:s38–s40.

147. Kayasut K, Le Touzrneau A, Rio B et al. Are multicentric Castleman's disease with cutaneous plasmacytosis and systemic plasmacytosis the same entity? Histopathology 2006;49:557–558.

148. Shimizu S, Tanaka M, Shimizu H, Hanyaku H. Is cutaneous plasmacytosis a distinct clinical entity? J Am Acad Dermatol 1997;36:876–880.

149. Hafner C, Hohenleutner U, Babilas P, Landthaler M, Vogt T. Targeting T cells to hit B cells: successful treatment of cutaneous plasmacytosis with topical pimecrolimus. Dermatology 2006;213:163–165.

150. Weber F, Schmuth M, Fritsch P, Sepp N. Lymphocytic infiltration of the skin is a photosensitive variant of lupus erythematosus: evidence by phototesting. Br J Dermatol 2001;144:292–296.

151. Haniffa MA, Wilkins BS, Blasdale C, Simpson NB. Cutaneous extramedullary hemopoiesis in chronic myeloproliferative and myelodysplastic disorders. J Am Acad Dermatol 2006;55:s28–s31.

152. O'Malley DP. Benign extramedullary myeloid proliferations. Mod Pathol 2007;20:405–415

153. Rieger E, Soyer HP, LeBoit PE *et al.* Reactive angioendotheliomatosis or intravascular histiocytosis?: an immunohistochemical and ultrastructural study in two cases of intravascular histiocytic cell proliferation. *Br J Dermatol* 1999;**140**:497–504.

154. Lazova R, Slater C, Scott G. Reactive angioendotheliomatosis: case report and review of the literature. *Am J Dermatopathol* 1996;**18**:63–69.

155. McMenamin ME, Fletcher CD. Reactive angioendotheliomatosis: a study of 15 cases demonstrating a wide clinicopathologic spectrum. *Am J Surg Pathol* 2002;**26**:685–697.

156. Okamoto N, Tanioka M, Yamamoto T, Shiomi T, Miyachi Y, Utani A. Intralymphatic histiocytosis associated with rheumatoid arthritis. *Clin Exper Dermatol* 2008;**33**:516–518.

157. Bryant A, Lawton H, Al-Talib R, Wright DH, Theaker JM. Intravascular proliferation of reactive lymphoid blasts mimicking intravascular lymphoma – a diagnostic pitfall. *Histopathology* 2007;**51**:401–402.

158. Baum CL, Stone MS, Liu V. Atypical intravascular CD30+ T-cell proliferation following trauma in a healthy 17-year-old male: first reported case of a potential diagnostic pitfall and literature review. *J Cut Pathol* 2009;**36**:350–354.

159. Flaig MJ, Rupec RA. Cutaneous pseudolymphoma in association with Leishmania donovani. *Br J Dermatol* 2007;**157**:1042–1043.

160. Gibney MD, Penneys NS, Nelson-Adesokan P. Cutaneous eruption of lymphocyte recovery mimicking mycosis fungoides in a patient with acute myelocytic leukemia. *J Cutan Pathol* 1995;**22**:472–475.

161. Requena L, Santonja C, Stutz N *et al.* Pseudolymphomatous cutaneous angiosarcoma: a rare variant of cutaneous angiosarcoma readily mistaken for cutaneous lymphoma. *Am J Dermatopathol* 2007;**29**:342–350.

162. Menasce LP, Shanks JH, Howarth VS, Banerjee SS. Regressed cutaneous malignant melanoma mimicking lymphoma: a potential diagnostic pitfall. *Int J Surg Pathol* 2005;**13**:281–284.

Section 8: The cutaneous "atypical lymphoid proliferation"

23 The cutaneous "atypical lymphoid proliferation"

In spite of better classification schemes, powerful ancillary techniques, and adequate clinicopathologic correlation, some cutaneous lymphoid proliferations defy precise diagnosis and classification. Sometimes this may be due to the use of inadequate material (e.g. crushed specimens, superficial biopsies or specimens that show drying artefacts – see Chapter 1), and a repeat biopsy may allow the correct diagnosis. At other times, however, an individual case cannot simply be put unambiguously into a given category of cutaneous lymphoma or pseudolymphoma. We use for such cases the working term "cutaneous atypical lymphoid proliferation." These cases show some overlap with those published in the literature as "borderline" between cutaneous pseudolymphomas and cutaneous lymphomas, and reported under various names including cutaneous lymphoid dyscrasia or clonal dermatitis, among others.

The term "cutaneous atypical lymphoid proliferation" is mainly a histopathologic one, and two main patterns can be identified: the first characterized by superficial infiltrates of lymphocytes (main differential diagnosis: mycosis fungoides vs simulators), the second by nodular proliferations of small lymphocytes admixed with reactive cells (main differential diagnosis: pseudolymphoma vs low-grade B- or T-cell lymphoma). A typical example of the second pattern is represented by lesions that are suggestive of marginal zone lymphoma on clinicopathologic grounds, but where monoclonal expression of the immunoglobulin light-chain is lacking, thus casting doubts on the diagnosis. More aggressive cutaneous lymphomas may be difficult to classify with precision, but are usually readily identified as malignant, and should not be included in the group of lesions discussed in this chapter.

We hope that, by using the information contained in this book and in others for cutaneous and extracutaneous lymphomas, the number of such cases will be reduced to a minimum, but they nonetheless exist and represent a problem in daily routine, particularly in dermatopathologic settings. Many colleagues who send us biopsy specimens in consultation know this problem very well, as well as the frustration of receiving a diagnosis of "cutaneous atypical lymphoid proliferation." However, this is a descriptive term and it is useful to avoid a more precise but possibly incorrect diagnosis. In cases of cutaneous lymphoid infiltrates that cannot be classified accurately, the following guidelines may be used.

1 Cases with obvious malignant features, but which cannot be classified precisely, should not be included in the group of the "cutaneous atypical lymphoid proliferations" but rather be termed "cutaneous lymphoma, unclassifiable." Problems in diagnosis and classification may be due to several causes, including incorrect handling and/or fixation of the specimen, thus hindering morphologic, phenotypic, and molecular studies (see Chapter 1). In such cases repeat biopsies should be obtained, and all available ancillary techniques should be used. Complete staging investigations should be performed in these patients.

2 If there are no features of an aggressive cutaneous lymphoma (both clinically and histopathologically), a general term such as "cutaneous atypical lymphoid proliferation" may be better than a more specific diagnosis that may be wrong. Repeat and follow-up biopsies are often crucial for the final classification of given cases.

3 In most cases with ambiguous histopathologic features, correlation with the clinical picture allows determination of a precise diagnosis.

4 If correlation with the clinical picture is not possible, the histopathologic report should mention all differential diagnoses applicable to a given case (e.g. solitary T-cell pseudolymphoma vs small/medium pleomorphic T-cell lymphoma vs low-grade B-cell lymphoma). Sometimes the pattern of infiltration and the analysis of the cell population do not allow a clear-cut distinction of T- from B-cell proliferations. Remarkably, in many low-grade cutaneous lymphomas (as well as in pseudolymphomas) the infiltrate is mixed, comprising almost equal numbers of T and B lymphocytes.

5 Staining for proliferation markers may give some useful clues. A low proliferation rate in nodular infiltrates of lymphocytes is observed more frequently in reactive conditions. In addition, the arrangement of proliferating cells may provide information concerning the putative neoplastic population

Skin Lymphoma: The Illustrated Guide. By L. Cerroni, K. Gatter and H. Kerl. Published 2009 Blackwell Publishing, ISBN: 978-1-4051-8554-7.

(for example, in cutaneous marginal zone lymphoma, proliferating cells are observed often at the periphery of nodules of reactive lymphocytes).

6 If possible, obtain a second expert opinion. In this context, readers should remember that a second meaningful opinion can be given only when complete information and sufficient histopathologic material are available. Particularly in ambiguous cases, diagnosis of cutaneous lymphoid infiltrates requires the study of many immunohistochemical stainings and of molecular analyses, combined with accurate and complete clinical data.

7 Finally, a diagnosis of "cutaneous atypical lymphoid proliferation" does not imply the need to perform staging investigations; short-term follow-up suffices.

Management of patients with low-grade cutaneous lymphomas includes for many entities the option of a "watchful waiting" strategy, thus implying that a delay in the diagnosis is not crucial in these cases. Particularly in children, a diagnosis of cutaneous lymphoma should be made only upon compelling clinicopathologic evidence. In cases without clear-cut features, the term "atypical lymphoid proliferation" may be useful to prevent a potentially incorrect diagnosis, while not dismissing the patient from follow-up programs. Above all and of the utmost importance, precise and clear communication among all physicians involved in the management of patients with cutaneous lymphoproliferative disorders is crucial in order to avoid misunderstandings that may have tragic consequences.

Index

Note: page numbers in **bold** refer to tables, those in *italics* refer to figures

histopathology 4–5
see also individual conditions
HIV infection
anaplastic large T-cell lymphoma 74, 78
CD8+ cutaneous infiltrates **232**, 238
cutaneous lymphomas 185–6
plasmablastic lymphoma 182
HLA-DR **6**, 194
Hodgkin cells **6**, 66, 225, 226
Hodgkin lymphoma, cutaneous
manifestations 225–7
association with
anaplastic large cell lymphoma 67, 75
lymphomatoid papulosis 247
marginal zone lymphoma 142
mycosis fungoides 11, 17, 67
T-cell-rich B-cell lymphoma 164
clinical features 225, *226*
histopathology, immunophenotype and
molecular genetics 225–6, *226*
treatment and prognosis 227
HTLV-I *see* human T-cell lymphotrophic
virus I (HTLV-I) infection
HTLV-II 185
human herpes virus 7 (HHV-7) infection
142
human herpes virus 8 (HHV-8) infection
anaplastic large T-cell lymphoma 74
cutaneous plasmacytosis 252
follicle centre lymphoma 131
HIV-associated cutaneous lymphoma 185
large B-cell lymphoma, leg type 156
marginal zone lymphoma 142
plasma cell granuloma 251, *251*
human T-cell lymphotrophic virus I
(HTLV-I) infection
in adult T-cell lymphoma/leukaemia
114, 115
in HIV infected patients 185
in mycosis fungoides 11, 115
human T-cell lymphotrophic virus II
(HTLV-II) infection 185
hydroa vacciniformis-like lymphoma 97,
107–9
and epidermotropic CD8+ cutaneous
T-cell lymphoma 97, 98
hypereosinophilic syndrome 69

idiopathic generalized follicular mucinosis
see follicular mucinosis
idiopathic pseudo-T-cell lymphoma 117
IFN-γ 72
IFN-α *see* interferon-α (IFN-α)
imiquimod 40, 72
immune response modifiers 40
immunocytoma 141
acrodermatitis chronica atrophicans
and 147
anetoderma 147

Borrelia burgdorferi infection 127, 231
marginal zone B-cell lymphoma and
141, 147
immunodeficiency
anaplastic large T-cell lymphoma 74
common variable 238
see also HIV infection; post-transplant
lymphoproliferative disorders
immunoglobulin heavy-chain (J_H) genes
5, 125, 145, 159, 164, 177, 196,
200, 209, 231
immunohistology of cutaneous lymphoid
infiltrates 5
immunophenotype 5
see also individual conditions
immunosuppression and cutaneous
lymphomas 182–7
indolent CD8+ lymphoid proliferation of
the ear 118
inflammatory myofibroblastic tumour 251
inflammatory pseudotumour, cutaneous
251
infliximab 186
interchromosomal translocation *see under
specific translocations*
interface dermatitis
cutaneous γ/δ T-cell lymphoma 99,
101, 102
lupus panniculitis 242
mycosis fungoides 20, *20*, 33, 101
subcutaneous T-cell lymphoma 90
interferon α (IFN-α)
actinic reticuloid 233
angio-immunoblastic T-cell lymphoma
125
bullous lesions in mycosis fungoides
and 35
follicle centre lymphoma 136
large B-cell lymphoma, leg type 160
lymphocytoma cutis 246
lymphomatoid granulomatosis 167
lymphomatoid papulosis 72
marginal zone lymphoma 146
mycosis fungoides 35, 40, 41
pegylated 40
post-transplant lymphoproliferative
disorders 183
Sézary syndrome 60
small-medium pleomorphic T-cell
lymphoma 119
subcutaneous T-cell lymphoma 92
interferon regulatory factors 25, 134
interleukin-2 (IL-2) 60
fusion protein 41, 92
interleukin-10 (IL-10) 57, 104
interleukin-12 (IL-12) 41, 60
intranuclear inclusions
cutaneous immunocytoma 141
plasmacytoma 148, *149*

intravascular angioendotheliomatosis
see histiocytosis, intravascular;
angio-endotheliomatosis
intravascular histiocytosis *see* histiocytosis,
intravascular
intravascular large B-cell lymphoma **1**, **3**,
4, 158, 175–8
association with haemangiomas 175
clinical features 176, *176*
histopathology, immunophenotype and
molecular genetics 176–7, *176*, *177*
treatment and prognosis 177–8
intravascular large NK/T-cell lymphoma
178–180, 208
intravascular proliferation of lymphoid
blasts, benign 253

Jessner-Kanof disease **232**, 252, *252*
J_H gene rearrangement **136**, 147, 149,
151, 160, 161
germline configuration 196
monoclonal 165, 166, 167, 169, 170,
178, 185, 186, 202, 203, 209
pseudomonoclonal 5

Kaposi's sarcoma 156, 175, 185
see also human herpes virus 8 (HHV-8)
infection
keratoacanthoma
in lymphomatoid papulosis 71
Ketron-Goodman disease *see* pagetoid
reticulosis, generalized
Ki-67 *see* MIB-1

large B-cell lymphoma, intravascular *see*
intravascular large B-cell lymphoma
large B-cell lymphoma, leg type **1**, **3**, **4**, **6**,
7, 129, 135, 156–61
association with Kaposi sarcoma 156
Bcl-2 expression and prognosis 160
Borrelia burgdorferi infection 156
Burkitt lymphoma-like 158
CD30 expression 74
clinical features 156–7, *156*, *157*
differential diagnosis with follicle centre
lymphoma 135
diffuse 132, 135, *135*, 159, 167
EBV-associated of elderly 168–9
epidermotropism *158*
histopathology 157–8, *157*, *158*
HIV infection 185
human herpes virus 8 (HHV-8)
infection 156
immunophenotype 158–9, *158*, *159*
microarray studies 159
molecular genetics 159–60
polycomb-group genes expression 160
prognosis 160
sentinel lymph node biopsy 160
treatment 160

Index